Choices in

Breast Cancer Treatment

Choices in

A JOHNS HOPKINS PRESS
HEALTH BOOK

Breast Cancer Treatment

Medical Specialists and Cancer Survivors Tell You What You Need to Know

Edited by

KENNETH D. MILLER, M.D.

THE JOHNS HOPKINS UNIVERSITY PRESS
Baltimore

Note to the Reader: This book is not meant to substitute for medical care of people with cancer, and treatment should not be based solely on its contents. Instead, treatment must be developed in a dialogue between the individual and his or her physician. This book has been written to help with that dialogue.

Drug dosage: The editor and publisher have made reasonable efforts to determine that the selection and dosage of drugs discussed in this text conform to the practices of the general medical community. The medications described do not necessarily have specific approval by the U.S. Food and Drug Administration for use in the diseases and dosages for which they are recommended. In view of ongoing research, changes in governmental regulations, and the constant flow of information relating to drug therapy and drug reactions, the reader is urged to check the package insert of each drug for any change in indications and dosage and for warnings and precautions. This is particularly important when the recommended agent is a new and/or infrequently used drug.

The Johns Hopkins University Press
2715 North Charles Street
Baltimore, Maryland 21218-4363
www.press.jhu.edu

Library of Congress Cataloging-in-Publication Data

Choices in breast cancer treatment : medical specialists and cancer survivors tell you what you need to know / edited by Kenneth D. Miller.
    p. cm. — (A Johns Hopkins Press health book)
  Includes bibliographical references and index.
  ISBN-13: 978-0-8018-8684-3 (hardcover : alk. paper)
  ISBN-13: 978-0-8018-8685-0 (pbk. : alk. paper)
  ISBN-10: 0-8018-8684-8 (hardcover : alk. paper)
  ISBN-10: 0-8018-8685-6 (pbk. : alk. paper)
  1. Breast—Cancer—Treatment—Decision making. I. Miller, Kenneth D., 1956–
RC280.B8C493 2007
362.196′99449—dc22   2007020366

A catalog record for this book is available from the British Library.

Freelance writer Kathleen Pascal helped write and edit the chapters in Part III. The editor gratefully acknowledges her contributions.

Figures 2.2, 2.3, 2.4, 2.5, 2.6, 6.1, 6.2, 8.1, 10.2, 10.3, 10.5, 10.6, 10.7, 12.1, 12.2, 12.3, 12.4, 12.5, 12.6, 12.7 are by Jacqueline Schaffer.

Special discounts are available for bulk purchases of this book. For more information, please contact Special Sales at 410-516-6936 or specialsales@press.jhu.edu.

Contents

Acknowledgments

I have many people to thank for contributing to *Choices*. Putting the book together has been a challenge and a passion.

Twenty-two years ago, we learned that our eldest daughter, Cara, was deaf. We needed to decide whether to use sign language or to use an oral approach to communicate with Cara, and we read a wonderful book, *Choices in Deafness* by our friend Dr. Sue Schwartz, which was incredibly helpful to us in making these difficult choices. At the same time, professionally, I was training in Oncology at the Johns Hopkins University in Baltimore and I developed an interest in breast cancer. It was at that time that I first thought about writing this book, *Choices in Breast Cancer Treatment*. I am thankful to Sue for writing her book about choices many years ago and I credit her with the title of this book. Similarly, I want to thank Drs. John Fetting and Laura Siminoff, whose research at Johns Hopkins on how women make choices kindled my own interest in this subject.

I also want to thank my wife, Joan, for making some of those difficult choices along with me then and throughout our life together. Joan has also been my editor, constructive critic, and cheerleader throughout this project. My family is the best! My parents, Dan and Cipie Miller, sparked my interest in medicine many years ago. My three daughters—Cara, Julie, and Kim—have enthusiasm, creativity, and compassion that inspire me as well.

Assembling and writing this book has been a team effort. Above all I want to thank the large number of women who shared their stories, insights, experiences, and hearts with me and with the people who will read this book. I admire each of them for their courage in their own journey and thank them for teaching me so much. I also want to thank a team of friends and colleagues who sensitively and skillfully interviewed some of the women. This team includes, Rick Weaver, Karen Eschow, Suzanne Adelman, and Donna Damico. Appreciation also to Marilyn Foster who helped me organize and edit the chapter on "What Is Breast Cancer?" and Kathleen Pascal who creatively worked on the four chapters that summarize the experience women have when learning about the diagnosis and then the decision-making process.

A special place of honor also to my friends and colleagues Drs. Joseph Kaplan and Chitra Rajagopal as well as to Suzanne Krikawa, R.N., Mary Bowen, and Rhonda Schoem, who provide such incredibly good care to women with breast cancer. They were of tremendous help to me in this effort.

A heartfelt thank you to my editor, Jacqueline Wehmueller, at the Johns Hopkins University Press, for encouraging and helping me throughout the process to convert the idea of a book about choices into a reality. I was incredibly fortunate that Jackie introduced me to Jean Silver-Isenstadt, M.D., Ph.D., who is a gifted and talented physician and writer. Jean helped take assorted chapters and contributions and craft them into the book that you see today.

Understanding the Choices

Kenneth D. Miller, M.D.

I am a medical oncologist. I am also the husband of a cancer survivor and the father of three daughters, the oldest of whom was born deaf. The emotional and intellectual weight of navigating treatment choices has pervaded most days of my adult life. I have sat on one side of the desk, in the guiding role of physician, and have also sat on the other side of the desk, as the desperate family member of a woman facing life-threatening disease — in the case of my wife, Joan, acute leukemia.

I specialize in the care of people with cancer. Over my years in practice, I have worked with hundreds of women diagnosed with breast cancer. A tremendous amount of literature is available to inform women about this disease. Medical information abounds in bookstores and on the Internet. Lengthy personal narratives detail individual struggles. What has been missing is a book that provides newly diagnosed women with the medical facts they need, while also allowing survivors — women who have walked this difficult terrain — to serve as guides. The patients' voices are too quiet in breast cancer literature. They illustrate certain points but do not flow unimpeded. They have been spliced out and overedited. Yet these most expert voices need to be heard. These are people who have been there.

Not all women want to attend support groups, but most women want to know what to expect. This book, built on interviews with and contributions written by dozens of breast cancer survivors and medical experts, provides honest accounts of what it is like to chart a course through these frightening waters, weather the storms, and live to tell the tale.

Unlike many other medical conditions that have a single best plan of action presented by the doctor, breast cancer is a disease that requires each patient to make many decisions about her treatment plan. Initially, most women feel totally unequipped to face this challenge. Most are very scared, and the complexities of the treatment choices can seem overwhelming at first. Support may come from many places (sometimes even unexpected places). This book describes how others have managed to build effective treatment plans against the terrible emotional undertow that pulls at almost every cancer patient.

In the United States, more than 200,000 women are diagnosed with breast cancer *each year.* For some, the disease is picked up by mammogram and diagnosed early, when cancer cells can barely be detected under a microscope. For others, tumors are found only after they have grown large enough to be seen or felt. And for a small group, breast cancer is first discovered only after it has already spread to other parts of the body. Each of these scenarios leads to different treatment options.

Historical trends in breast cancer treatment reflect our ever-improving medical understanding of the disease, as well as the availability of improved medicines and less disfiguring, less debilitating, surgical options. Approaches to treatment planning also reflect new respect for a woman's role in the decision-making process and a relatively new recognition of every patient's right to give informed consent. The doctor-patient relationship has become more balanced over the past twenty years.

In the early 1900s, the scientific understanding of breast cancer wrongly held that this was a disease that began in the breast, grew larger, and then spread in an orderly fashion, first to the lymph nodes and only then to other parts of the body. We now know that the process is more complicated than that. Back then, doctors had little effective medical therapy to offer. Because mammograms did not yet exist, cancers were rarely diagnosed early. As a result, the primary treatment was an extensive surgery called the Halsted radical mastectomy, which involved removal of the breast, the chest wall muscle beneath the breast, and all the lymph nodes under the arm on the affected side.

Times have changed dramatically. Today, breast cancer is better understood. It is diagnosed much earlier, it is treated with less radical surgery, and it faces a powerful arsenal of medications, with many more under development.

Understanding the Choices

Breast cancer is not one simple disease. There are different kinds of breast cancer, some more aggressive than others. There are also known risk factors for developing breast cancer. This book considers treatment options from four different perspectives:

1. the perspective of women without cancer but who have been identified as possessing a higher-than-average risk of developing the disease;
2. the perspective of women with non-invasive cancer—called ductal carcinoma in situ, or DCIS—which is present only inside the breast ducts;
3. the perspective of women with invasive cancer, which has penetrated through the cell walls of breast ducts and has a greater chance of spreading;
4. and the perspective of women with metastatic cancer, which has spread outside the breast.

Both within and among these four diagnostic categories, women make different treatment decisions.

Women at High Risk

The known risk factors for developing breast cancer include a strong family history of the disease, especially in "first-degree" relatives such as sisters, mothers, or aunts. It is also known that any woman who carries the breast cancer–related gene known as BRCA has a higher-than-average risk of developing breast or ovarian cancer. Women known to be at high risk for breast cancer but who do not have the disease often choose to increase their self-surveillance by conducting more frequent breast self-exams, by scheduling regular mammograms and MRIs, and by having more frequent breast exams done by their doctors. Some choose to go beyond close observation and begin taking a preventative medication called tamoxifen. Others adopt the most aggressive approach to prevention: mastectomy. None of these choices is inherently right or wrong; each decision is highly personal — made in response to medical data and individual needs. Each decision affects life differently.

Women with Non-Invasive Breast Cancer

Women with DCIS are faced with different surgical options, including removal of only the tumor (lumpectomy); lumpectomy with subsequent radiation therapy; or mastectomy. A woman in this situation might also need to decide whether or not to take tamoxifen, a medicine that may increase long-term survival but that also produces side effects. Again, knowledgeable people make different choices, for different reasons.

Women with Invasive Cancer

For anyone whose cancer has demonstrated the ability to invade outside the ducts, surgical options are usually lumpectomy with radiation, or mastectomy. Surgeons also must know whether to perform a limited (and less disfiguring) sampling of lymph nodes or whether to remove all the lymph nodes that drain fluid from the affected breast. Women with invasive cancer must decide whether or not to take postoperative therapy to reduce the risk of recurrence; this may include chemotherapy, hormonal therapy, or both. This book provides many accounts by those who have been down this path of hard decisions; they share what they learned, how they chose, where they found strength, and what, if anything, they would do differently now.

Women with Metastatic Cancer

Any woman who learns that her breast cancer has spread to other parts of her body is thrown into a frightening place. Her situation is serious, but it is not without hope. Medical treatment for advanced cancer brings many side effects and takes many months, but it also saves lives. These treatments include chemotherapy, hormonal therapy, radiation, and surgery. Women balance the expected benefits of these often harsh treatments with the challenges they bring to quality of life. Different women make different wise choices. Age, faith, work, temperament, general health, support networks, family structure, obligations, and values all influence the direction they take.

The Treatment Team

The control of breast cancer involves a team approach among care providers. Ideally, this care is coordinated among empathic, accessible specialists who have experience working together. Seeking second opinions and additional referrals is common, and it is smart.

Generally speaking, second opinions are valuable but can be confusing. They are most helpful when it comes to confirming a diagnosis, refining a treatment plan, exploring alternative approaches, or transferring care to a new physician. It is important to think through your purpose for seeking a second opinion and to express that goal to the physician offering the opinion. Once you have received a second opinion, it is also useful to look first at how the opinions you have heard are similar, instead of how they differ. At times, doctors' terminology may differ enough to make similar opinions sound quite distinct. Ask if the perceived differences between opinions are meaningful, because sometimes trivial details seem important.

It may help to have the doctors confer, and asking them to do so is entirely reasonable. Rarely can a meaningful treatment decision be made by simply tallying doctors' votes for or against a particular approach. Finally, realize that seeking *too many* second opinions can also delay a difficult decision, which may not be helpful either medically or emotionally. But, as many women in this book describe, it is enormously important to find health care providers you feel good about.

These providers include primary care physicians, gynecologists, surgeons, medical and radiation oncologists, radiation therapists, nurses, and psychotherapists. This book includes chapters written by experts in many of these fields — several of whom are themselves breast cancer survivors. Here, you will learn about the disease, meet highly regarded practitioners who work to cure it, gain an understanding of breast cancer treatment options, and, most importantly, learn from the experiences of other women.

How This Book Is Organized

Our purpose is to help readers not only to understand and map out their options but also to weather the difficulty of treatment planning. Doing so requires good medical information, and it also requires emotional strength. To impart information and support, we have divided the text into five sections. The first provides a general overview of breast cancer as a disease to be reckoned with. There, we present the anatomy of breast cancer, an overview of individual risk factors for developing cancer, recent treatment trends, and the nature of the patient-doctor relationship.

The second part provides detailed chapters on each aspect of treatment, with contributions from nationally recognized leaders in each of the relevant medical specialties of surgery, oncology, radiation therapy, and plastic surgery. Treatment options are clarified by those who prescribe and provide them. Surgery is explained by surgeons, chemotherapy by medical oncologists, and so on. For those unable to travel to the nation's leading cancer centers for private consultations, these chapters deliver the experts to you.

The last three sections of the book include personal voices. Part 3, interweaving excerpts from personal narratives written by women with breast cancer, follows the steps of diagnosis and treatment in order. Part 4 offers these women's extended personal narratives without interruption or commentary, grouping their unique stories according to the type of cancer each woman faced and survived. These are the patients' recollections of their experiences and feelings. While their stories are very important, it is possible that some of their information and advice is not medically sound, and readers should not make decisions about their own care based solely on these patients' stories. Last, part 5 offers three chapters written by breast cancer experts who themselves have had the disease.

If you or someone close to you has been diagnosed with breast cancer, this book will help you through what thousands of women describe in retrospect as a frightening, stormy episode safely navigated with the help of many others.

PART ONE

The Big Picture

CHAPTER 1

Making Decisions

Laura A. Siminoff, Ph.D.

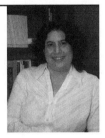

For most people a diagnosis of breast cancer is initially terrifying, and clear thinking seems impossible. First there is the diagnosis. Then there are all these medical terms coming at you, all these statistics. And there are so many *options*.

You are immediately given choices, and you are asked to make decisions. All you want is a guarantee of good health, but you are asked to navigate a path through a strange landscape. Last week, you gave no thought to this path. Today, you must decide which direction to take and who will be your guide. When asked to choose the best surgical option, many women say they feel ill equipped, uninformed, and emotionally strained.

The authors of this book hope to help women avoid feeling this way. This chapter explores the essential relationship between a woman with breast cancer and her physician. It also begins the process of helping the reader to identify her own values and priorities. Once you know what you want from treatment—and what you don't want—then you will be able to make decisions much more easily and confidently.

For all women, the initial intense emotions of the diagnosis eventually resolve into a story that includes decisions made and paths taken. Unlike the reader of a story, however, the woman with breast cancer must help write the script. That script generally begins with some kind of surgery, and for some women surgery is all the treatment that's needed or wanted. For other women, radiation therapy, chemotherapy, and hormonal therapy are options. These treatments pose risks, but they also offer increased survival.

Wait, you think. Wait. I know how to manage real estate, sew my own clothes, practice law, or home-school my children, but how in the world can I be expected to make crucial medical decisions about breast cancer? I'm no doctor. I need an experienced consultant for this one. (Even doctors need help making decisions when they have breast cancer.)

It's natural for you to feel this way because treatment decisions are complex. You are processing a lot of new information at once, while you're under terrific stress. And good communication between patient and doctor, although extremely important, is sometimes not easy to achieve. The patient is usually learning about breast cancer from a basic starting point, and the doctor is trying to provide technical background and data to someone who is still shaken from receiving frightening news. Patients want to be cured, but concerns about possible side effects from treatment and the difficulty in knowing what treatment is best make decisions more difficult.

Doctors Talking with Patients, Patients Talking with Doctors

The oncology (cancer) consultation shares most of the features of any doctor-patient interaction, but it is burdened with its own set of problems. Research has shown that three issues often complicate discussion: first, the stigma and fear associated with a diagnosis of cancer; second, the complexity of the medical information itself; and third, uncertainty regarding the course of the disease and the benefits of treatment. If communication falters for any reason, patients can be left with incomplete information or even with fundamental misunderstandings about treatment risks, benefits, and alternatives.

Stigma and Fear

Years ago, a diagnosis of cancer caused a person to experience intense shame. The origins of the disease were not understood, and many people believed that cancer was contagious. People would hide the diagnosis to avoid being shunned. Even today, many people are uncomfortable or embarrassed talking about private parts of their bodies. Breast cancer was once treated with disfiguring and often disabling surgery that left women feeling stigmatized by their post-surgical physical limitations. This radical surgery, where the entire breast and the muscles underneath the breast were removed, is almost never performed today.

Although some stigma still clings to certain cancers and the disease remains a source of embarrassment within some communities, today the most common reaction to a cancer diagnosis is fear. Americans dread cancer more than all other medical diagnoses. In surveys, Americans have repeatedly identified cancer as a disease both painful and fatal. In fact, most American women are more concerned about breast cancer than about heart disease, even though heart disease kills far more women each year.

Then there are the stories. Some people believe that surgery will cause the cancer to spread. Others fear chemotherapy. In studies we have conducted with cancer patients, people tell us that they personally know of someone whose cancer seemed to get worse when treatment was received. Thus, many people enter the cancer-care arena with misinformation and enormous dread. (Cancer treatments sometimes make people feel sick before they feel better, but it can also save lives. Generally, the side effects of treatment can be well controlled.)

Complexity of Medical Information

Cancer is complicated, and knowledge about one form of cancer does not necessarily translate to other forms. Prognosis depends on the type, location, and stage of cancer at the time of diagnosis, as well as on the general health of the patient. With breast cancer treatment decisions, the most important variables to consider are the type of cancer;

the size of the tumor;

the number of lymph nodes positive for cancer;

whether there are hormone receptors within the tumor; and

whether the tumor has spread beyond the breast.

Understanding each of these variables helps you make informed treatment decisions. Once you have the information, you will have many decisions to make:

What type of biopsy should I have?

Should I consider breast conserving surgery?

Should I consider reconstructive surgery?

Should I take adjuvant therapy (hormone or chemotherapy) after the tumor has been removed?

It is a lot to deal with.

Medical Uncertainty

Making decisions would be easier if physicians could simply tell their patients what the future holds. But physicians can base their recommendations only on statistics. A doctor can only tell a patient the *likelihood* of the cancer returning after surgery and can only say what added value a treatment will *likely* have on survival. No one can predict the *actual* outcome for a specific patient.

To illustrate this point, let's assume that Ms. Smith, a 65-year-old woman in average health, is diagnosed with breast cancer. Let's further assume that her tumor is small (say, 2.0 centimeters), that it is found only in the breast, and that only one of the nodes sampled from under her arm has cancer in it. Finally, let's assume that Ms. Smith's tumor is hormone-receptor positive, meaning that it responds to the female hormones estrogen or progesterone, and thus that it still acts somewhat like normal breast tissue. Can her oncologist tell her precisely whether she will be cancer free and well in ten years? No.

What the physician can tell Ms. Smith is based on data collected from

The Big Picture

other patients: of 100 women with Ms. Smith's characteristics who opted for surgery only, without radiation or chemotherapy, 61 would be expected to be alive in ten years, but 22 would be expected to die from their breast cancer, and 17 to die of other causes. The physician cannot know whether Ms. Smith is likely to be one of the 61, the 22, or the 17, but can promise that the chances of ten-year survival are in her favor.

How might Ms. Smith improve her chances of being alive in 10 years? Medical oncologists can offer several different types of adjuvant therapy to be taken after surgery. Again, the oncologist cannot predict outcomes with certainty but can only look at past data. For example, the oncologist cannot know if Ms. Smith was completely cured by the surgery—that is, if she is one of the 61 women who do not need further treatment. However, the doctor can provide statistics about how many more women are cured by taking various additional treatments and how many are not. The challenge of making decisions about cancer is that no one can know with certainty how Ms. Smith will respond to therapy.

Giving and Getting Information

Doctors' approaches to patient education vary widely. Not all doctors communicate as *much* information as they should, and not all doctors have good communication skills—they may be fine clinicians but don't interact well with patients. Some physicians still hesitate to disclose details of treatment, such as associated risks, prognostic information, and potential treatment alternatives. A patient needs to think about how much she wants to know and how she will let her doctor know her wishes regarding communication.

Research reveals the following information about doctor-patient communication:

- Physicians often fail to relate information in a comprehensive or comprehensible way.
- Most patients continue to display significant gaps in their recall and understanding of the treatment-related information that they have discussed with their doctors.
- Physicians sometimes change their style of conveying information

to patients in response to the personal characteristics of patients. Notably, older patients, persons with less education, and minority women sometimes receive less information and less social and emotional counseling than other patients.

It has been repeatedly shown that providing detailed information about prognosis and treatment risks has generally *not* been associated with negative psychological outcomes. In other words, statistical information generally does not upset patients. In fact, some studies have found that these discussions diminish patients' anxiety and increase their adherence to treatment regimens.

Thus, a breast cancer consultation with a medical oncologist should include a discussion of the *rationale* for any proposed treatment or procedure, the associated *benefits and risks,* and available *treatment alternatives.* If communication has been effective, then the patient will recall and understand what the physician has said. She will be less anxious and more satisfied, and will follow through better on treatment regimens and will keep scheduled appointments. Studies have also shown that she will have a better quality of life after the diagnosis of breast cancer.

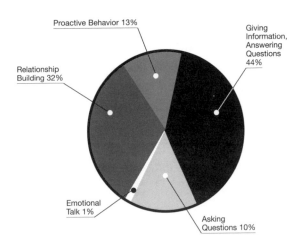

Patient Talk

Proactive Behavior 13%

Giving Information, Answering Questions 44%

Relationship Building 32%

Emotional Talk 1%

Asking Questions 10%

FIGURE 1.1. Women talk about a number of things during a consultation with a medical oncologist about postoperative chemotherapy or hormonal therapy.

The Big Picture

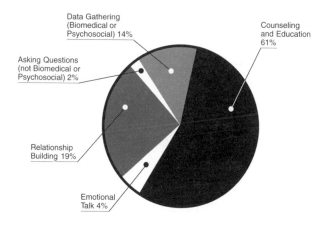

FIGURE 1.2. During a consultation with a woman about postoperative chemotherapy or hormonal therapy, oncologists generally focus on education.

Unfortunately, most consultations between patient and physician are less than ideal. Patients initiate only 10 to 20 percent of the conversation. Moreover, patients spend much of their time trying to build a relationship with the physician, while the physician spends about 80 percent of the time discussing medical topics. It is a problem. The patient is trying to engage the doctor in the social and emotional aspects of the diagnosis, often with limited success. The doctor is trying to educate the patient, also with less than perfect results. Figures 1.1 and 1.2 illustrate what percentage of the doctor-patient interaction is spent engaged in various activities. These two charts reveal a gap between patients and doctors, even during critical conversations. But the situation is even more challenging than that.

Studies have shown that oncologists calculate the likelihood of treatment benefit idiosyncratically rather than systematically. For example, most physicians speak in terms of general relative risks and benefits. Following surgery, adjuvant chemotherapy, for example, is often said to bestow a 30 percent survival advantage on patients. This number is an *average*, however—the actual results vary greatly depending on the specific characteristics of the patient. For one group of women, the benefit of adjuvant therapy may be so small that it enables only one additional woman out of 100 to survive. For another group of women, as many as 35 out of that 100 may survive because they received chemotherapy. Because it is an average, the general statistic "30 percent additional survival benefit" may underestimate or overestimate the benefit for a specific patient. It is not a terribly useful number to communicate unless it is put in context for the specific patient.

Unless they have accurate information about treatment outcomes as a point of reference, patients cannot be properly informed partners with their doctors in deciding whether to take adjuvant therapy and, if so, what kind. The doctor is obliged to convey enough information for the patient to be able to make informed, satisfying, and medically sound decisions. What constitutes "enough" is often a judgment call by the doctor, based on perceptions of the patient's knowledge about her prognosis and on her desire for more detailed information.

For patient-doctor communication to be effective, the patient and the physician must be "on the same page" when treatment decisions are discussed. But many studies of oncology patients show the opposite to be true. Oncology patients often have misperceptions about the meaning of numbers. They overestimate their risk of a negative outcome without therapy, and they overestimate the positive impact of therapy.

Many studies have shown that patients did not have a clear, full understanding of the risks and benefits of adjuvant therapy, for example. Why? First, most patients were not prepared for what the medical oncologist had to tell them. They were overwhelmed by the information. Even when the physician encouraged them to participate, most patients were reactive rather than active and were unable to shape the course of the conversation.

Second, most oncologists did not impart specific information about benefits and risks when patients did not ask for it. Physicians may have been reluctant to provide patients with potentially distressing information, while patients may have been reluctant to hear it.

Third, given the lack of specific information exchanged, it is understandable that patients, compared to their physicians, overestimate treatment benefits. This is a significant problem because if patients have an inflated estimate of the benefit of standard treatment, they may be less interested in participating in clinical trials that involve experimental therapy that may be beneficial for them.

Fourth, the decision-making process is often compressed. The overwhelming majority of patients make final decisions about treatment during the first meeting with their physicians. The average patient-physician encounter usually lasts no longer than fifty minutes. After obtaining a medical history and performing a physical exam, relatively little time is left for the doctor to discuss adjuvant therapy. But while treatment cannot be delayed indefinitely, and treatment should not be delayed at all in some circumstances, often there is time for the patient to consider her options and gather more information before making a decision. (If you need more time to make a decision, ask your doctor whether you can take more time, even if it's only overnight. It's best to come to an agreement that the decision will be made by a specific date.)

What Patients Need to Know

While doctors disagree about how much information to share with patients, it is well known that patient understanding of the information that is given can be poor. Several studies have found that current practice yields low patient retention of information. For example, studies report that only 60 to 70 percent of all cancer patients can correctly recall what their treatment entailed; that about 40 percent cannot list even a single major treatment side effect; and that 70 to 75 percent cannot name one treatment alternative. A study of breast cancer patients also found little accurate recall or understanding of chemotherapy's risks and benefits. A separate study of radiation oncology patients found that patients exhibited limited knowledge about treatment alternatives. Notably, 80 to 90 percent of patients can correctly identify their diagnosis.

One challenge is that patients and physicians often define a given problem differently and hold different ideas about what a desirable outcome would be. The use of medical jargon and a lack of a shared context can cause or exacerbate communication failures.

To overcome these problems, patients need to ask themselves:

How much information about the disease and its treatment do I
want to know?

What role do I want to play in making the decision?

What are my values concerning the balance of treatment benefits
and risks?

How Much Do You Want to Know?

The standards of communication between physicians and cancer patients
have changed enormously in the last twenty years. In the past, information as fundamental as the cancer diagnosis itself was routinely with-
held; now it is conveyed to patients as a matter of course.

Research shows that most breast cancer patients report a desire for
maximum information. In a survey of people who had been treated for
breast cancer, patients were asked what additional information they
would have liked to receive. Fifty-two percent of the respondents indicated that they would have wanted to know about research programs.
Moreover, many patients expressed a desire for more specific personalized information. One study found that women who had been provided
with specific estimates of outcome with and without therapy reported
less need for information about risk of relapse (i.e., the cancer coming
back). Thirty-two percent of women received specific, numeric information from their physicians about the chances of their cancer coming
back. Of these, 48 percent reported wanting more information about
relapse. Among the women who received no information of any kind
about the chances of the cancer coming back, 55 percent wanted to know
more about risk of relapse.

As noted earlier, studies have found that breast cancer patients consistently overestimate the benefit of adjuvant therapy. (In one study, this
benefit was estimated at about twice its actual value.) At the same time,
recent studies affirm earlier findings that many women substantially overestimate their risks of recurrence. Patients with very early stage breast
cancer wrongly estimate their risk of recurrence at five years to be 30 to
39 percent. In fact, this estimate is more than double the actual risk for
most of these women. The picture is not as bleak as many patients think.

How much do *you* want to know? About 20 percent of patients cope by seeking only the minimum information they need; a lot of information causes anxiety and makes them feel overwhelmed. Other people—again, a minority—want to know absolutely everything. They cope by seeking as much information as possible. Finally, the majority of patients want to know a great deal of information, but they often want to pace their learning, and they may not want to know every single detail.

Studies show that if the patient does not take charge of the discussion with her doctor, her doctor will rely on her or his own personal style, which varies little from patient to patient. Some doctors are natural "information withholders"; they rarely elaborate unless pressed to do so. Patients who want a lot of information will be more likely to get what they need from these doctors if they prepare a question list in advance and if they explicitly ask for numerical information.

In one study evaluating quality of care, a large group of physicians was asked to report what they told patients about diagnosis and treatment; their replies indicated that detailed information about surgery was given to 11 percent of the patients; a moderate amount of information was given to 55 percent; and vague information was given to 13 percent. Women were given thorough information on diagnosis 39 percent of the time, with 35 percent receiving vague information, and 7 percent receiving no information. When asked what prevented them from giving a satisfactory disclosure of information, 58 percent of the doctors did not answer the question. Of those who did, 80 percent referred to the patients' psychological problems and 11 percent to the patients' limited education. It was also found that younger and more educated women were about 50 percent more likely to receive thorough information. In addition, this study found that the patient's age, education level, and tumor size were each independent, significant predictors of the quality of information she received. These study findings show that patients must be explicit with their doctors about how much information they want to receive. Do not assume that the doctor will share everything unprompted.

What Role Do You Want to Play in Making Decisions?

Today, patients are more active participants in treatment planning than ever before. Breast cancer patients in particular appear to want to have

Patient leaves all decisions to doctor	4.6%
Doctor makes final decision but considers patient's opinion	19.7%
Doctor and patient share responsibility for decision	46.3%
Patient makes final decision but considers doctor's opinion	26.6%
Patient makes final decision	2.8%

Note: Based on a sample of 395 women.

a "working relationship" with their physicians—a relationship that allows for synergistic interaction between information sharing and relationship building. This increased patient role allows for shared decision making, an approach now considered the ideal. The "doctor-knows-best" model has fallen from favor; it does not satisfy most patients, and it does not result in better health outcomes. Nonetheless, women's preferences still range from wanting full decision-making power to wanting the doctor to take complete charge. Our own research has shown that well over 50 percent of breast cancer patients want to make decisions in partnership with their physicians. Smaller numbers want to be either the sole decision maker or want to leave the decisions to their doctors (see table 1.1).

If patients do not lay out their preferences clearly, then the physician should ask. However, this rarely happens. Most doctors perceive a patient's silence as signaling either satisfaction with the information received or a lack of desire for information. Understandably, given the circumstances, patients tend not to express their information needs during the consultation process.

Different women have different information needs and different decision-making styles. One study of cancer patients found that over 90 percent of patients said they wanted full information about their condition, but about 25 percent wanted the physician alone to make the decision concerning treatment. In contrast, another study of cancer patients found that older patients and those who are sicker want less information than younger, healthier patients. They also have less desire to be the primary decision maker. This information has special significance for

The Big Picture

oncologists and other physicians who treat patients with life-threatening illnesses or who provide care to older patients. It may in part explain why some doctors provide less information to older patients.

There is also evidence that patients with chronic illness may, over time, become more participatory and better informed than their less seriously ill counterparts. Most studies highlight patients' generally strong preferences for having information but differentiate between information needs and patient decision-making styles. Even patients who do not wish to be the primary decision maker seem to benefit from a detailed exchange of information and open communication with their physicians.

What Are Your Values Concerning the Balance of Treatment Benefits and Risks?

All cancer treatments entail risks and benefits. "Risks" refers to side effects. In the case of adjuvant therapy for breast cancer, patients most commonly experience hair loss, weight gain, nausea, and vomiting. The benefits of treatment are cancer cure or a delay of cancer's recurrence (delay of the cancer coming back).

Some studies suggest that doctors and patients disagree about the value of the benefit offered by adjuvant therapy, with patients considering even a modest amount of increased survival worthwhile. As shown in Figure 1.3, nearly *half* of all women consider adjuvant therapy worth the risk, discomfort, and inconvenience if it results in even *one-half of one percent* increase in survival.

What are *your* values concerning risks and benefits of treatment?

How Much of a Reduction in Breast Cancer Would Make the Adjuvant Worthwhile?

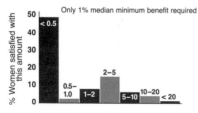

FIGURE 1.3. Women generally indicate that even a less than 1 percent reduction in the risk of dying of breast cancer would justify treatment with chemotherapy, even when they are informed about the side effects and risks of treatment.

Think about what you want, and then make sure you have all the information you need—and that you understand the information—before making a decision. The stories of women with breast cancer related in this book illustrate a wide range of values when it comes to the risks and benefits of treatment. Their stories may help you identify your own values.

Building the Alliance

Trying to devise one magic formula for what all physicians should tell their patients would be futile. Describing the behavior of the "perfect patient" is an equally ill-conceived undertaking. There are too many variables for any single approach to meet all of the individuals' needs in this difficult situation. Generally speaking, however, here is what a physician should be doing:

- Adopting flexible communication styles that encourage patient involvement and respect patient differences
- Showing empathy, giving reassurance, and encouraging questions
- Adjusting their flow of medical information to respond to patient preferences
- Seeking clarity about how much the patient wants to know and how active the patient wants to be in developing a treatment plan
- Pausing frequently during an initial consultation to make sure the patient is taking in what is being said

And here is what a patient should be doing:

- Guiding her doctor into an alliance that meets her medical, physical, and emotional needs
- Thinking about what she wants to know and when she wants to know it
- Keeping her values in mind when weighing the risks and benefits of treatment
- Understanding that not all treatment decisions need to be made immediately

• Asking if there is some time for reflection and additional information gathering before a decision is made

In the next chapter, we begin at the beginning of all of this information by describing what cancer is.

CHAPTER 2

What Is Breast Cancer?

Kenneth D. Miller, M.D.

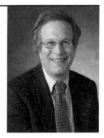

First, please understand that you did nothing to cause breast cancer. Some women worry that coloring their hair, using certain cosmetics, getting too much sun (or not enough sun), or having once injured their breast may have caused them to develop breast cancer. It really has nothing to do with any single thing that you might imagine. And there is nothing you could have done to prevent breast cancer. At this time, there is no universal, 100 percent reliable medical or holistic strategy that can prevent breast cancer.

The truth is that the medical profession does not know exactly what causes breast cancer, but we do know that it is incredibly common. Certainly, there are some families whose risks are higher, but for most people diagnosed with breast cancer, there really is no known cause.

How Common Is Breast Cancer?

Breast cancer occurs too frequently. Approximately 240,000 women are diagnosed with this disease each year in the United States. The incidence of breast cancer increases with age, so it is more common in women over age 60 than in those under 40. Figure 2.1 shows the number of women diagnosed with breast cancer for every 100,000 women per year in the United States. Rates of breast cancer have been fairly steady for many age groups over the past several decades, though they have risen slightly for women over age 60. Stated another way, a woman's chance of developing breast cancer between the age of 20 and the age of 40 is 1 in 200; between 40 and 60, 1 in 20; and between 60 and 80, 1 in 11.

What Exactly Is Breast Cancer?

The breast—also called the mammary gland—is designed to make and deliver milk. The nipple receives milk from a fan of multiple, branching ducts that spread throughout the breast (Figure 2.2). The walls of every duct are made up of millions of cells, all lined up in a very orderly fashion. Every day, millions of these cells are shed, and millions more take their place. They all look pretty much the same, and they are continuously being replaced.

Cells in the breast grow and divide, or are replaced. If a cell does not divide correctly, an abnormal cell is created. We don't really know why. This unwanted change can occur in two separate areas of the breast: in the ducts (where most problems occur), and in the milk glands, called the *lobules*.

Figure 2.3 shows a cross section of normal duct tissue as it would

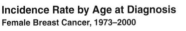

Incidence Rate by Age at Diagnosis
Female Breast Cancer, 1973–2000

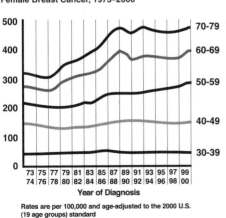

Rates are per 100,000 and age-adjusted to the 2000 U.S.
(19 age groups) standard

FIGURE 2.1. From 1973 to 2000 the incidence of breast cancer increased. The increase was greatest in woman over age 50.

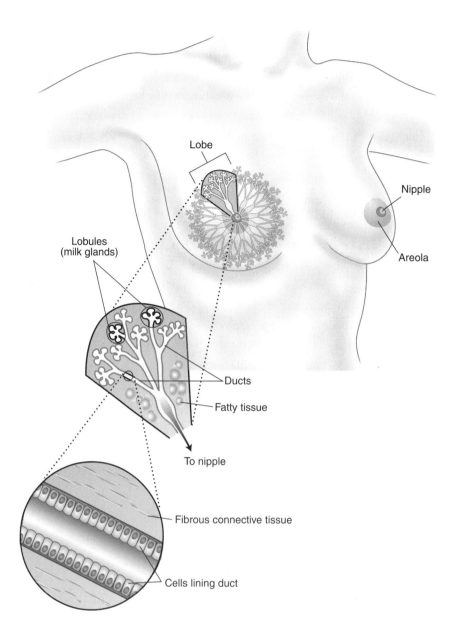

Lobe

Nipple

Lobules
(milk glands)

Areola

Ducts

Fatty tissue

To nipple

Fibrous connective tissue

Cells lining duct

FIGURE 2.2. The normal breast has milk glands known as lobules that produce milk, which is then carried to the nipple through the ducts in the breast. This illustration of an abnormal breast shows the structure of the lobules and the ducts and the anatomy of the normal duct tissue. Each duct is typically lined by a single layer of cells that are called ductal cells and are uniform in their size and appearance.

appear under a light microscope. (This tissue and the other tissue pictured in this section can be obtained through a biopsy.) A number of cellular changes can occur in the duct. If the normal process of cellular replication gets carried away, then the duct can fill up with too many cells, all of which appear normal. This is referred to as *hyperplasia*. Or, the duct can fill with too many cells that have an abnormal shape or unusual internal features. This is referred to as *atypical ductal hyperplasia* (see Figure 2.3). While the condition itself is not cancer, it is associated with a greater risk of developing cancer in either breast. A similar situation in which cells with a different abnormal appearance proliferate in the lobules of the breast is called *lobular neoplasia*. Women with this condition are also at higher risk of developing breast cancer in either breast.

Atypical cells can also start to pile up on each other, rather than growing in an orderly way. This massing of atypical cells is the defining characteristic of cancer. If the cancer cells are confined within the duct or lobule, the condition is referred to as *non-invasive breast cancer*. On the other hand, if the cancer cells penetrate through the walls of the duct or lobules and infiltrate into the surrounding tissue, the diagnosis is *invasive breast cancer*. Typically, breast cancer is classified as either ductal or lobular, which leads to the impression that some cancers develop in the duct and others in the lobules. In fact, it is the pattern of cell growth that distinguishes ductal and lobular breast cancers from one another.

Non-Invasive Breast Cancer

When cancer cells are confined within the duct or lobule, the breast cancer is considered non-invasive. If the cells have certain features, the diagnosis is *ductal carcinoma in situ* (DCIS). On the other hand, other features of the cancer cells lead the pathologist to the diagnosis of *lobular carcinoma in situ*. Both types of non-invasive breast cancer require treatment, which is described later in the book.

Invasive Breast Cancer

In some women, the cancer cells invade through the walls of ducts or lobules and infiltrate surrounding tissues. If the cancer cells have specific features, this condition is called *infiltrating ductal breast cancer*. Women

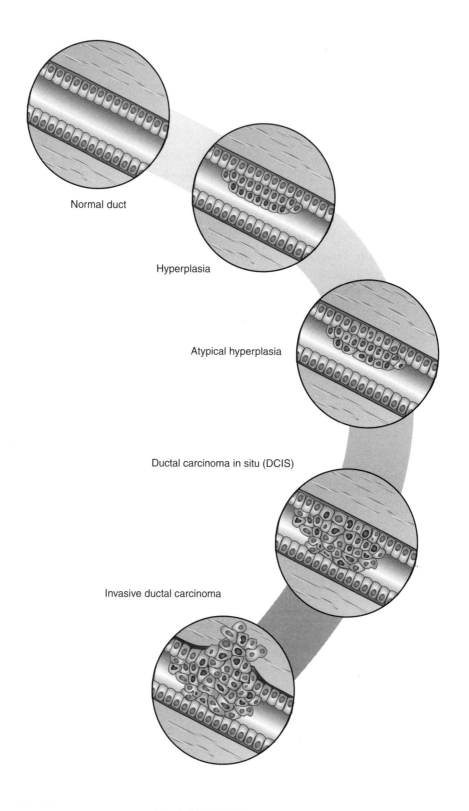

Normal duct

Hyperplasia

Atypical hyperplasia

Ductal carcinoma in situ (DCIS)

Invasive ductal carcinoma

can also develop *invasive lobular breast cancer.* Here again the abnormal cells pile up in the lobules and the surrounding tissues of the breast. While invasive lobular breast cancer exhibits different characteristics from ductal cancer, it poses a similar risk for developing recurrent disease in the breast and elsewhere in the body.

To summarize, when a tissue biopsy is done of a suspicious lump or abnormality on a mammogram image, it is classified into one of five diagnostic categories:

1. Normal ducts and lobules.
2. Benign changes, including fibroadenomas.
3. Atypical hyperplasia and lobular neoplasia. (These are associated with an increased risk for the development of breast cancer.)
4. Non-invasive breast cancer—ductal carcinoma in situ and lobular carcinoma in situ.
5. Invasive breast cancer—Infiltrating ductal and infiltrating lobular breast cancer.

What Does the Biopsy Show?

A biopsy is a procedure that retrieves a sample of suspicious tissue for examination under the microscope. It is a critical first step in accurate diagnosis and, if necessary, in treatment planning. (The various biopsy procedures are discussed in detail in chapter 7.) Sometimes a breast-tissue biopsy reveals more than one type of cellular change. In that case, a woman may receive diagnoses of invasive cancer and non-invasive can-

---

FIGURE 2.3. Ductal cells in the normal duct appear uniform in size, shape, and appearance. In hyperplasia, the basic appearance of the cells is normal, but there is an increased number of cells. Regular hyperplasia is not associated with an increase risk for the development of breast cancer. In contrast, in atypical ductal hyperplasia the number of cells is also increased and the cells may have an abnormal appearance. This condition itself is not breast cancer but is associated with an increased risk of developing breast cancer.

In intraductal breast cancer (ductal carcinoma in situ) the ductal cells are very abnormal in appearance and fill the duct, although they do not have the ability to invade through the duct into the normal tissues. In infiltrating ductal cancer, however, the cancer cells invade out from the duct into the fatty tissues of the breast.

cer at the same time. Other changes may be seen as well, including atypical hyperplasia, as noted above.

Pathologists who review biopsy slides after biopsy and other cancer surgery assess multiple factors, including the nature of the cellular change, the size of the lesion, and the margin, which is the area immediately surrounding the identifiable lesion. A margin that tests negative for cancer cells indicates that the entire tumor was successfully removed and that its measured size is most likely accurate. On the other hand, if a margin tests positive for cancer cells, then the breast tissue may still contain additional cancer, and the final size of the tumor may be larger than was first anticipated. Other pathology findings that affect treatment planning are the status of the underarm lymph nodes, which drain fluid from the breast; the presence or absence of estrogen and progesterone receptors; and the presence or absence of a protein called HER-2-Neu, which may provide information about the growth rate of the tumor. The estro-

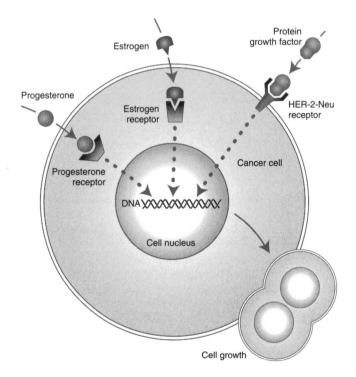

FIGURE 2.4. Breast cancer cells may have special receptors for estrogen and progesterone and may have a special surface receptor known as HER-2-Neu.

The Big Picture

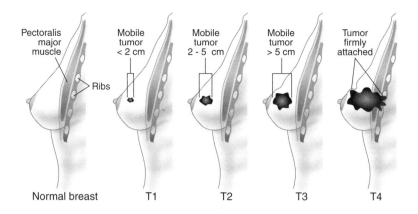

FIGURE 2.5. The stage of a breast cancer is related to three factors including the tumor size (T), involvement of lymph nodes (N), and the presence of cancer outside of the breast and nodes (M). The "T" aspect of staging is related to the size of the tumor and whether it is fixed to the skin or the underlying chest wall. If the tumor is fixed to the skin or the muscles of the chest wall, it is regarded as a higher "T" stage.

gen or progesterone receptors are special receivers in the breast cancer cell that bind estrogen or progesterone and then signal the cell to grow. HER-2-Neu is a protein on the cell surface which is stimulated when it binds a specific protein. The "activated" HER-2-Neu receptor then stimulates the breast cancer cell to grow. The presence of the estrogen or progesterone receptor is generally considered to be a favorable feature, while the presence of the HER-2-Neu receptor protein is considered to be less favorable because typically this type of cancer acts more aggressively (see Figure 2.4).

Cancer Staging

Staging is the term used for assessing how far a cancer has spread at the time of diagnosis. A well-established "TNM" staging system for breast cancer has been universally accepted. It involves analysis of the tumor's size (T), the degree of lymph node involvement (N, for node), and the presence or absence of metastatic spread (M).

Tumor Size

The tumor is measured in centimeters at its widest point and is then classified as T1 through T4 (see Figure 2.5).

- T1 refers to a tumor two centimeters (about three-quarters of an inch) or smaller.
- T2 refers to a tumor between two and five centimeters.
- T3 refers to a tumor greater than five centimeters but mobile.
- T4 refers to a tumor of any size that is fixed to the skin or chest wall.

Lymph Node Involvement

In the TNM staging system, "N" refers to the number of lymph nodes containing cancer cells (see Figure 2.6).

- N0 means no lymph node involvement.
- N1 means 1 to 3 lymph nodes are involved.
- N2 means 4 to 9 lymph nodes are involved.
- N3 means ten or more lymph nodes are involved or refers to a situation in which any of the nodes involved are located above the collarbone.

Metastatic Breast Cancer

There are only two possible options for the "M" status.

- M0 indicates the absence of metastatic disease.
- M1 indicates the presence of metastatic disease.

The TNM status determines the diagnostic staging of the breast cancer, which can range from stage 0 to stage IV, with sub-stages. The details can get complicated. Here is how the National Cancer Institute's web site explains the different stages:

> *Stage 0* (in situ) is breast cancer that has not invaded through the duct or lobule into the connective tissue of the breast, and there has been no spread to the lymph nodes.

FIGURE 2.6. In addition to "T," the stage of the tumor is also related to the possible spread of cancer cells to the lymph nodes under the arm. A higher "N" in the staging system indicates involvement of a larger number of nodes and the involvement of the nodes above the collarbone.

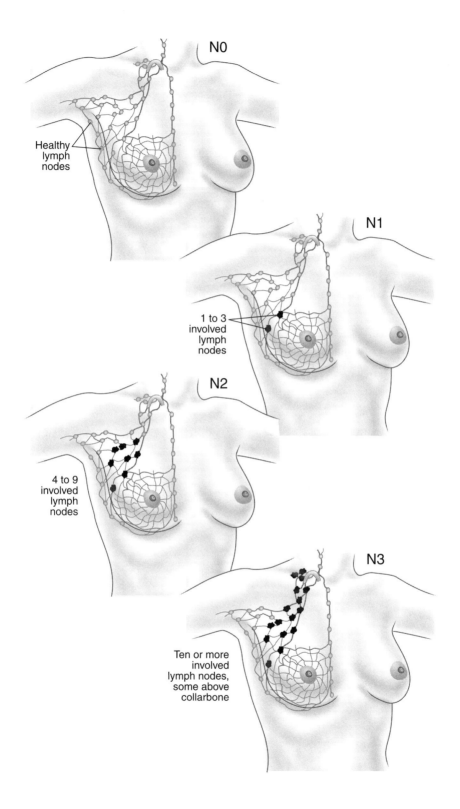

N0

Healthy
lymph
nodes

N1

1 to 3
involved
lymph
nodes

N2

4 to 9
involved
lymph
nodes

N3

Ten or more
involved
lymph nodes,
some above
collarbone

Stage I is an early stage of invasive breast cancer. Stage I means that the tumor is no more than 2 centimeters (less than three-quarters of an inch) across, and has not spread to the lymph nodes.

Stage II is any one of the following: the tumor in the breast is no more than 2 centimeters (less than three-quarters of an inch) across, and the cancer has spread to the lymph nodes under the arm; or the tumor is between 2 and 5 centimeters (three-quarters of an inch to 2 inches), and the cancer has spread to one, two, or three lymph nodes under the arm; or the tumor is larger than 5 centimeters (2 inches) but has not spread to the lymph nodes under the arm.

Stage III is also called *locally advanced cancer.* There are several sub-categories in stage III, which include the findings that the cancer has spread to four or more underarm lymph nodes; that the lymph nodes are attached to one another ("matted") or to other structures ("fixed"); that the tumor is large (more than 5 centimeters across) and the cancer has spread to the underarm lymph nodes; that the tumor may have grown into the *chest wall* or the skin of the breast; or that the cancer has spread to lymph nodes under the breastbone or to the lymph nodes under or above the collarbone.

Stage IV is distant metastatic cancer. The cancer has spread to other parts of the body such as the lungs or bones.

The Three Major Treatment Decisions

There are three major areas of concern that women with breast cancer must address when considering treatment. Each is important.

- Achieving local control
- Achieving regional control
- Minimizing the risk of recurrent metastatic disease

Sometimes women ask, "If I have chemotherapy, does that mean I don't have to have a mastectomy?" or "If I have the lymph nodes removed, does that mean that I don't need to have radiation?" These issues are interrelated, but often the decisions women make about one issue may be separate and very different from their decisions on the other issues.

Achieving Local Control

Local control of the cancer relates to the tumor itself: how do you assure that the tumor is gone from the breast? There are currently three options: (1) lumpectomy alone, (2) lumpectomy followed by radiation therapy to the breast, or (3) mastectomy. Years ago, the majority of women underwent mastectomy for almost all types of breast cancer, but current practice favors breast conservation because studies consistently indicate that women who choose lumpectomy and radiation therapy have an equal chance of long-term survival as those who choose mastectomy. Physicians are obligated to tell a patient if one treatment is even slightly superior — even by a small percentage point — but in most cases lumpectomy with radiation and mastectomy are equally excellent forms of treatment.

When making a choice between lumpectomy and mastectomy, additional factors must be considered. These factors are unique to each individual, and she should discuss them with her surgeon and oncologist. For example, a very small percentage of women are diagnosed with *noninvasive* breast cancer that is extremely small and well differentiated (meaning that the cancerous cells resemble normal cells) and has a wide margin of normal tissue around the tumor, and they could consider choosing a lumpectomy alone with no radiation. The decision for most women is whether to have the lump removed and followed with radiation therapy, or whether to undergo mastectomy. Because long-term survival rates are equivalent for these two options, this decision truly becomes a choice dictated by a woman's personal feelings.

Some women feel strongly that they do not want to have a mastectomy. They choose to have the lump surgically removed, with a wide margin around where the tumor was, and then to receive radiation to the breast. This treatment usually involves going for radiation treatment five days a week for approximately six weeks. The first few visits with the radiation oncologist may take one or two hours, so that doctor and patient can become acquainted and the radiation sessions can be carefully planned. The individual radiation treatments themselves, however, take a relatively short time. Newer techniques may shorten the duration of radiation treatments.

Women who choose radiation should recognize that there is a small risk of developing a local recurrence at the site of the previous cancer, so ongoing surveillance with breast self-exams, mammograms, and examination by the doctor throughout their lives will be important. The chance of a local recurrence is low, typically only between 3 and 15 percent over a woman's lifetime. Should cancer recur, however, she would need to undergo mastectomy.

Some women decide to undergo mastectomy at the outset; they prefer to forgo the possibility of recurrence and the inconvenience or side effects of radiation. When choosing this option, the woman needs to select a surgeon, and together they should discuss her options and schedule a date with the hospital. Once admitted to the hospital, she undergoes a surgical procedure that takes approximately one to two hours, during which her surgeon removes the breast and, often, one or more lymph nodes. If a woman undergoes mastectomy, she will also want to consider whether or not to undergo breast reconstructive surgery, a subject addressed in chapter 13.

The following brief scenarios are intended to highlight the variables that influence treatment decisions for achieving local control.

Lumpectomy Alone

Ms. Morales is a 40-year-old woman whose mammogram revealed suspicious calcifications, a sign of possible breast cancer. A biopsy demonstrated a benign adenoma (a tumor), but also in the biopsy sample there was a two-millimeter focus of a very well-differentiated, non-invasive intraductal breast cancer. The biopsy was otherwise negative, and her mammogram, breast exam, and ultrasound revealed no suspicious changes. She was given several options, including lumpectomy alone, lumpectomy with radiation, or mastectomy. She met with a radiation oncologist who advised her that, given the very small size (2 mm) of the low-grade tumor, lumpectomy followed by observation (regular checkups and self-exam) would be a reasonable approach for her. She is being followed carefully without radiation treatment.

The Big Picture

Lumpectomy and Radiation

Ms. James had a two-centimeter infiltrating ductal breast cancer and was concerned that she would have to undergo mastectomy. After talking with her doctor and reviewing the evidence, which shows that lumpectomy followed by radiation therapy results in the same chance of long-term survival as does mastectomy, she chose lumpectomy and radiation to preserve as much of her breast as possible.

Modified Radical Mastectomy

Ms. Perry underwent a breast biopsy that located several tumors (infiltrating ductal breast cancer), each measuring approximately 1.5 centimeters. Ms. Perry wanted to undergo lumpectomy and radiation treatment. However, given the multifocal nature of the disease, the risk of local recurrence would be greater after radiation than it would be for women who have a single tumor focus. She and her surgeon therefore decided to proceed with mastectomy.

Treatment with Tumor-Reducing Therapy Prior to Surgery

Ms. Jones had a very large mass in her breast, measuring approximately eight centimeters in size, with positive lymph node involvement. The cancer had also spread elsewhere in her body. Ms. Jones initially wanted to proceed with mastectomy, but as she began to understand that the cancer had spread beyond the breast, she decided to be treated first with "systemic therapy," which involves taking medication that acts throughout her body, as well as in the breast. She responded very well to treatment with hormonal therapy (tamoxifen). The lesions in her lung and bone improved dramatically, and the nodule in her breast was reduced in size by more than 80 percent. She subsequently underwent a lumpectomy followed by radiation therapy.

Achieving Regional Control

For women with non-invasive breast cancer, the risk of having cancer in the lymph nodes is so small that the lymph nodes often are not sampled at the time of surgery. For women with invasive breast cancer, though, examining the lymph nodes during initial surgery is an important and common practice. Typically, this procedure involves making an incision underneath the arm and then removing one or more of the lymph nodes, which are then examined under a microscope by a pathologist.

The number of lymph nodes removed is determined by the procedure performed. In the last several years, there has been growing interest in trying to pinpoint which lymph nodes actually drain the tumor or are closest to the tumor, and thereby to minimize the number of nodes removed. This process, called *sentinel lymph node biopsy*, is done frequently; it usually brings a lower risk of side effects. Removing the lymph nodes, in general, is not part of the cancer therapy but instead is one of the diagnostic procedures done to determine the stage of the tumor.

Minimizing the Risk of Recurrence

Typically, the greater a woman's risk of developing recurrent metastatic (advanced or spreading) disease, the more likely it is that her doctor will recommend systemic therapy. (Systemic therapy is medicine that circulates throughout the bloodstream.) Here again, a number of factors are taken into account to determine the need for systemic therapy. These include:

- the type of breast cancer (ductal, lobular, inflammatory);
- the size of the tumor;
- the status of the lymph nodes under the arm;
- the results of special studies, including studies of the estrogen or progesterone receptors;
- the presence or absence of the protein known as HER-2-Neu.

Any woman who has had an invasive breast cancer does have some risk of developing recurrence. For example, statistics show that for all premenopausal women who have had node-negative invasive breast cancer, the risk of developing recurrent metastatic disease and then dying from breast cancer is approximately 20 percent (one in five). The individual risks for women can be assessed by analyzing the factors described above. For some women, the risk of recurrence is exceptionally low, so potentially no systemic treatment would be suggested. But for almost all women with invasive breast cancer, it is realistic to expect some form of adjuvant (preventative) therapy.

Systemic Therapy

Women who have non-invasive breast cancer usually do not have a significant risk of the cancer metastasizing or shortening their life. Therefore, chemotherapy would not be given to reduce the risk of recurrence elsewhere in the body. But these women, if they choose lumpectomy and radiation, are at risk for local recurrence of cancer within the breast or for the development of cancer in the other breast. For this reason, there has been growing interest in the use of hormonal therapies like tamoxifen for some women who have had non-invasive breast cancer.

Women who have had infiltrating (invasive) ductal or infiltrating lobular breast cancer are at risk for recurrence of cancer elsewhere in the body. During the past fifty years, there has been a tremendous amount of research done on strategies to reduce this risk.

For many women with estrogen-sensitive tumors, hormonal therapy significantly reduces the risk of recurrence and the risk of death. Tamoxifen, which blocks the hormone receptors, has become a common treatment because it has proven effective in premenopausal and postmenopausal women. A newer class of drugs called aromatase inhibitors reduces the production of estrogen by the adrenal gland and other tissues and can also be effective, but these drugs are used only for treating postmenopausal women.

Adjuvant chemotherapy is important for women who are at higher risk of recurrence or who have tumors that do not respond to hormonal therapy. Multiple types and combinations of adjuvant chemotherapy are available; they are discussed in detail in chapter 17. To begin, however, consider the following three scenarios, which summarize the major variables guiding treatment decisions about adjuvant therapy.

Adjuvant Chemotherapy

Ms. Davis is a 35-year-old woman who has a 1.5-centimeter breast cancer that is hormone-receptor negative. She would not benefit from treatment with tamoxifen, and so she decides with her oncologist to undergo a course of treatment with chemotherapy.

Adjuvant Treatment with Tamoxifen

Ms. Lewis is an 85-year-old woman with a large tumor and positive nodes. Her tumor is hormone-receptor positive. She might benefit from treatment with chemotherapy, but at her age she would most likely face greater risks and more burdensome side effects. Given these concerns and the promise of hormonal therapy, she and her oncologist decide she will take Arimidex and not have chemotherapy.

Adjuvant Chemotherapy and Then Hormonal Therapy

Ms. Smith is a 59-year-old woman whose post-lumpectomy biopsy revealed a three-centimeter infiltrating ductal breast cancer. The lymph node sampling reported that four lymph nodes were positive for cancer, and tests demonstrated that the tumor would likely respond to hormonal therapy. After considering the treatment options, Ms. Smith chose to receive chemotherapy followed by a hormonal therapy. Because she is postmenopausal, her doctor chose to treat her with an aromatase inhibitor (Arimidex) instead of tamoxifen.

Putting It All Together

Most people reading this book are in unfamiliar territory: the medical jargon is probably new, and personal anxiety is likely to be at an unprecedented extreme. For many women facing a breast cancer diagnosis, initial panic makes it difficult to focus on textbook information.

One of the soothing mantras of overwhelmed new medical students is this: "If it's important, I'll hear it again." This reassuring fact is true here, as well. Treatment options are presented by many voices throughout this book, and the most important considerations are reiterated. Medical information is illuminated by the personal narratives that constitute the human core of this book.

CHAPTER 3

A Statistic of One

April Fritz, RHIT, CTR

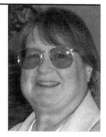

My dad was a doctor, so I grew up around medical terminology and numbers. When I was about 25, I began working in a hospital's medical records department, coding the records of discharged patients and compiling statistics on types of diseases and other medical information. For the last thirty years I have been a cancer registrar, a health professional who gathers data on cancer patients and then converts that information into useable statistics. Needless to say, it was a total surprise when I felt a mass in my breast that turned out to be cancer. The first breast cancer statistic I encountered that affected me personally came from my surgeon, who said that the odds were 80 percent that my mass was benign.

But guess what? I was in the other 20 percent.

Once I got past the shock of not being in the 80 percent, I went into research mode. If you are reading this book, you probably are doing the same thing. Research mode is when you go on the Internet or ask friends and other people you know who have had cancer what they would do if they were in your shoes, how they would handle their treatment choices, and what they know about survival rates. But do you really want to know your likelihood of surviving five or ten years? As a cancer data specialist, I know how misleading some statistics are—not because they are wrong but because they don't exactly apply to me.

If I were to go into research mode today, I would be confronted with a huge array of figures about breast cancer, like these:

1. One woman in seven will develop cancer in her lifetime. (Who are the other women in my group and how can I trade places with one of them?)
2. Women have more treatment choices than ever. (Fine, but do some choices work better than others?)
3. The number of women choosing breast conservation surgery has risen more than 300 percent in two decades. (OK, but what's breast conservation surgery?)
4. Caucasian women have the highest rate of breast conservation surgery in recent years. (That's good information, but I'm . . . *fill in the blank*.)
5. Women in New England have higher rates of lumpectomy and radiation therapy than any other area of the country. (Good for them, but I live in . . . *fill in the blank*.)
6. Disadvantaged women have lower rates of lumpectomy. (What does this mean?)

You're probably thinking: *There are so many facts and numbers and rates and trends out there—how can I figure out what is useful and important to me?* Well, as a health professional used to working with numbers, and as a woman who has been where you are today, let me be your guide through the statistical swamp.

Let's start with some definitions.

Demographics is the term used to refer to the characteristics by which people are commonly grouped and differentiated, such as age, race, ethnic heritage, sex, marital status, and place of residence. Also among these characteristics are personal beliefs, personal choices, and cultural aspects, but these factors are harder to put into neat categories.

Breast conservation surgery is surgery that seeks to preserve as much of the breast as possible. Only the tumor is removed, along with a minimal amount of surrounding tissue. The rest of the breast is spared or conserved (hence, the names *breast sparing* and *breast conservation* surgery). There are a number of different technical names for surgery that spares the breast: lumpectomy, quadrantectomy, partial mastectomy, excisional biopsy (when there is no tumor left in the breast after the biopsy), segmental mastectomy, wedge resection, and other procedures where the primary tumor but not the entire breast is surgically removed. Breast conservation surgery is usually combined with either radiation therapy to the axillary (armpit) lymph nodes or with complete removal of the axillary lymph nodes (lymph node dissection).

Breast removal surgery or *mastectomy* is surgery that removes the entire breast. There are three different surgical techniques for removing the entire breast: (1) simple, (2) modified radical, and (3) radical. The differences are in the amount of additional tissue removed. Simple mastectomy removes just the breast. Modified radical mastectomy usually removes some lymph nodes, and radical mastectomy removes breast, lymph nodes, and muscle.

Stage at diagnosis is a shorthand way of saying how far a cancer has spread at the time of diagnosis. There are four basic categories with regard to breast cancer:

In situ refers to cancer arising in a breast duct and just sitting there, incapable of spreading; it is also called intraductal or non-invasive.

Localized refers to cancer arising in a breast duct but spread into the supporting breast tissues, where it has the *potential* to spread to lymph vessels or blood vessels; it is also called invasive; still, it is confined to the breast with no axillary node involvement.

Regional refers to cancer involving structures adjacent to or beyond the breast, such as the axillary lymph nodes and/or the skin over the breast.

Distant, also called *metastatic,* refers to cancer that has spread to other organs away from the breast such as the liver or lungs; these distant sites of cancer are sometimes called *mets.*

While these terms are still in common use, a newer medical shorthand for cancer staging is the TNM system, which is explained in detail in chapter 2. For most of this chapter, we don't need that level of detail. For now, understand that Stage 0 is equivalent to in situ. Stage I refers to localized disease (meaning a tumor less than three-quarters of an inch in diameter with no involved lymph nodes). Stage II refers either to tumors up to two inches in diameter with involved lymph nodes *or* to tumors larger than two inches across without involved lymph nodes. The stages go all the way up to IV, which refers to distant metastasis.

A Bit of History

Today, all women have the luxury of treatment options, but the evolution of these choices spans only a few decades. The fundamental choice between breast sparing surgery and breast removal dates only to the mid-1970s, a time of vast change not only in medicine but also in politics, mores, and attitudes about women's and patients' rights.

For most of the twentieth century, treatment choices for breast cancer were shaped by two assumptions: first, that breast cancer was a localized disease that could be cured only by complete removal of the breast, the underlying chest wall muscles, and the underarm lymph nodes; and second, that the doctor, not the patient, should make the treatment decisions.

The first assumption, initially championed by Dr. William Halsted in 1894, led to the wide acceptance of radical mastectomy by the medical community, a field dominated by men. For fifty years, surgeons believed that the more tissue removed, the better the chances of cure. Thus, with few female physicians to question its necessity and virtually no input from patients, the surgery recommended by doctors remained the disfiguring Halsted radical mastectomy.

However, world events changed part of that picture when women went to work in support of the war effort in the early 1940s. In the next decade, more and more women entered the work force full time, and more women sought higher education. Increasingly conscious of their positions in the world outside the home, women grew more aware of the life—and medical—choices available to them. The 1960s saw women becoming politically organized, participating in protests on college campuses and even during the Miss America beauty pageant. By the early 1970s, women's voices were being heard more clearly than ever before.

In 1971, breast cancer research gained momentum when the federal government funded clinical trials to evaluate the survival differences between women treated with radical mastectomy and those treated with the less disfiguring *modified* radical mastectomy. The results of that landmark study were published in 1977 and showed that there was no statistically important difference in overall survival, in the occurrence of distant metastases, or in the overall success of treatment between the two study arms. These results have held true through twenty-five years of follow-up evaluation.

The next question was how *much* less surgery could be done while maintaining the same success rates. A subsequent clinical trial initiated in 1976 compared the modified radical mastectomy to lumpectomy with radiation. Those results, initially published in 1985 and updated in 2002, confirmed that even over many years, there is virtually no difference in disease-free survival (meaning rates of recurrence either locally or as distant metastases) between modified radical mastectomy (breast removal) and lumpectomy (breast sparing) surgery. This second major breast cancer treatment trial confirmed what many clinicians had believed for a decade or more—that comparatively minimal surgery followed by radiation is a good treatment option. When this scientific evidence entered clinical practice in community hospitals, the results were dramatic: breast removal rates began to fall and breast sparing surgery rates began to rise. Today radical mastectomy is hardly ever performed, and women often have the choice of breast sparing surgery rather than more disfiguring breast removal surgery.

The choice of breast cancer treatment is a personal one, involving not only a woman's age, race, ethnicity and other demographics but also her cultural background and such basic things as how far she lives from a treatment facility. That's why a lot of new patients in research mode get bogged down in the statistics swamp. They grasp at generalities and try to apply them to their own specific cases. It would take millions of cases to identify just a few (if any) patients who match *your* exact demographics and beliefs. So we have to come up with a way to sort out what is important to *you* and what you can set aside while you are in research mode.

All Those Numbers

First of all, if you are going to research statistics, get them from a reliable source, like the National Cancer Institute (cancer.gov) or the American Cancer Society (cancer.org), trusted national women's health organizations like the Susan G. Komen Breast Cancer Foundation, or your local health care facility. Avoid places like personal web sites or web sites that are obviously commercial in nature. While the stories on these sites may be interesting, there are underlying motives behind what the web site chooses to display. Your doctor can recommend other professional web sites that provide reliable information.

I work with breast cancer statistics on a daily basis, and I have gathered some statistics especially for this chapter. This information comes from the Surveillance, Epidemiology and End Results (SEER) Program of the U.S. National Cancer Institute.[1] (All the technical information is in the notes at the end of the chapter.) This is called *descriptive* data—it includes proportions of cases in various categories extracted from an extremely large database. This database includes women from many backgrounds, but for the sake of simplicity, I am going to keep my remarks general.

The Rise in Popularity of Breast Sparing Surgery

Between 1983 and 2001 (the database range), breast removal surgery ceased to be the treatment of choice. The procedure's frequency dropped by half in nineteen years. That is, it went from being chosen by more than eight in ten women to being chosen by barely four in ten. Meanwhile, the popularity of breast sparing surgery more than tripled (or, in other words, increased by 300 percent, as this statistic reads above). Figure 3.1 shows how rapidly breast removal surgery declined and breast sparing surgery increased. Today, breast sparing surgery is the treatment of choice for most women with breast cancer.

You may be thinking, *But I'm not "most" women, and maybe I don't want to have breast sparing surgery. I just want to get that thing out of me and get on*

The Big Picture

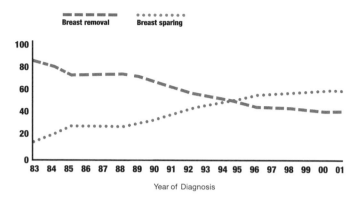

Breast Sparing Surgery Trends, 1983–2001

▬ ▬ ▬ ▬   • • • • • • • • •
Breast removal   **Breast sparing**

Year of Diagnosis

FIGURE 3.1. In 1983 over 80 percent of women with breast cancer were having a mastectomy (breast removal surgery). By 2001 less than 40 percent were having this same procedure and more were having lumpectomy (breast conserving surgery).

with my life. People have different reactions. Fortunately, you can look at the trends in breast cancer surgery in a number of ways. When the information is available, it is useful to examine statistics that are more relevant to your unique situation, rather than data that aggregates the treatment choices of women with the entire range of diagnostic scenarios, from miniscule tumors to distant metastases.

There are differences in how frequently breast sparing surgery is used in each stage. Women with in situ cancer were among the earliest to accept breast sparing surgery. This is the group in which the rise in conservation surgery was the greatest, increasing from 30 percent in 1983 to more than 70 percent in 2001. Women with localized disease were initially less likely (19%) to undergo breast conserving surgery but by 2001 were almost at the same level as the group with in situ disease (64.5%). Only about 11 percent of those with lymph node disease were treated with breast sparing surgery in the early 1980s; this rate increased 44 percent by 2001. That figure is much smaller than for lower-stage cases, because once cancer has been found outside the breast (in the lymph nodes), patients are more likely to be treated with complete removal of the involved breast. Breast conservation is still a good option medically for women who have cancer in the lymph nodes.

Breast sparing surgery may be ideal for in situ cancers and invasive localized cancers, but that kind of treatment may not be adequate for larger tumors. On the other hand, if a woman with involved lymph nodes prefers not to lose her breast to this disease, breast sparing surgery can be supplemented by other types of treatment, such as radiation therapy. Treatment is a matter of *informed* choices on the part of the woman, based on—but not mandated by—the recommendations of her doctor.

Demographics

Demographic data enable us to describe large populations, but they do not differentiate in close detail among individuals. Demographic categories cannot do full justice to any person's psychological complexity. Being a certain age and race, for example, does not mean that you will think the same way as everyone else of your age and race. Yet traits such as age, race, ethnicity, and marital status do play their roles in how many women feel about their bodies and about their diagnoses.

Marital Status

In the SEER database, single women who either had never been married or who were divorced at the time of diagnosis preferred breast sparing surgery 2 percent more than married women did ("married" status also included common-law wedlock, separation, and widowhood). This is not a large difference. The actual or imagined feelings of a woman's current or potential partners may influence her thinking about surgical options.

Age at Diagnosis

You may have heard that breast cancer is predominantly a disease of mature women; more than three-fourths of the women with breast cancer are age 50 and older. The midpoint of the age range (median age) at diagnosis is 63 for white women and 56 for black women. If you sort patients into three age ranges—30–49, 50–69, and age 70 and higher—some interesting findings appear. In 1983, the young women had higher acceptance of breast sparing surgery, and their rate of breast conservation surgery tripled by 2001. In the middle group, the initial proportion opting for breast sparing surgery was only slightly less than for the younger group, but their rate of breast sparing surgery *quadrupled* over the same period. Women in the oldest group initially chose breast sparing surgery at a rate similar to the youngest patients but by 2001 had rates comparable to those of the 50- to 69-year-olds.

You really can't make statements about women in general! No matter how old you are chronologically, the decision to have breast sparing surgery is personal. It is based on how young you feel, on your general health, on your attitude toward your body and your health, and on your doctor's recommendation. Breast sparing surgery can be considered by women of virtually any age. Your doctor should not second-guess how important your breasts are to you.

Race and Ethnicity

More striking than the differences in surgical choice made by women of various ages are the differences in choice made by distinct racial and ethnic groups. Although some people dislike the collection of racial and ethnic data, such statistics enable the federal government to monitor whether all citizens have access to the same level of health care. The organizations that provide data for the SEER database have been carefully selected to sample population groups of special interest,[2] providing good information on trends in breast cancer surgery by race.

Figure 3.2 shows the differences in acceptance of breast sparing surgery by four major categories of women: (1) white, (2) Hispanic/Latina, (3) black, and (4) those of "other races" (which includes Native Americans and Alaska Natives, Hawaiians, Pacific Islanders, and Asian U.S. residents reported as being of Chinese, Japanese, Korean, Filipino, or other Asian descent).

All race groups had virtually the same rate of acceptance for breast sparing surgery in 1983—just under 20 percent. Over time, however, the breast sparing surgery rate for patients in the "other race" group and for Hispanics did not rise as quickly as for white and black women.

Cultural differences are one of many variables affecting women's choices about breast sparing surgery. In some cultural communities, it may be difficult for a woman to speak up and express her personal pref-

Breast Sparing Surgery Trends, 1983–2001

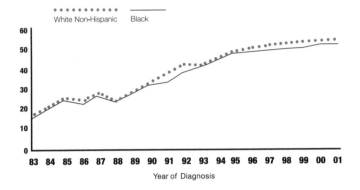

FIGURE 3.2. From 1983 to 2001 there was a steady increase in the percentage of women who had lumpectomy (breast conserving surgery). But the percentage of black women who had breast conserving surgery was consistently smaller than the percentage of white women having this surgery.

erences to a male doctor. In this situation, the doctor may have greater influence over the ultimate choice his patient makes. The data on treatment choices show that cultural differences are reflected in different treatment decisions. If you were raised in a culture that did not encourage you to express your own wishes (especially to a doctor), then it is important for you to know now that you really do have a say in how you are treated.

Socioeconomic Status

The authors of a large study conducted by the National Cancer Institute found that for each of the several cancers studied, patients in high-poverty areas tended to be diagnosed at later stages and had lower survival rates than patients living in low-poverty areas. In addition, residents of high-poverty areas were less likely to receive the most up-to-date type of treatment, such as breast conservation surgery, for their cancers.

Socioeconomic status had a clear relationship to surgical treatment patterns in breast cancer, regardless of patients' racial or ethnic background. Overall, and consistently among the race categories, patients in high-poverty areas had a lower rate of breast sparing surgery compared to patients in low-poverty areas. There are many reasons for these lower rates of breast sparing surgery. For one thing, breast sparing surgery is less likely to be the treatment of choice for patients diagnosed at higher stages, which unfortunately is the case for a greater proportion of women in the high-poverty-area group. Another possible reason is that patients in high-poverty areas may not realize or understand that they do have a choice in how they are treated and that there are different surgical options.

Regional Factors

There were notable regional differences in the rate of breast sparing surgery in 2001. Eastern states had the highest rate of breast sparing surgery (66.1%). The eastern states include New England, where women chose breast sparing surgery an amazing 73 percent of the time. For the central states, the rate was considerably lower, 58.3 percent. Western states (a mix of Pacific Rim and mountain states) had a rate of 61.3 percent. Even considering the stage at diagnosis within each region, figures were consistently higher for breast sparing surgery in the East than in other regions, both for in situ cancers and for small localized cancers with no involved lymph nodes.

It is not clear why there are such regional differences. But what do the differences mean to you as a patient? Like cultural differences, regional or geographic differences are simply something you should be aware of. Why is the rate for breast sparing surgery so much higher in the East? Possibly because the early clinical trials were conducted by a research group in Pennsylvania and the word spread from there. Access to treatment facilities may also account for the differences. Good cancer care after a breast sparing surgery includes radiation therapy, which involves returning to the hospital five days a week for five or six weeks. If a patient lives too far away, all that daily travel can be a real burden for the patient and her driver. In those cases, the patient may decide to have a mastectomy instead.

In addition to issues of physical access, personal attitudes and work responsibilities may account for regional differences. A woman working on a farm, for example, or managing a large family may not be able to take the time to drive to a treatment facility five days a week for several weeks and may prefer mastectomy for that reason. Alternatively, some women do not see the preservation of breast tissue as critical to their body image or self-worth. For others, it may be the desire to have the treatment "over and done with" that motivates the choice of mastectomy. Patient preference and physician attitudes toward various types of treatment are difficult to measure, but the data show that there are regional differences.

The bottom line is that treatment preference varies across the country; it varies among patients, and it can also vary among physicians. It is always okay to seek out a doctor who will listen to you and treat you according to your wishes. This may involve getting a second opinion. You don't have to "follow the crowd" in your region if you choose not to. Know that you do have options and that you can seek your preferred treatment close to home.

Lymph Node Procedures

While it may seem difficult enough to weigh the choice between breast sparing surgery and breast removal surgery, it is not the only challenging decision that must be made. Diagnosis of the axillary lymph nodes also involves making a choice about surgery. In the last ten years, a new technique has been developed for identifying involved lymph nodes. It is called sentinel node dissection or sentinel node biopsy. This technique uses liquid dye and radioactive material to track the flow of lymphatic fluid away from the area of the tumor and into the first receiving lymph nodes outside the breast. If those first lymph nodes (the "sentinel" nodes) are removed and found to be free of tumor, then the odds are very high that no other "downstream" nodes in the axilla are involved. This technique minimizes surgery because it enables doctors to identify healthy lymph nodes without having to remove them or others. Prior to the advent of sentinel node biopsy, it was necessary to remove and examine most of the axillary lymph nodes to be sure that the cancer had not spread. Sentinel lymph node surgery can be performed with either breast sparing surgery or breast removal surgery.

The percentage of women choosing sentinel node biopsy has been rising, and the percentage of women having full axillary lymph node dissection has been decreasing. These trends are apparent even when the data are subdivided by stage at diagnosis. This is good news for a woman who wants minimal surgery, since sentinel lymph node biopsy goes hand in hand with her choice of breast conservation surgery.

Survival

"What are my chances of living a long, healthy life after breast cancer?" is undoubtedly the one-billion-dollar question. When I was first diagnosed, I had access to the same powerful databases that I have used in writing this chapter, but I chose not to work the formula that would tell me survival odds. I thought that piece of information might be frightening and self-limiting. I want to lead you to the other side of the statistical swamp by using some numbers to demonstrate that you *will* get through all this. For example (sound the trumpets!): *for early stage disease, the relative survival rates for patients with breast cancer are equivalent to those for patients of the same age and demographics who do not have breast cancer.*

The landmark breast treatment comparison studies of the 1970s and 1980s greatly expanded the range of surgical options for women with breast cancer. Those studies were scientifically constructed and carefully managed, and the findings were backed up by additional studies. The results of those studies demonstrated that survival after breast conserving surgery was the same as survival after mastectomy. The same results are also evident in descriptive statistics based on larger groups of breast cancer patients from a much wider range of demographics and tumor characteristics.

Table 3.1 shows that five- and ten-year relative survivals are comparable by type of surgery and for each stage at diagnosis. In fact, for noninvasive (in situ) cancer, the relative survival rate is the same as the survival of the general population. Diagnosis and treatment for in situ cancer does not affect overall survival. For localized cancers that have the potential to spread undetected to other parts of the body, the survival rates are similar whether women opt for breast sparing or breast removal sur-

TABLE 3.1. FIVE- AND TEN-YEAR RELATIVE SURVIVAL
Breast Sparing versus Breast Removal Surgery, by Stage

	5-Year Relative Survival (%)		10-Year Relative Survival (%)	
	Breast Sparing (n = 98,412)	Breast Removal (n = 90,302)	Breast Sparing (n = 98,412)	Breast Removal (n = 90,302)
In situ	100.0	100.0	100.0	100.0
Local	96.0	94.7	92.2	90.1

Source: Surveillance, Epidemiology and End Results (SEER) Program, available at www.seer.cancer.gov.
SEER®Stat Database: Incidence—9 SEER Registries 1983–2001, November 2003 submission, National Cancer Institute.

gery. And even though those rates are somewhat lower than for the general population, they are no reason to stop living now.

Conclusion

I want to leave you with one primary message: the choice of treatment should be a mutual decision between each woman and her doctor. This chapter documents trends based on data collected over more than nineteen years on the medical experience of half a million women with breast cancer. Yet every woman with breast cancer is unique; every woman is her own set of statistics. It may not be possible to find one graph or table that predicts with 100 percent accuracy what any personal outcome will be. However, understanding this information can help inform your personal treatment decision.

We can see where trends in treatment differ by race, ethnicity, stage at diagnosis, age at diagnosis, marital status, socioeconomic status and other variables. While most women now choose breast sparing surgery, it may be that you prefer to make a different choice. Remember that you are a statistic of ONE. No person in any database is an exact match for you and your unique demographics. Right now your survival rate is 100 percent. After twelve years, my personal survival rate is still 100 percent. I know I am beating the odds this time. It is very possible that you too can beat the odds—that's why the statistics on breast cancer are improving every year!

PATIENT RESOURCES

Cancer database: Surveillance, Epidemiology, and End Results (SEER) Program.
    SEER*Stat Database: Incidence-SEER 18 Regs, November 2003 Submission
    (1973–2001), National Cancer Institute, DCCPS, Surveillance Research Pro-
    gram, Cancer Statistics Branch, released April 2004, based on the November
    2003 submission. Available at www.seer.cancer.gov

Statistical software: Surveillance Research Program, National Cancer Institute
    SEER*Stat software, version 5.1.11-beta. Available at www.seer.cancer.gov/
    seerstat.

Fisher, B. "Breast-Conserving Surgery in the Treatment of Invasive Breast Can-
    cer: Its Validity and Outstanding Issues." *Breast Journal* 1 (1995). Reprinted by
    permission of Blackwell Science, Inc., and available at www.asri.edu/bfisher/
    br_conserving_surgery.html.

Ries, L. A. G., M. P. Eisner, C. L. Kosary, B. F. Hankey, B. A. Miller, L. Clegg, A.
    Mariotto, M. P. Fay, E. J. Feuer, and B. K. Edwards, eds. *SEER Cancer Statis-
    tics Review, 1975–2000*, National Cancer Institute. Bethesda, MD. Available at
    http://seer.cancer.gov/csr/1975_2000, 2003.

Singh, G. K., B. A. Miller, B. F. Hankey, and B. K. Edwards. *Area Socioeconomic
    Variations in U.S. Cancer Incidence, Mortality, Stage, Treatment, and Survival, 1975–
    1999.* NCI Cancer Surveillance Monograph Series, no. 4. Bethesda, MD: Na-
    tional Cancer Institute, August 2003. NIH Publication No. 03-5417.

Web Sites for Women's History

www.marybold.com
www.cwluherstory.com
www.nsabp.pitt.edu

SOURCES AND NOTES

1. The SEER Program is a federally funded health surveillance program that has been collecting data about new diagnoses of cancer since 1973. Nine population-based cancer registries have participated in the surveillance program since the late 1970s, covering approximately 9.5 percent of the U.S. population. After program expansion in 1992 and again in 2000, the SEER Program now covers 26 percent of the population. The data in this chapter are based on the nine population-based registries for the years 1983–1991 and are augmented by data from five additional registries for the years 1992–2001.

SEER Program participants are carefully selected for their ability to provide high-quality, detailed, timely information on populations of special interest. More than 3 million cancer cases are included in the SEER database. SEER data are collected on patient characteristics, primary tumor site, type of cancer, stage at diagnosis, first course of treatment, and vital status at annual intervals after diag-nosis. Research interests, treatment patterns, and data-collection methods have evolved over the thirty years of the SEER Program; therefore, the amount and detail of information gathered has changed as well. Detailed data about the type of surgery performed for breast cancer, which form the basis for this analysis of trends, have only been available since 1983, roughly corresponding to the beginning of the change in attitudes about breast sparing surgery. Data were extracted from the November 2003 SEER Public Use Data File (1973–2001) using the SEER*Stat statistical software developed by the National Cancer Institute and provided in the public domain. The data described in this chapter are based on the medical histories of over 513,000 women with breast cancer who were diagnosed between 1983 and 2001 and received some form of surgery to the breast.

2. In 1980, the U.S. population was about 83 percent white; according to the 2000 census, the United States is now 75.1 percent white. Based on the 2000 census, the SEER data used in this review represent 23 percent of the total U.S. population, including 20.3 percent of whites, 17.5 percent of blacks, 39.9 percent of Hispanics, and 47 percent of other races due to oversampling of smaller populations.

CHAPTER 4

"Why Me?"

A Discussion of Risk

Mark Robson, M.D.

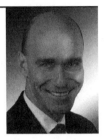

It is important that women in the United States know that over one in eight women will be diagnosed with breast cancer. Organizations such as the American Cancer Society and the mass media in general have been instrumental in educating the public about this disease that struck more than 200,000 women in 2006 and caused over 40,000 deaths. Among women, breast cancer is second only to lung cancer as a cause of cancer-related death.

Public awareness of breast cancer is even higher than awareness of a bigger killer: cardiovascular disease. Nearly everyone knows someone who has been diagnosed with breast cancer, and many women feel vulnerable. It is only natural, then, that women seek information to help them assess their own personal risk. The quest is a challenging one because medical science cannot determine with certainty the specific factors that cause breast cancer in an individual woman. In fact, the most common "risk factors" actually cause only a mild increase in risk. It is true that researchers have identified a few risk factors that present a very high risk and may be said with reasonable certainty to be the cause of cancer in a particular woman, but these factors are fortunately quite rare. So how should people begin to think about personal risk?

Risk can be described in a number of different ways. Perhaps the most common scientific approach is to consider "relative risk." If a characteristic is more common in women with cancer, then the relative risk from that factor will be greater than one, which suggests that the given characteristic may, in fact, increase the risk of cancer. The characteristic will then be called a "risk factor." For instance, if the ratio is 1.2, it is said that the factor increases risk by 20 percent. Note that this does *not* mean that 20 percent of the women with the factor get cancer. It means that the factor is roughly 20 percent more common in those with cancer than in those without, though it may be present in a large number of women who never develop cancer. Such a factor may increase risk in a *group* of women, but it cannot be said to have caused cancer in any *particular* woman. (There are many examples of such factors, including those that are the best known, discussed below.)

Other ways of expressing risk are more straightforward. Studies may simply describe the percentage of women (number per 100) with a given pattern of risk factors who develop cancer in a specified time. When you are looking at the results of studies that describe risk factors, it is important to know exactly *how* risk is being described, so you can understand how significant each factor may be.

Risk Factors

Age

The number-one risk factor for breast cancer is increasing age. The annual risk of invasive breast cancer in women under age 40 is less than 1 of every 1,000 women. For women over age 70, that number increases to nearly 1 of every 200 women each year. Looked at another way, less than 15 percent of all cases of breast cancer are diagnosed in women under age 45. For many women, increasing age may be their only identifiable risk factor.

Reproductive Risk Factors

A number of factors related to a woman's reproductive life have an influence on her breast cancer risk, including age at menarche (the age at which a woman has her first menstrual period). Women who begin having regular periods at a later age have a lower breast cancer risk than women who begin having their periods early. However, the difference is modest. Women who begin having their periods at age 15 or older have an approximately 20 percent lower risk than women who begin their periods before age 12. At the other end of the reproductive life cycle, women who enter menopause before age 45 have nearly half the breast cancer risk of women who continue to have menstrual cycles past age 55.

A woman's age when she first gives birth also influences breast cancer risk. A woman who has her first child before the age of 20 has about half the risk of a woman who never gives birth. Having children is not uniformly protective, however. Women who have their first children after the age of 30 to 35 actually have a slightly higher breast cancer risk than women who never give birth. Risk decreases with increasing numbers of live births. Breast feeding also appears to reduce risk, although the benefit is again modest. For each year of breast feeding, breast cancer risk is reduced by about 4 percent.

There has been considerable controversy over the effect of abortion on breast cancer risk. Some studies have suggested a mild increase in breast cancer risk, but a large analysis of all available studies concluded that there was no increased risk among women who have had early termination of pregnancy, either spontaneous or induced.

Finally, there does not appear to be any increase in breast cancer risk among women who have undergone ovarian stimulation for infertility compared to women who have never undergone such treatment. There may be a small increase in risk in the year following treatment, however, and this increase is probably related to the growth of previously undetected cancers that were stimulated by the hormonal treatment.

Environmental Exposures

Hormonal treatments (for example, oral contraceptives or post-menopausal hormone replacement therapy) are the environmental exposures of greatest concern to women considering their breast cancer risk. An aggregate analysis of fifty-four studies examining the influence of birth control pills on breast cancer risk suggested a mild increase in risk among women taking combination oral contraceptives, and other studies have suggested that this increase in risk may be greater among women who have a strong family history of breast cancer. However, different pills may pose different risks, as suggested by observations of lower risks among women taking the Pill after 1974, when the amount of estrogen in most formulations was reduced. In addition, the risk posed by so-called progestin-only contraceptives is still not clearly defined. The breast cancer risk from oral contraceptives seems to return to baseline once women have been off the Pill for about five years.

What's less clear is the relationship between postmenopausal hormone replacement therapy (HRT) and breast cancer risk. A combined analysis of fifty-one studies indicated a 21 percent increase in breast cancer risk among current users of hormone replacement therapy, as compared to nonusers. Risk appeared to increase by approximately 2 percent per year of use. These aggregate data were recently confirmed by the large Women's Health Initiative (WHI) study, in which women who received combination hormone replacement therapy had a substantially greater breast cancer risk than those who did not. Although the relative increase in risk was significant, the actual excess number of breast cancers among women receiving hormone replacement was modest. So, although the risk of breast cancer in women using combination hormone replacement is higher than in women not using replacement, it is not possible to attribute an individual woman's cancer definitively to HRT, as she might have developed the cancer even if she was not taking the drug. In the WHI studies, there was no obvious increase in breast cancer risk among women receiving estrogen-only replacement, suggesting that the progestin component of the therapy may play a significant role in increasing breast cancer risk. However, women who have a uterus (women who have not had a hysterectomy) need the progestin component of therapy to help prevent uterine cancer if they take HRT.

A number of other environmental factors have been suggested as possible causes of breast cancer. These include breast implants; exposure to deodorants, hair dyes, or electromagnetic fields related to cell phones or power lines; and *in utero* exposure to the drug diethylstilboestrol (DES). Researchers have found no clear association between any of these exposures and risk of developing breast cancer. Numerous studies have examined whether exposure to pesticides may increase breast cancer risk, and, again, there is no conclusive evidence that this is the case. Trauma to the breast and breast reduction surgery were once thought to be associated with an increase in breast cancer risk, but this association is no longer considered valid.

The *only* environmental exposure clearly associated with an increased risk of developing breast cancer is excess radiation. However, the amount of radiation required to increase risk is substantial—much more than most women ever receive. The studies showing an increase in risk included women who had undergone multiple X-ray examinations for scoliosis or for follow-up of tuberculosis, and in survivors of the nuclear explosions at Hiroshima and Nagasaki. Most women never receive nearly this much radiation in their lives. The one group of women who are at significant risk from radiation exposure are those who receive therapeutic radiation to their chests for Hodgkin's Disease or other types of cancer. These women have a dramatically increased risk for breast cancer and need to be monitored carefully.

Lifestyle Factors

Doesn't it seem as if there's a new report released every day about how the way we lead our lives affects our risk of cancer? Many of these lifestyle studies are contradictory, which leads to considerable confusion among women who are seeking to minimize their own breast cancer risk. Adding to the confusion is that many of the lifestyle factors that have been studied may influence the risk of breast cancer differently in premenopausal women and postmenopausal women. Generally speaking, the impact of modifiable lifestyle factors on breast cancer risk has not been clearly established, and, even when some effect is suggested, its magnitude appears to be small.

A number of studies suggest mild reductions in breast cancer risk among women who engage in recreational or occupational exercise, for example. And it may be that taller, heavier women have an increased breast cancer risk, particularly after menopause. This increased risk has been hypothesized to result from an increase in circulating estrogen produced by fat cells, but this association has not been clearly established. Of course, maintaining an ideal body weight has a number of health benefits in addition to reducing breast cancer risk.

Although maintaining an ideal body weight may help reduce breast cancer risk, there is no clear evidence that breast cancer risk is affected by particular changes in diet. One area of significant focus has been dietary fat. While there have been some studies showing a mild association between total dietary fat and breast cancer risk, it is not clear that modifying dietary fat intake reduces that risk to a significant degree. Similarly, there is no evidence that avoiding specific types of fat, such as dairy or animal fat, is helpful.

Other dietary components, such as coffee or food hormones, have not been associated with an increased risk. The influence of soy products and phytoestrogens on breast cancer risk is under investigation. To date, there is insufficient evidence to determine whether dietary supplementation with soy products is helpful in reducing risk—though there is no evidence to suggest that soy products should be avoided. Some studies have suggested mild reductions in breast cancer risk with increased consumption of dietary fiber or fruits and vegetables, but these studies are not sufficiently convincing to support dramatic dietary modification for this goal. In terms of supplements, some studies have suggested mild reductions in risk in women whose diet includes more foods containing vitamin C or vitamin A, but this finding does not necessarily mean that taking supplemental vitamins is helpful. Other supplements, such as vitamin E and selenium, have not proven beneficial.

Two other lifestyle exposures of importance are tobacco and alcohol. Numerous studies have failed to show a connection between smoking and breast cancer risk. Studies have shown that smoking increases the risk of lung cancer—the number-one cause of cancer death among women. Excess alcohol exposure, on the other hand, *has* been linked in a number of studies to an increase in breast cancer risk. An aggregate analysis of fifty-three studies concluded that the risk of breast cancer increases by approximately 7 percent for every ten grams of daily alcohol intake. This is approximately the amount of alcohol contained in a glass of wine. A can of beer contains about thirteen grams of alcohol, and a shot of liquor about fifteen grams. Therefore, a woman who has a glass of wine each night may increase her breast cancer risk modestly, and heavier drinking may pose an even greater risk.

Family History

The one breast cancer risk factor that nearly everyone knows about is family history. But before talking about the influence of family history on breast cancer risk, it is important to note that most women with breast cancer have no other family member with breast cancer. Although studies differ, only 10 to 15 percent of women with breast cancer have a first-degree relative (mother, sister, daughter) or second-degree relative (aunt, grandmother, granddaughter) with breast cancer. A slightly greater proportion may have a more distant relative affected.

In general, women who have a family history of breast cancer have about twice the breast cancer risk of women without such a history. The risk is higher for women with an affected first-degree relative (mother, sister) than for those whose only affected relative is more distant. In addition, the risk is higher for women whose relative was diagnosed before age fifty. Women who have more than one affected relative are at higher risk than those with only one affected relative.

Most women with a family history of breast cancer have only a single affected relative. In these families, the family history may be due to chance (breast cancer is a common disease that may easily strike more than one woman in a large family) or it may be due to shared environmental exposures. Rarely, the family history may be more striking, with multiple women over several generations affected with breast cancer, usually at younger ages and sometimes in both breasts (bilateral). Such women are said to be at risk for hereditary breast cancer.

Hereditary Breast Cancer

Hereditary breast cancer results from inheriting an abnormal (mutated) gene from one parent. It is important to note that either parent can pass along a gene that predisposes to hereditary breast cancer, so a history of breast cancer among one's father's relatives is just as important as a history among one's mother's relatives. Hereditary breast cancer accounts for less than 10 percent of all breast cancer. Even among women with a family history of breast cancer, only a small number are at risk for hereditary breast cancer. Several different genes can cause hereditary breast cancer, but the most common ones are called *BRCA1* and *BRCA2*.

The breast cancer susceptibility gene, *BRCA1*, is located on chromosome 17q. Mutations in this gene account for up to 45 percent of hereditary breast cancer cases. Individuals with such mutations are at increased risk for breast, ovarian, or prostate cancer, and possibly for other cancers. It is reported that women from high-risk families who personally carry mutations in the *BRCA1* gene have up to an 85 percent lifetime risk of developing breast cancer and up to a 40 to 60 percent lifetime risk of developing ovarian cancer. This can be compared to the 12.5 percent lifetime risk of breast cancer and 1 to 2 percent lifetime risk of ovarian cancer for women in the general population. Some studies suggest that cancer risks may be lower in some families. Men with *BRCA1* mutations may also be at increased risk for breast cancer. The degree to which male breast cancer risk is elevated is not well defined, but the absolute risk appears to be small. Men with *BRCA1* mutations are also at increased risk for prostate and probably pancreatic cancer.

Mutations in the *BRCA2* gene, located on chromosome 13q, account for up to 35 percent of families with hereditary breast cancer. Early studies suggested that the breast cancer risk associated with *BRCA2* was similar to the risk associated with *BRCA1*, but more recent studies suggest breast cancer risk may be lower in certain families. The ovarian cancer risk for those who carry *BRCA2* mutations is estimated to be between 16 and 27 percent by age 70. Men who carry mutations in *BRCA2* have a 5 to 10 percent lifetime risk of breast cancer. Cancers of the pancreas, prostate, skin (melanoma), and other sites have also been associated with

BRCA2 mutations. Research continues to identify the risks of specific diseases.

Women with a mutation in either *BRCA1* or *BRCA2* who have been diagnosed with breast cancer are at increased risk for developing a second breast cancer. Evidence suggests that 25 to 30 percent of such women will develop cancer in the other breast (called the *contralateral breast*) in the ten years following their first diagnosis.

Inherited mutations in *BRCA1* and *BRCA2* have been detected in individuals of all races and ethnic groups. In most cases, the mutations are specific to a particular family. However, individuals from certain populations have a greater risk of inheriting specific *BRCA1* and/or *BRCA2* mutations. In such populations, these specific mutations have existed for many generations. For instance, in the Ashkenazi Jewish population, approximately one out of every forty individuals has inherited one of three mutations in *BRCA1* or *BRCA2*.

Histologic Risk Factors

Histology is the study of the microscopic structure of tissue; in this section we refer to the findings observed through the microscope by a pathologist who is examining tissue taken from the breast. Some women who undergo a breast biopsy after discovering a suspicious lump or having an abnormal mammogram are found not to have cancer, but, as noted in chapter 2, they are diagnosed with conditions known to be associated with a higher risk of developing breast cancer. Two such conditions are atypical ductal hyperplasia and lobular carcinoma in situ (lobular neoplasia). Women with these diagnoses have annual breast cancer risks of between 1 and 1.5 per 100 women. In these women, the cancer may be diagnosed in either breast, not just on the side in which the diagnosis of atypical hyperplasia or lobular carcinoma in situ was made.

Options for Women at Increased Risk for Breast Cancer

Screening

Women who are known to be at increased risk for breast cancer may wish to pursue more careful screening to detect any potential cancer at its earliest and most curable stage. Unfortunately, screening tools are relatively limited. Monthly breast self-examination is recommended, but studies in average-risk populations have failed to demonstrate significant benefits from self-examination, and many women at increased risk feel uncomfortable with self-exam. Breast examination from an experienced breast health care provider is recommended two to four times a year. Annual mammography is also recommended, beginning at an age that is five to ten years younger than the youngest breast cancer diagnosis in the family. For women with *BRCA1* or *BRCA2* mutations, breast cancer screening, including mammography, is recommended to begin at age 25, since that is the age at which risk starts to be higher than it is for the general population.

It is important to remember that the program described here is intended not to prevent cancer but to catch it early if it does develop. Unfortunately, the effort is not always successful. Mammograms are less sensitive in younger women for two reasons: younger women tend to have denser breasts, and cancers that develop in younger women often grow quite rapidly. As a result, between one-third and one-half of the breast cancers diagnosed in women undergoing increased surveillance are found as palpable (meaning they can be felt with the hand) lumps within one year of a mammogram reported as normal. In most of these cases, the mass cannot be seen on a mammogram even when it can be palpated. In other cases, it is clear that the tumor grew between the time of the last mammogram and the time the lump was felt.

In order to combat these "interval cancers," additional screening has been recommended. One proposed method is breast ultrasound. While ultrasound can clearly identify cancers that are invisible on mammogram when a woman has a palpable lump, no benefit has been established for ultrasound screening in women without palpable masses. Another technique that has recently been investigated is breast magnetic resonance imaging (MRI). This is a lengthy, expensive, and complicated examination. It appears to be highly sensitive in detecting breast cancer, but often it also shows abnormalities which, after further evaluation (often including biopsy), turn out to be benign. For this reason, breast MRI is currently only appropriate for women who are at the highest levels of risk (such as those with a *BRCA* mutation in their family). Even then, it should be done only after a careful description of the risks and benefits.

Other techniques that have been proposed for breast cancer screening include thermography, positron emission tomography (PET) scanning, Sestamibi scanning, ductal lavage, and transcutaneous electrical impedance. Although these techniques are the subject of ongoing studies, none has yet proven to be useful in breast cancer screening.

Women who carry a *BRCA1* or *BRCA2* mutation should also receive ovarian cancer screening, including pelvic examinations, transvaginal color-Doppler sonography, and CA-125 screening biannually starting around age 35. Unfortunately, this type of screening may not detect ovarian cancer at a curable stage, as ovarian cancer screening has not been proven to be beneficial in any population. Women with the *BRCA* mutation should be offered oophorectomy after they have finished having children.

Prevention

Efforts at early detection are not an attempt to prevent cancer from developing but rather to catch it early if it does develop. These efforts are not always successful, no matter how well the screening is performed, and so there is considerable interest in preventing breast cancer. Unfortunately, few methods have proven effective. As noted in the discussion of risk factors, there are no lifestyle changes, dietary modifications, or supplements that have been conclusively shown to reduce the risk of breast cancer. One exception is the drug tamoxifen, which, in a large study, was shown to reduce the incidence of breast cancer in women at increased risk. In these women, taking tamoxifen for five years decreased the risk of developing breast cancer during that time by nearly half. However, similar studies from the United Kingdom and Italy did not demonstrate a clear benefit, and most women in the U.S. study did not develop breast cancer whether or not they took tamoxifen.

In addition, tamoxifen has a low but measurable risk of significant side effects, including cancer of the uterus and deep venous thrombosis (blood clots in the legs which can travel to the lungs). Women taking tamoxifen sometimes complain of hot flashes, vaginal discharge, weight gain, and depression. A newer medication, raloxifene, appears to be as effective as tamoxifen at reducing breast cancer risk, at least in post-menopausal women. The greatest advantage of raloxifene (also known as Evista) is that it does not appear to cause uterine cancer. Many of its other side effects, however, are similar to those experienced by women taking tamoxifen. A new class of drugs called aromatase inhibitors may be effective in reducing breast cancer risk in postmenopausal women. Studies to evaluate such a benefit are being performed. It is unlikely, however, that these medications will help premenopausal women.

While tamoxifen and raloxifene appear to reduce risk in some women at increased risk, it is not clear whether they do the same for women with mutations in *BRCA1* or *BRCA2*. The only studies looking at the benefits of tamoxifen for breast cancer prevention in these women have been inconclusive.

Because screening is imperfect and because available medications to reduce risk are not completely effective, women at the highest risk often consider prophylactic mastectomy: the removal of the breasts without a diagnosis of cancer, in order to prevent the disease from occurring. To some people this may seem like an overreaction. However, many women who choose to undergo prophylactic mastectomy have had terrible experiences with family members dying of breast cancer, or they have already had cancer themselves. For these women, the risk of having a cancer go undetected by screening is simply unacceptable. They are willing to lose both breasts to avoid that possibility.

Studies have shown that prophylactic mastectomy reduces the incidence of breast cancer by 95 to 98 percent and also reduces the chances of dying of breast cancer. No randomized study has compared the outcomes in women who undergo prophylactic mastectomy versus surveillance to prove that there is an overall survival benefit to surgery, but mathematical models called decision analyses predict significant gains in life expectancy in groups of women at highest risk who undergo the surgery. It is important to note that prophylactic mastectomy may not be completely preventive, as some women have microscopic amounts of breast tissue remaining after surgery which may give rise to cancer. The risk of this happening is thought to be small, but it is not zero, which is why some physicians refer to the procedure as a *risk-reducing* mastectomy rather than *prophylactic.*

For almost everyone, the decision to have a prophylactic or risk-reducing mastectomy is a difficult one. It should only be made after detailed consultation with an expert in cancer risk assessment, a breast surgeon, a reconstructive (plastic) surgeon, and a psychologist. Genetic testing is not necessary before one can undergo risk-reducing surgery, but it is often helpful in defining a woman's individual risk. Many women overestimate their breast cancer risk; after gaining a clearer understanding of their own chances of developing breast cancer, they may no longer want to consider surgery.

For women who are at risk for hereditary breast cancer, there is also a significant ovarian cancer risk. Many women choose to address this risk by prophylactic removal of the ovaries and fallopian tubes (salpingo-oophorectomy), with or without removal of the uterus (hysterectomy). As is the case for prophylactic mastectomy, this procedure does not completely eliminate the risk of cancer, as there is a small remaining risk of peritoneal carcinoma (cancer of the lining of the abdomen). Nonetheless, studies show that salpingo-oophorectomy reduces ovarian cancer risk by approximately 95 percent. As an additional benefit, women who enter premature menopause as a result of ovary removal experience a reduction in breast cancer risk. For these reasons, most women with *BRCA1* or *BRCA2* mutations undergo salpingo-oophorectomy as soon as they are finished having their children.

Conclusion

Thanks to extensive media coverage and professional efforts at public education, many people know that breast cancer is a common disease. People are also generally well educated about many of the risk factors for breast cancer. Unfortunately, many do not realize that for most women with breast cancer, no single factor or combination of factors can clearly be said to have caused the disease.

Women without a strong family history of breast cancer can estimate their cancer risk using a variety of widely available models, such as the Gail model (an example is available at http://bcra.nci.nih.gov/brc/). These models underestimate the risk for women with a strong family history and for women whose family history is on their father's side. In addition, the models do not take into account environmental exposures such as radiation or hormone replacement. Despite these drawbacks, such models can provide a general idea of risk for the majority of women.

Women with stronger family histories of breast or ovarian cancer, or who may have other risk factors increasing their personal risk, may benefit from consulting with a cancer risk assessment specialist, who will take a careful personal and family history to provide the most accurate possible estimate of individual risk. This consultation may include discussion of genetic testing, but such testing is only helpful for a minority of women. Interpretation of the results may be complex, and testing should only be done after a thorough discussion of the risks and benefits. If testing is ultimately pursued, it involves a simple blood test. Results are usually available after five to six weeks, at which time a follow-up meeting is held and the results are discussed in detail. Other than cost, there are few risks to genetic testing. Although many people have concerns about the possibility of discrimination on the basis of the test result, especially in the area of health insurance, to date there is no evidence of systematic health insurance discrimination, and thousands of women have been tested without suffering any adverse consequences with respect to health insurance.

Once the risk assessment is complete, with or without genetic testing, the risk counselor will devise an individualized plan for managing a woman's cancer risk. This plan may involve intensified surveillance with additional radiographic tests, the use of medications such as tamoxifen, and, for a small minority of women, surgical prevention strategies.

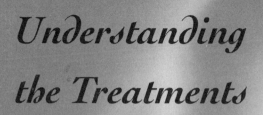

PART TWO

Understanding the Treatments

The Doctors' Perspectives

CHAPTER 5

Assembling the Treatment Team and Charting a Course

Kenneth D. Miller, M.D.

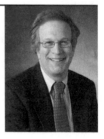

Assembling the Treatment Team

Many women have one primary care physician—either an internist, a gynecologist, or a family practitioner—whom they have known for some time. Over the years, many women have also seen a specialist or several specialists, such as an endocrinologist about a thyroid problem, a dermatologist who removed a mole, or an orthopedic surgeon regarding knee pain. In most cases one physician becomes responsible for treating that specific problem while (ideally) communicating information about the patient and the medical problem to the primary care physician.

The treatment of breast cancer is different, however, because cancer care is almost always a team effort involving and coordinating multiple physicians, including

- A primary care physician
- A gynecologist

- A radiologist
- A surgeon
- A medical oncologist
- A radiation oncologist
- A plastic surgeon or reconstructive surgeon
- Nurses with special training in medical and radiation oncology

The cancer care team also includes your family, friends, neighbors, and possibly clergy, as well as a large support network of knowledge-able nurse clinicians and potentially a psychologist or social worker and a nutritionist.

Who Is the Team Leader?

Each woman with breast cancer is the team leader. Each woman, with help from those around her, makes decisions about her treatment and then gives the consent to proceed. But in the group of physicians noted above, the team leader is often the medical oncologist or the primary care physician, who coordinates the efforts of the other physicians and the team. In some circumstances a surgeon may perform the biopsy, per-form the follow-up surgery, and then coordinate a woman's follow-up care, even though the medical oncologist serves as the team leader.

Who Are the Team Members?

Primary care physician or gynecologist. Usually when a woman has felt a lump in her breast, she turns to her primary care physician or gynecol-ogist. A lump may also be found when the primary care physician or the gynecologist orders a routine mammogram or performs a routine breast examination. If this physician finds something suspicious during a phys-ical examination, he or she may order a mammogram and then notifies the patient of the results. When a lump has been discovered, this physi-cian usually refers the woman to a surgeon for further evaluation or a biopsy.

Radiologist. The radiologist is the physician who reviews the mammo-gram and writes a report on his or her findings. A radiologist may also perform an ultrasound or MRI of the breast and may perform a breast biopsy.

Surgeon. Surgeons train in general surgery for five or more years following medical school; some surgeons then do additional fellowship training in breast surgery. These are the surgeons who usually see a woman after an abnormal mammogram or after a lump is noticed during a physical examination. The breast surgeon is usually responsible for making a diagnosis by performing a simple biopsy using a fine or thin needle, or using a larger needle to take a core biopsy, or making a surgical excision to sample or remove the mass. This doctor correlates the findings of the physical exam and the X-rays with the biopsy results and reviews them with the patient.

If the biopsy is negative, a plan for follow-up care is important. If the biopsy reveals cancer, this doctor shares the result with the patient and usually presents treatment options including lumpectomy with radiation or mastectomy. This same doctor usually performs this follow-up surgery.

For women who undergo a mastectomy, the breast is removed; with a lumpectomy, only a portion of the breast is removed. In either case, the surgeon is responsible for obtaining clear margins (meaning that the tumor is removed along with a rim of normal tissue surrounding the tumor). Some women choose lumpectomy followed by radiation treatments. For women who undergo a mastectomy, the surgeon is usually the first physician to talk about the possibility of reconstructive surgery. If a woman is interested in this option, the surgeon usually refers her to a plastic or reconstructive surgeon.

Medical oncologist. The medical oncologist is a physician who trained in internal medicine and then spent additional years training to treat people who have cancer or blood problems. The medical oncologist often meets with a woman after the diagnosis of breast cancer has been made and before surgery takes place, to discuss the treatment options, including lumpectomy or mastectomy, and also to begin the discussion of the possible use of chemotherapy or hormonal therapy.

Radiation oncologist. A radiation oncologist is a physician who has spent years training in the use of radiation to treat cancer. The radiation oncologist will prescribe and supervise radiation treatments for women who have undergone a lumpectomy, as well as for women who have undergone mastectomy and require radiation either because of the size of the primary tumor or because many of their lymph nodes contained cancer.

Plastic surgeon or reconstructive surgeon. A reconstructive surgeon (also sometimes called a plastic surgeon) is a doctor who trained in general surgery and then spent two or more additional years training in reconstructive surgery. These physicians specialize in reconstructing a breast following mastectomy. Reconstruction may involve placing a breast implant under the skin or moving skin and muscle from one area to another to replace the breast that has been removed. (This procedure may be a TRAM flap procedure, which is described in chapter 13.)

Nurses and other health care professionals. Nurses, social workers, psychologists, and nutritionists offer information, advice, and support based on their expertise in coping strategies, practical matters, healthy diet programs, and other areas.

Choosing Your Physicians and Your Team

A large number of physicians are brilliant and technically excellent, and a large number of physicians are kind, compassionate, supportive, and good listeners. These two skills (technical ability and empathy) often go hand-in-hand. Ideally, you want physicians who are knowledgeable *and* compassionate *and* who will give you the time and attention you need during this process. If you have a primary physician whom you know and trust, you usually can rely on his or her recommendations for a surgeon whom he or she has gotten to know over time. Similarly, if you see a surgeon whom you trust, you usually will find that the surgeon and your primary care physician will direct you to an excellent medical oncologist, radiation oncologist, and reconstructive surgeon.

It is an excellent idea to ask friends, neighbors, and other health care professionals for feedback as you assemble your treatment team. Certain criteria are essential. Your physicians should be board certified in their fields, which indicates that they have met certain criteria and passed certain examinations to obtain these credentials. It is okay to ask these physicians how often they treat women who have the specific type of cancer that you have. Also, you can create a list of questions about your specific condition and treatment options, about how often you can expect to see them over time, and about any personal treatment strategies or philosophies that they have concerning treatment.

The doctor-patient relationship is exactly that—a relationship. And it starts with the first meeting. The first meeting is an opportunity to get to know these doctors and also for them to hear from you about your concerns, worries, and expectations.

During the days and weeks after the diagnosis of breast cancer, a woman may meet more new physicians than she has met in her entire life. These specialists can offer their opinion and advice based on a review of a woman's history, her physical examination, the X-ray findings, and biopsy results, if available. During this time, a woman has the opportunity to decide whether she has confidence in each doctor and is comfortable with him or her.

A Second Opinion?

Seeking a second opinion is usually not a rule or a requirement, though some insurance companies encourage or require a second opinion before treatment begins. For some women, a second opinion can be helpful; it allows them to review the results, confirm the diagnosis and treatment plan, and perhaps to consider other treatment options. Other women, for many reasons (including her own confidence in the initial treating physicians, their recommendations, and their ability), choose not to seek a second opinion.

Suppose, for example, that the surgeon who performs a breast biopsy discusses mastectomy or lumpectomy with radiation as treatment options with a woman who has a diagnosis of invasive cancer. If that patient is clear that she definitely wants to undergo a mastectomy, then she may choose to proceed with her surgery with that surgeon and not seek a second opinion. Suppose, though, that she then finds it difficult to make a decision regarding postoperative chemotherapy or hormonal therapy. She may decide to consult two or three medical oncologists for guidance about that part of her treatment.

If you want to have a second opinion, then ask for this opportunity. Often it is useful to call your primary care physician to ask him or her which physicians to see for a second opinion. Alternatively, you can ask your surgeon, radiation oncologist, or medical oncologist to tell you who serves as local or regional resources for women who want to have a second opinion regarding their treatment.

If you go for a second opinion, it is helpful (and often required) to have materials relating to your breast cancer diagnosis forwarded to the consulting physician before or at the time of your appointment. You can ask the doctor's office staff ahead of time what specific materials the doctor will want to review. These materials may include your mammogram films and the radiologist's reports, a pathology report of the biopsy and possibly the microscope slides, and reports from other tests or consultations. At a second opinion appointment, the consulting physician generally will review your history, examine you, and then review any additional materials that you bring. He or she can then make recommendations to you and also discuss how these recommendations may be the same as or different from what you discussed with the first physicians you consulted.

Second opinions often agree with the first opinion, or the differences are small. You need to review with the second doctor whether his or her thoughts are essentially the same as the first doctor's views or are different in a meaningful way. If they are significantly different, it is helpful to clarify why.

If the two doctors' opinions are very different, then your primary care physician may be able to help you reconcile the differences and make decisions regarding your care. Women often choose to continue their care with the first physicians they saw, although some women decide to transfer their care to the doctor who offered the second opinion. This decision is often based on many factors, including personal comfort with the doctor's interpersonal style.

University Hospital or Community Hospital?

When you have cancer, the care that you receive largely depends upon the knowledge, dedication, and ability of the members of your treatment team. Most community hospitals have many excellent doctors who have wide experience in the treatment of breast cancer. Some major university cancer centers can offer the advantage of a team of physicians who see a large number of women who have breast cancer.

Some women have a clear desire to seek a second opinion at a major medical center or to receive their care at this type of facility. Other women prefer to receive care closer to home, in their own community.

At a major medical center and in your community, it is perfectly reasonable to ask the physicians on your team how much experience they have in treating women with breast cancer in general and your specific type of breast cancer in particular. Asking these and other specific questions is not an insult. The best physicians, those who are excellent at their craft and are compassionate, will respond with honesty and humility, regardless of their age, experience, position, or status.

Other Team Members

Much of the day-to-day support for women with breast cancer comes from family, friends, neighbors, the extended community, and clergy. But the role of oncology nurses in the care of women with breast cancer is immense. The nurse often sees a patient more frequently than the physician and often gets to know her better and more personally than the physician does. Women frequently feel more comfortable telling their nurses more details than they tell their doctors about their response to treatment and side effects. Oncology nurses and nurses in the surgeon's office and radiation centers as well as technologists can become good friends and important allies in the treatment process.

Other team members can also provide invaluable help and support. Some women choose to see a psychologist, social worker, or other counselor during treatment. The support and guidance of these professionals can make a difficult time easier for the patient. Some women also benefit from seeing a nutritionist during their treatment, welcoming the chance to grow stronger and feel better through dietary choices.

The Changing Team

During the first few months following the diagnosis of breast cancer, a woman will often see many new physicians on a regular basis. The participation of the team members changes over time, however. For example, after a lumpectomy, a woman may undergo chemotherapy and see her medical oncologist each week. When radiation follows surgery, she is seen at the radiation center daily.

Then, later, when radiation therapy is completed, she may see the radiation oncologist every six months but see the medical oncologist every three months and the surgeon yearly. The pattern of follow-up care varies depending upon the nature of the breast cancer that was treated and the preferences of the physicians on the treatment team.

Charting a Course

A woman with breast cancer has many decisions to make. These decisions regard three categories of concern:

1. Local control of the cancer. This means making sure that the cancer has been fully removed from the breast.
2. Regional control of the cancer. When a woman has invasive breast cancer, it is important to find out whether the cancer has spread to the lymph nodes and to perform additional treatment if it has.
3. Systemic control of the cancer. Systemic treatment is performed to reduce the risk of the cancer recurring elsewhere in the body.

To a large extent, these three concerns need to be addressed separately. For example, a woman might believe that undergoing a mastectomy allows her to forego adjuvant chemotherapy, but because the mastectomy only deals with local control, chemotherapy would still be helpful to reduce the risk of the cancer recurring elsewhere in the body. Or, a woman may have received chemotherapy following mastectomy, but the chemotherapy does not produce enough of a change in the risk of recurrence in the breast to allow her to forego treatment with radiation therapy. Keeping these three issues—local, regional, and systemic control—separate and distinct can sometimes simplify the decision-making process.

Local Control of the Cancer

For women who have non-invasive breast cancer, we are not greatly concerned about the risk of the cancer recurring elsewhere in the body. But there is a risk of local recurrence, and some women choose to undergo a mastectomy, while others choose breast conserving surgery followed by radiation. This is a very important decision, and ultimately it relates to a woman's personal preference and concern regarding the risk of the cancer recurring in the breast if they choose breast conservation. The risk of a local recurrence after radiation is approximately 3 to 10 percent over a lifetime. Most women consider this risk comfortable and acceptable, while others choose mastectomy because they feel that this 3 to 10 percent risk is too high.

For women with invasive breast cancer, the issue of local control is similar. Some women choose lumpectomy followed by radiation, while others choose to undergo a mastectomy. There are multiple factors that undoubtedly contribute to this decision, including the objective risk of a local recurrence and an individual woman's concern regarding this risk. Multiple studies have shown that the chance of long-term survival is the same for women who undergo mastectomy or lumpectomy.

A woman's personal feelings about the cosmetic changes with either mastectomy or lumpectomy can contribute to her decision as well. Decisions based on physical appearance should not be considered as just trivial issues of vanity. If a woman knew that a mastectomy would improve her chances of living a normal life, then she might choose this procedure unequivocally over lumpectomy. The data, however, indicate that for most women, lumpectomy followed by radiation is equivalent to mastectomy in terms of long-term survival, so both are good options.

Regional Control

Typically, the lymph nodes are not biopsied for women who have non-invasive breast cancer because the nodes are almost always uninvolved. For women who have invasive breast cancer of almost any size, however, there is a risk that the nodes may contain breast cancer cells. Today, surgeons generally favor a limited (sentinel) node biopsy of the lymph nodes from the armpit (axillae). If the sentinel node does contain cancer cells, then the surgeon may perform another procedure to remove additional nodes. (See chapter 6.)

Systemic Therapy

Women who have non-invasive breast cancer are at a very low risk of developing a recurrence of their breast cancer, and postoperative chemotherapy is not recommended for them. Hormonal therapy such as tamoxifen may be helpful in reducing the risk of a second cancer developing, and this treatment may be a good preventive strategy for women with non-invasive disease.

Any woman who has invasive breast cancer has some risk of the cancer recurring elsewhere in the body in the future. This risk is related to many factors, including the size of the cancer, the type of cancer, the involvement of lymph nodes, and several characteristics of the tumor (including the estrogen receptors, for example). The medical oncologist is often the best person to assess the degree of risk and to review treatment options with you. Options include no additional treatment, if the risk is low, or chemotherapy or hormonal therapy.

Decisions on adjuvant therapy to reduce the risk of recurrence are often based on the medical oncologist's recommendations, but it is important for women to have the opportunity to participate in this process. For some women the choices are relatively clear-cut. For example, a woman who is 40 years old and has a five-centimeter-sized invasive breast cancer that is estrogen receptor negative will not benefit from treatment with tamoxifen, while chemotherapy will improve her chance of long-term survival. In contrast, a 75-year-old woman who has a tumor one centimeter in size that is estrogen receptor positive would likely derive more benefit from treatment with tamoxifen or Arimidex and relatively less added benefit if chemotherapy is given as well.

Often, the situations are less clear. For example, for some women, the greatest reduction in risk is due to the use of hormonal therapy (such as tamoxifen or Arimidex), though chemotherapy may yet add one, two, or three percentage points of advantage for long-term survival without breast cancer. Some women in this situation would clearly want chemotherapy to improve their chances a few percentage points, even given the risks and side effects. Other women might choose to forego chemotherapy unless the advantages of adding it are greater. In these situations the medical oncologist can review the information and make recommendations, but, again, the input of the woman who has the cancer is essential in this process.

Standard Therapy or Clinical Trials

Multiple clinical trials are available for women who have breast cancer, and they are being conducted to increase our knowledge about surgery, radiation, and postoperative chemotherapy and hormonal therapy. The trials that were conducted in the past are the basis of our practice of medicine today, and the trials of today will improve the treatment of women in the future. With all of this in mind, many women are pleased to have the opportunity to participate in a clinical trial, even if they ultimately choose not to do so. Here are some considerations to take into account when making this decision:

1. Is there a trial that offers me an opportunity to obtain a treatment that would not be available otherwise? What are the risks and benefits of both the standard treatment and the new treatment?
2. Does the trial offer me new treatments that are at least as good as the existing standard of care?
3. If this is a trial of a new drug, am I one of the first patients on the trials (in which case I may be receiving a very low starting dose of the drug, a dose that may not be effective)? Or will I be receiving one of the higher dose levels, where more side effects might be expected?

As noted earlier in this chapter, breast cancer treatment is a team effort. The team you have assembled will help you arrive at decisions for your treatment based on information about you, your preferences, your breast cancer, and what is known about your situation from the research studies that have been done in the past.

CHAPTER 6

Facing Surgery

Peter J. Deckers, M.D. *&* Theodore N. Tsangaris, M.D.

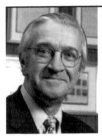
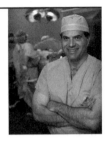

A slide that is used in teaching medical students depicts four types of patients. The first patient comes in and says, "Doctor, do whatever you want to do. I just want to live." The second patient says, "Doctor, I demand this of you." The third says, "I just can't make up my mind." And the fourth says, "Doctor, based on your clinical judgment and recommendation, and on my own personal understanding and desire, I think we'll go with . . . " It's a good slide because it demonstrates a range of starting points, a range of perspectives from which to seek a meeting of the minds between a woman and her doctor. The first patient is relinquishing too much authority and power. As surgeons, we are here to offer guidance to our patients, not to make all the decisions. At the opposite end of the range is the fourth patient, who is empowered by her own care plan.

Historically, patients had few rights and almost no role in decision making. Times have changed. Today's medical students are trained to respect patients' rights and always to seek informed consent. Patients too have changed, often doing extensive independent research and seeking multiple medical opinions. When it comes to breast cancer, this activism is wise and fortifying.

Impulsive decisions are usually not beneficial. Women should consider getting second opinions and talking to their families before making final decisions. Often they respond, "Well, shouldn't I do something immediately if it's cancer?" The answer is no. It's not going to make much difference if we act right away, or next week, or in three weeks, though a surgical decision should generally be made within three to four weeks of diagnosis. Some patients feel that if this is cancer, we ought to be doing something within the next twenty-four hours. But the statistics have shown that this is not true.

Take a deep breath. Take the time to learn about your options.

Begin with a Biopsy

Whenever a breast lump is discovered or an uncertain finding appears on a mammogram, then a biopsy procedure must be done to determine a diagnosis. Is this cancer or is it not? If this is cancer, then what do the cancer cells look like? What part of the breast anatomy do they occupy? Will the cells respond favorably to hormone therapy? A biopsy can answer all of these questions and is a critical first step in mapping out a treatment plan. And negative biopsies reassure women that they don't have cancer at all.

Because there are three different biopsy procedures, the patient, along with her surgeon, is faced with a surgical choice right from the start. The choice of biopsy technique is influenced by whether the abnormal finding can be felt by the examiner (is "palpable") or whether it is only detectable by mammogram. (If the mass is clearly a fluid-filled cyst, then it must be drained through a needle and the collected fluid may be sent to a laboratory for analysis. Later, a follow-up mammogram and/or ultrasound can confirm that the cyst has completely resolved.) The breast surgeon discusses all mammogram and physical examination results with patients when helping guide decisions about biopsy techniques.

The three biopsy procedures are known as fine needle aspiration, needle localization, and stereotactic core biopsy.

Fine Needle Aspiration

This kind of biopsy can often be done as soon as a solid mass is first felt in the breast, at the same outpatient office visit. It is a straightforward procedure. The breast tissue is simply numbed with lidocaine, and a thin needle is inserted into the lump to draw out a sampling of cells from the mass. This cell sample is then sent to a laboratory for evaluation by pathologists. Even if the biopsy results come back negative for cancer, the surgeon may still recommend that the patient have the lump removed. If the result is positive for cancer, the doctor will definitely recommend further surgery. For some women, a surgeon may recommend skipping this tissue-sampling step and instead scheduling a time for the whole lump to be completely removed in the operating room and then sent for lab analysis.

Stereotactic Core Biopsy

Stereotactic core biopsies are usually performed in the radiology department, not in an operating room. They rely on computer-assisted, mammogram- or ultrasound-guided visualization of the lesion. A special needle is used to obtain larger tissue samples. This needle can take up to twenty tissue samples, each two-to-three millimeters wide and about two centimeters long. A metallic clip is left in the biopsied area to mark the region of concern for future mammograms.

Excisional or Incisional Biopsy

Usually, a surgeon performs this kind of biopsy in the operating room. When the breast lesion cannot be felt on physical exam and finding it requires visual guidance, a special mammogram is performed. A needle is inserted into the numbed breast tissue; the needle guides the surgeon to the abnormal area, which is then sampled or removed. This is called needle localization. If, on the other hand, the abnormal area can be felt by the surgeon during the physical examination, then the biopsy of this area is performed without a needle localization. If the entire lesion is removed, this procedure is called an excisional biopsy, but if only part of the lesion is sampled (because of its large size), the procedure is called an incisional biopsy.

Removing Cancer

What happens when a biopsy result comes back positive for cancer? It is time to make treatment decisions, and these decisions almost always involve surgery. As noted in chapter 5, the first goal of breast surgery is to reduce or eliminate the risk of a recurrence of the cancer in the breast, known as local recurrence. The second goal is to determine whether the cancer has spread beyond the breast. This is done through biopsy and, often, removal of lymph nodes under the arm (called the *axillary* area, or *axilla*).

Many factors influence surgical planning, including:

- The type of cancer
- The size of the tumor
- Whether there are multiple areas of cancer in the breast
- The size of the breast in relation to the tumor
- The psychological response of the patient to each option
- The patient's general medical condition, surgical history, and age

At one time, all breast cancer was treated with extremely aggressive surgery. Now we know that there is *no survival advantage* to this choice. This is an extremely important point that may seem to fly in the face of logic, so it bears repeating: *Clinical studies have consistently shown that women who opt for total breast removal do not live longer than women who choose to remove only the cancerous lump and then have radiation therapy.* The important reasons to choose one surgical approach over another will become clear as each surgery is described, but choosing between total breast removal (mastectomy) and tumor removal (lumpectomy) should not be viewed as a life-or-death decision.

Why isn't a woman safer just removing all the breast tissue? Because if the cancer is limited to only a defined small area of the breast, then either approach can effectively eliminate all the cancer cells. However, if the cancer has invisibly spread to other parts of the body, then neither mastectomy nor lumpectomy will kill every cancer cell in the body. The

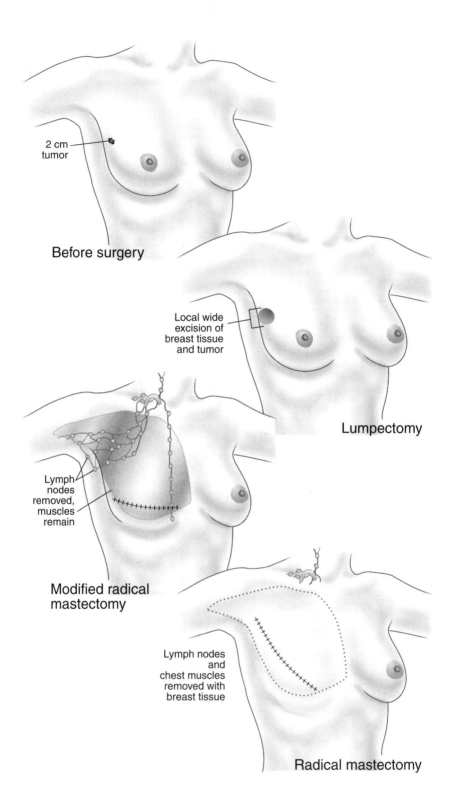

2 cm tumor

Before surgery

Local wide excision of breast tissue and tumor

Lumpectomy

Lymph nodes removed, muscles remain

Modified radical mastectomy

Lymph nodes and chest muscles removed with breast tissue

Radical mastectomy

treatment that attacks and kills cancer throughout the body is chemotherapy. And it does its job with increasing effectiveness.

Thanks to mammograms and early detection, most breast cancer is found and removed before it has spread. "Women who have cancer that is not palpable — that is, not perceptible by touch — but that is visible on X-ray and whose biopsies are positive have a very, very high cure rate," says breast surgeon Jerome Sandler (author of part of chapter 7). "That is the reasoning behind having regular mammograms done. Mammograms can pick up early carcinomas before they have spread." Thanks to advances in drug therapy, even some breast cancers that have spread can be defeated. Oncologists prescribe powerful anti-tumor drugs and hormones. Drug regimens are individualized, as much as possible, based on information in the biopsy results.

With this background in mind, in this chapter we describe the different surgical options (see Figure 6.1).

Preventing Local Recurrence

The history of breast surgery reveals an evolution from very aggressive treatment to one of minimal if any disfigurement.

The Halsted Radical Mastectomy

Named after Dr. William Halsted, who is recognized as the "father of breast surgery," the *Halsted radical mastectomy* was a drastic and highly disfiguring operation used to treat breast cancer patients long before the development of effective cancer-screening techniques. Women arriving at Dr. Halsted's clinic generally had very advanced cancers, many of which were large enough to see on exam and all of which were large enough to feel. Their cases were desperate, and radical action seemed to offer the only hope for survival.

FIGURE 6.1. The Halsted radical mastectomy was the standard of care for many years. The modified radical mastectomy is less deforming and just as effective as the radical mastectomy and gradually replaced it. In the past thirty years, a more limited procedure, lumpectomy, has become the procedure of choice for most women with breast cancer.

Halsted's procedure involved surgical removal of the breast, the muscles of the chest wall under the breast, and the contents of the armpit to excise any cancer cells that may have traveled to the lymph nodes. Because axillary lymph nodes are also important for draining fluid from the arms, women who underwent this surgery were often left with severe arm swelling that greatly impaired their quality of life. Halsted believed that breast cancer developed within the breast, grew larger in the breast, spread over time to the lymph nodes, and then late in the disease metastasized elsewhere in the body. We now know that cancer can metastasize early in the course of the disease, and we fortunately have medicines to fight cancer effectively throughout the body.

Transition from Radical to Modified Radical Mastectomy

During the 1960s and 1970s, many surgeons concluded that the radical mastectomy was not necessary for every person with breast cancer. Almost overnight (and without any significant scientific or clinical evidence to support the change in protocol) it seemed, surgeons stopped performing Halsted's radical mastectomy and began treating patients with a new operation: the *modified radical mastectomy*. This procedure also involved removing the breast and the axillary lymph nodes, but unlike Halsted's procedure, it preserved the muscles of the chest wall. This change made the operation safer, easier to perform, and less disfiguring. Most important, it did not diminish the chance of long-term survival or increase the risk of local recurrence when compared to the historical results of the radical mastectomy.

Transition to Breast Conserving Surgery with Radiation

Unlike the sudden transition from radical mastectomy to modified radical mastectomy, which took place without solid clinical evidence supporting the change, the transition from modified mastectomy to breast conserving surgery with subsequent radiation therapy required solid proof of radiation's merits. The first research studies of breast conserving surgery (also called breast conserving therapy, or BCT) were conducted in Italy in the early 1970s. These studies demonstrated that removal of a quadrant of the breast (approximately one-fourth of the breast) followed by radiation to the remaining breast tissue resulted in survival rates that equaled those following mastectomy. This was an exciting finding.

Yet surgeons were puzzled by the sad fact that some women still died of breast cancer after having a mastectomy, including removal of the breast and removal of axillary lymph nodes, even when no cancer cells had been found in their lymph nodes! Why did these deaths happen?

A clinical trial established by the National Surgical Adjuvant Breast and Bowel Cancer Program (NSABP) in the 1970s sought to solve this mystery. It was called the B-04 Trial. In this study, women in whom the surgeon did *not* feel enlarged or abnormal lymph nodes were randomly assigned to undergo one of the following treatments:

- mastectomy without node dissection (removal),
- mastectomy with excision of the axillary lymph nodes, or
- mastectomy without node dissection but with radiation to the regional nodes.

After twenty-five years of follow-up, the NSABP found that all three groups had the same rate of survival. Women lived just as long whether doctors had removed the lymph nodes, radiated the nodes, or left the lymph nodes alone. It was a surprising result.

In women who underwent radiation therapy to the axillary lymph nodes, the risk of a recurrence of the cancer in the axilla was the same as for women who had the lymph nodes removed surgically. However, this similar rate of local recurrence was lower than the risk of recurrence in women whose lymph nodes had been left in place and were not treated with radiation. (Any woman later found to have local recurrence of cancer in her lymph nodes had those nodes surgically removed.)

This same trial, the B-04 Study, also followed women in whom surgeons *did* feel abnormal lymph nodes on physical examination. These women were randomly assigned to undergo either lymph node excision or lymph node radiation. Here again, the study found no difference in survival rates between the two groups.

This landmark study demonstrated the effectiveness of radiation therapy in reducing the risk of local recurrence of cancer in the axilla. It also reaffirmed that reducing the risk of local recurrence does not increase the rates of long-term survival. Thus radiation was shown to be an extremely important treatment but not a magic bullet.

The wonderful result is this: these studies proved that lesser surgical procedures do not reduce a woman's chance of long-term survival. This comforting evidence has enabled thousands of women to undergo safer, less disfiguring operations at no increased risk.

A New Operation: Lumpectomy

What about simply removing the tumor from the breast, rather than removing the whole breast, or a whole quadrant of the breast? In the late 1970s and early 1980s, a new study called the B6 Trial of the NSABP compared three different surgical options for treatment of invasive breast cancer:

- Mastectomy
- Lumpectomy
- Lumpectomy with radiation

Ultimately, this and other studies found absolutely no difference in survival or disease-free survival rates among the three options. But it did find differences in the rates of local breast cancer recurrence among the three groups. For women who had a mastectomy, the recurrence rate on the chest wall was extremely low. For those who underwent lumpectomy alone (without radiation), the risk was close to 40 percent, while for lumpectomy followed by radiation it was 6 to 9 percent. Clearly, the study showed that radiation helps prevent local recurrence. It also further illustrated that the real life-threatening problem for women with breast cancer is the risk of the cancer recurring elsewhere in the body and that this risk is not significantly reduced by more radical surgery.

Can Lumpectomy Suffice without Radiation?

A number of good clinical trials have shown that lumpectomy alone is an inferior treatment to lumpectomy followed by breast radiation. A study published in 1996 followed a group of women whose invasive breast cancers shared all of the following characteristics:

- the invasive cancer was less than two centimeters in size (less than one inch),
- there was little non-invasive cancer in the breast,
- there were wide margins of normal tissue surrounding the tumor that was excised along with the tumor itself (known as "negative margins of excision"), and
- there was no lymph node involvement.

For those women who opted for lumpectomy without radiation, the risk of local recurrence within three years was slightly higher than 9 percent, and beyond three years additional recurrences could be anticipated. Radiation reduced the risk of local recurrence within three years to only 2 percent.

Research also shows that tamoxifen can lower the risk of the cancer recurring after radiation, but it does not replace radiation. The best outcome after lumpectomy often includes treatment with a combination of radiation first and then tamoxifen.

In summary, lumpectomy alone has proven less effective in preventing local recurrence than lumpectomy followed by radiation, lumpectomy followed by tamoxifen, or especially lumpectomy followed by the combination of radiation and tamoxifen.

There is ongoing interest in defining which group of women may be effectively treated by lumpectomy alone. It seems reasonable that it will be elderly women who have very small invasive breast cancers that are well differentiated (less wild appearance), with negative margins and positive hormone receptors. There is also interest in the possibility of treating just a portion of the breast with radiation using one of several techniques (partial breast irradiation). We hope and expect that future clinical trials will provide more information about the appropriate course of treatment.

What about Surgery for Non-Invasive Breast Cancer?

The historical evolution of surgical treatment for non-invasive cancer (called ductal carcinoma in situ, or DCIS) has followed a similar path from first-line mastectomy to breast conserving approaches. In the past, it was thought safer to simply remove the whole breast because any increased risk of local recurrence might mean a chance that the next cancer would be invasive. Also, doctors feared that radiation might be less effective with DCIS because radiation acts most effectively against aggressive cancers.

But no! The study that showed DCIS could be effectively treated with breast conservation was called the B-17 Trial of the NSABP. It compared the results of lumpectomy with and without radiation for all types of DCIS. As with studies of invasive cancer outcomes, the B-17 Trial showed no difference in survival rates among the two treatment groups. It also showed a lower risk of local recurrence in the group that received radiation.

Another study, the B-24 Trial, has also shown that tamoxifen can further reduce the risk of local recurrence following lumpectomy and radiation therapy for women with DCIS. Tamoxifen reduces the risk of cancer in the other breast, as well.

Ongoing efforts are again being made to determine if there is a group of women who can be effectively treated with lumpectomy alone for DCIS. Several studies support this approach for a small group of women with very small areas of low-grade (less malignant) DCIS, in whom surgeons can obtain a generous margin around the tumor.

The Role of Lymph Node Dissection in Breast Cancer Treatment

Many women, when they learn that they have breast cancer, immediately want aggressive surgery because that approach seems to make intuitive sense. It is a rational response when viewed through the lens of mortal fear. But there is more to consider. There is no value to radical surgery if the cancer has already spread beyond the breast.

The lymph nodes under the arms were once thought to hold absolute answers as to whether a breast cancer had spread. Likewise, removing all the nodes was thought to be a reliable roadblock to the potential spread of breast cancer. These beliefs argued for aggressive surgery. Yet, over the past century, several key factors have resulted in a trend toward much more limited axillary surgery:

1. The diagnosis of breast cancer at an earlier stage and smaller size for many women
2. The reduced risk that the axillary nodes will contain cancer in this large number of women with early stage disease
3. An appreciation that breast cancer can metastasize elsewhere in the body without involving the nodes, so that even the most extensive node dissections may not be curative
4. Improvements in the use of chemotherapy and/or hormonal therapy that may reduce the risk of recurrence for women more effectively than extensive node dissection

The fact is that women with non-invasive breast cancer do not require an axillary node procedure because the chance that the cancer has spread to the nodes is negligible. For women who do have invasive breast cancer, axillary surgery is now viewed as a diagnostic procedure to determine the stage of the cancer. It is no longer considered therapeutic. This new framework has led to a new approach. Rather than subject all breast cancer patients to full axillary lymph node removal (which can lead to postoperative difficulties), surgeons now commonly rely on a far easier procedure called a sentinel node biopsy.

What Is a Sentinel Node Biopsy?

The cells of the body are bathed in a clear, colorless fluid called *lymph*, which drains into a web of structures called *lymphatics*, which in turn drain the fluid through the lymph nodes and then into the bloodstream. Lymph from most segments of the breast drains to lymph nodes in the armpit, but breast lymph can also drain to nodes located next to the breastbone (the sternum) or next to the collarbone (the clavicle).

In the 1990s an innovative technique was developed to map the flow

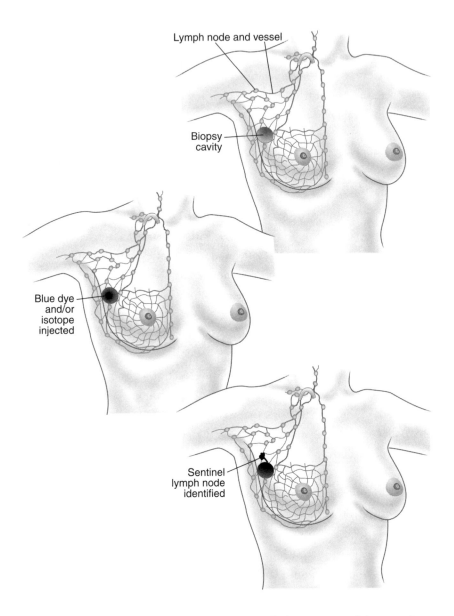

Lymph node and vessel

Biopsy cavity

Blue dye and/or isotope injected

Sentinel lymph node identified

FIGURE 6.2. To prepare for a sentinel node biopsy the breast surgeon injects a radioactive substance and/or a blue dye into the site of the tumor or around the nipple. The surgeon is then able to identify which lymph node or nodes in the axilla (armpit) is the sentinel node.

of lymph fluid from a given tumor—to follow where it drained. It became possible to see which lymph node received most of the lymph from the tumor. This lymph node came to be known as the sentinel node.

A sentinel node biopsy is performed by injecting a harmless radioactive fluid or a blue dye, or both substances, depending upon the surgeon's preference and experience, into the area around a tumor, into the area where the tumor was prior to its surgical removal (called the biopsy cavity), or into the tissue under the nipple or areola (see Figure 6.2). Then, using visual inspection for the blue dye or a special instrument similar to a Geiger counter for the radioactive fluid, the surgeon can confidently identify which node has received the most radioactive material traveling in the breast's lymph. The blue dye usually appears to the naked eye in that same node, though some dye may also be seen in another node. The surgeon removes the blue node or nodes, or the nodes containing the most radioactive material, and sends the tissue to the pathology department, where they are carefully examined under the microscope to see if they hold any cancer cells.

This procedure, the sentinel node biopsy, identifies cancer in 95 to 97 percent of women who would be found to have axillary cancer using a more extensive lymph node dissection. It is a very accurate procedure when performed by an experienced surgeon. The technique sometimes picks up axillary cancer that a more traditional lymph node dissection would miss. For this reason, a sentinel node biopsy should be considered for any woman undergoing a planned node dissection. If the sentinel node is found to be positive for cancer, many surgeons will perform an axillary lymph node dissection (removal) at a later date.

Though it is only 95 percent sensitive, the sentinel node biopsy is significantly less traumatic than an axillary node dissection and results in fewer complications. In some cases, however, a standard lymph node dissection is recommended.

When Should a Woman Consider Traditional Lymph Node Dissection?

Sentinel node biopsy is the surgery most commonly performed to determine whether axillary nodes are involved and to help determine the stage of breast cancer. However, there is still a role for standard node dissection in the following situations:

- If the surgeon feels any enlarged, suspicious lymph nodes on physical exam
- If the surgeon can not clearly identify a specific sentinel node using the procedure described above
- If a woman not previously suspected to have axillary spread has a positive sentinel node biopsy. Women in this situation may then undergo a limited node dissection, though this is a choice that needs to be made after thorough discussion between the surgeon and the patient.

The number of axillary lymph nodes varies from person to person. The nodes are thought of in three anatomic "groups" or "levels." Level 1 nodes are located toward the lower part of the axilla, while level 2 and level 3 nodes are higher up in the axilla.

The Halsted radical mastectomy included an extensive dissection of the nodes in all three levels. The flow of lymph fluid traveling through the axilla was disrupted, and, as a result, women often developed severe arm swelling called *lymphedema*. Today, lymph node dissection is usually limited to level 1, although the dissection may be more extensive if the surgeon can feel enlarged, hard, or suspicious nodes elsewhere in the axilla. Lymph node dissection is usually well tolerated and can be performed at the time of lumpectomy or mastectomy. It is very rare for a level 3 node dissection to be done anymore. Women who have malignant level 3 nodes are usually treated with radiation and chemotherapy.

An axillary lymph node dissection can quantify the number of lymph nodes harboring cancer. In some cases, medical and radiation oncologists use this number to guide their therapy. However, a retrospective study from Johns Hopkins of 200 patients demonstrated that the majority of decisions regarding whether or not to use chemotherapy had been made prior to lymph node dissection. If this finding is borne out by subsequent research studies and medical practice, then, in the future, lymph node sampling or dissection for staging and treatment planning may become less necessary.

Is Mastectomy Ever Recommended over Lumpectomy with Radiation?

Yes. But not because it increases survival. Usually, a doctor's decision to recommend mastectomy over lumpectomy involves one or more of the following situations:

- When a woman has a large tumor in a small breast, or multiple tumor sites within the breast
- When lumpectomy would result in a very poor cosmetic outcome, for example, if there is a large amount of tissue to be removed or if the surgery requires the removal of the nipple and areola
- When the surgeon feels that obtaining clear margins will not be possible
- When a tumor is present in a breast that also has multiple calcifications. (Calcifications themselves are not malignant, but because certain patterns of calcification are of unclear significance, they may make mammograms difficult to interpret. Mammograms are the centerpiece of long-term monitoring; without clear mammograms, it is impossible to recognize local recurrence quickly and confidently.)
- When women either do not want to undergo a six-to-seven week course of radiation therapy as an outpatient; feel uncomfortable with receiving radiation therapy at all; or have a contraindication to radiation, such as previous radiation to that area or certain medical conditions such as systemic lupus and other connective tissue diseases

Multidrug chemotherapy administered before surgery sometimes can effectively decrease the size of the tumor in a woman's breast so that breast conserving surgery (lumpectomy and radiation) may be possible. There is a growing trend toward the use of this type of pre-operative chemotherapy especially for women who have large breast cancers or where there is obvious spread of the cancer to the lymph nodes in the axilla. In making this decision, it is very important to realize that the choice between breast conserving surgery with radiation and mastectomy does not have any relationship to rates of cure. With either surgery, you are equally likely to survive. There is, however, a greater chance of local cancer recurrence after lumpectomy with radiation than after mastectomy, though in general this risk is low. If the cancer does recur in the breast, then mastectomy is usually necessary. Today, the standard approach in most centers is to offer breast conserving surgery, sentinel node biopsy, and then radiation therapy for treatment of invasive breast cancer.

Approximately 240,000 women are diagnosed with breast cancer each year in the United States. While surgery still remains an important weapon against this disease, major changes in the field may result from strategies that reduce the risk of breast cancer, better screening methods to detect tumors when they are small enough to be eliminated without the use of radiation, and systemic therapy so effective that breast surgery and axillary node sampling may no longer be needed.

Today, the risk of developing metastatic breast cancer, a major concern, is the same for women who choose breast conservation and for women who choose mastectomy. This risk is reduced by treatment with hormonal therapy, chemotherapy, or both. It is precisely because long-term survival rates are equivalent with the two surgical approaches that the choice between them becomes a highly personal one. Some women value an objective list of pros and cons to assist in making the choice. For other women, however, the decision is made at an emotional, "gut," level. Either approach is legitimate, and no matter which method feels most comfortable, most women find it helpful to consider the experiences of others who have faced this decision before.

CHAPTER 7

Profiles of Two Breast Surgeons

Interview with Jerome Sandler, M.D.

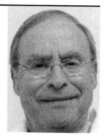

W hen a woman comes into my office, she has been referred
by her doctor because of a mass in her breast or an abnormal mammogram; she is upset and fearful for her life. Part
of my job is to allay her anxiety and to explain not only what I am planning to do but what I think about the lesion. When a patient comes in,
I try to relieve her anxiety either by telling her that I don't think it is
malignant or, if I *do* think it is malignant, that the chances for a cure are,
in most cases, reasonable. Occasionally, a patient has an advanced malignancy where the discussion goes differently.

The first step in management is to establish a diagnosis. We have a
minimally invasive procedure called stereotactic core biopsy. The procedure is performed in a special room at the hospital or outpatient facility. The patient lies face down on a padded table that has a hole in the
center, placing the affected breast in the hole. The breast is compressed,
and a picture is taken. The lesion is identified on the screen by moving
the camera fifteen degrees in one direction and taking a picture and moving the camera fifteen degrees in the other direction and taking a picture. Then both pictures are seen on a split computer screen. The cur-

sor of the computer is placed over the lesion in the positive view and on the lesion in the negative view. Then we feed that information into the computer, and the depth from the skin to the lesion is computed. At that point, we numb the skin of the breast tissue and attach a needle to the computer. By dialing the needle to the appropriate depth and moving it in a clockwise pattern, this special biopsy needle can take anywhere from three to twenty biopsies of the lesion in question. We generally take about fifteen biopsies, but we can take as many as we think are necessary. Stereotactic core biopsy is used primarily in those women in whom there is an abnormal mammogram and a nonpalpable abnormality. Most women who come in with a palpable abnormality can have a core biopsy performed in the office or pathology department at the hospital. Because we can feel the lesion, we can obtain sufficient tissue without the X-ray guidance. Some women prefer that we *not* do the core biopsies but just go ahead and excise the lesion. That is a patient-driven decision, and no method is better than another.

Recently, with the advent of newer biopsy instruments, ultrasound guided biopsy in the office has supplanted the need for biopsies in the operating room. This development allows surgeons to establish the diagnosis and discuss treatment options without a more invasive procedure. Also, MRI-guided biopsies are now possible in women with small lesions that cannot be felt or seen on mammogram or ultrasound.

A very difficult part of a surgeon's job is making the telephone call to tell the patient she has cancer. I dislike calling people on the phone to tell them the diagnosis, but it is important for them to prepare for our next meeting, where we discuss options. Over the years, a telephone call has become the way I do it only because if a woman comes in and hears me say, "Well, your biopsy was positive. You have cancer," that is the last thing she hears me say! At that point, nothing else registers because, understandably, the only thing the patient is thinking about is her life. By preparing the patient in advance and arranging for a family member or friend to be present at the treatment discussion, a meaningful discussion can take place.

I hope that having a family member or friend present makes it possible for all aspects of care to be remembered.

Having said that, I should add that what I say and how much I say depends on the patient and other factors. A 90-year-old woman usually does not have the attention span or concerns of a 40-year-old woman whose whole lifetime is ahead of her. So I try to tailor the discussion to the patient and her needs. One interesting difference in patients now, in the age of computers, is that many patients come with sheets of information that they picked up off the Internet. I think it is wonderful that they are seeking information on their own, although sometimes the generalities they read about are not applicable to their specific case.

A number of significant changes have occurred in the surgical treatment of non-invasive breast cancer. Our approach to the treatment of non-invasive breast cancer has changed, and I try to give women this perspective. A surgeon named Mel Silverstein studied every case of non-invasive breast cancer that came through the Van Nuys Cancer Center. Over time, he modified a system of grading ductal carcinoma in situ, which is now known as the Van Nuys Classification. His system uses the size of the tumor, the nuclear grade of the tumor, the amount of normal tissue around the tumor excised, and the age of the patient. These factors assign a grade of 1, 2, or 3, with Van Nuys-1 being the lowest. For instance, a Van Nuys-1 would be a very small tumor of low nuclear grade with at least one centimeter of normal breast tissue around it. The Van Nuys system allows us to quantify a number of parameters, assigning each possibility on a range of points. Using the three primary parameters, the lowest possible score would be 3; the highest possible score would be 9. Adding age into the mix, using the same 1–3 scale, up to a cut-off age of 50–55, the cumulative score can guide us toward recommending the optimal treatment for an individual. If you have a 3 or 4, the lowest score possible, we would treat very minimally, for example, just excising the tumor. A score of 4, 5, 6, or 7 might be considered an intermediate grade; we would remove the tumor and probably add radiation afterwards. And for a score of 8 or 9 we would recommend wide lumpectomy with radiation, or mastectomy. Though technically it is non-invasive cancer, women with advanced lesions should be treated as if they have invasive cancer.

Another major advance has been the increasing use of sentinel node biopsies. Numerous studies have shown that sentinel node biopsy is very accurate in determining if cancer has spread to the lymph nodes under

Interview with Robert Barnett, M.D.

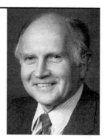

T he word *cancer* still evokes a tremendous amount of fear in most patients, and this fear can be hard to deal with emotionally and can cloud the decision-making process. Often women ask, "Shouldn't I do something immediately?" and I tell them that there is time to consider their options carefully—it's not going to make a difference if we do surgery this week or next. I usually encourage women to make a decision within three to four weeks following the diagnosis of breast cancer.

The physician has a large role in the ultimate decision that a woman makes. A physician must be honest in presenting options to the patient. Everybody has their own biases about how something should be managed, but I try to lay out the options to patients. Often patients decide to follow their surgeon's recommendations, but a low percentage—around 20 percent—prefer mastectomy if I recommend a conservative approach. And vice versa: about 20 percent of women decide on lumpectomy when I have recommended that they undergo a mastectomy because of the size or location of the tumor or because it is multifocal. Women need to have the information, and then they can make an informed choice. With this in mind, women who are similar in age and have a similar diagnosis of breast cancer will make different treatment decisions. I don't think we fully understand why this is so. A lot of it has to do with a woman's own beliefs, concerns, and fears but also with the influence of family and friends. We also need to recognize that we live in a multicultural society—people come from different cultures.

If a woman is making a choice that is very contrary to my own beliefs, I often encourage her to seek out a second opinion. Sometimes women themselves choose to seek a second opinion, and I always think that a good physician should be positive when a patient says, "I think I'll get a second opinion." The physician should say, "Absolutely, you should get a second opinion." In my experience, most of the time when a patient would get a second opinion, it would be in agreement with my opinion. Sometimes it would not be, but I think that happens a fairly small percentage of the time, and the difference of opinion may be small. It wouldn't be a 180-degree variance from what I would recommend, but it might be some thirty-degree variance. I think it is valuable for patients to be informed, and they can get information on the Internet, or by talking to other doctors, or by talking to other patients. I think it is valuable. And patients are well educated these days.

Family and friends usually mean well, but they can confuse the issue a lot. They have their own biases, and they may give advice that they think is good, but it may not be the best advice for the patient in question. I know some cases where the family put so much pressure on the patient. On the other hand, I know patients where the family members have been well informed and have had some valid experiences to lead them to give good advice, so it's a mixed bag. Surgical techniques are being refined constantly, and the best practice today would be very different from five years ago, so talking with a good friend who had breast cancer even five years ago may skew you to think toward what is now a dated approach.

Emotional counseling is important for some but not all women. Some patients come in, and they are so strong and so stable, you can tell by talking to them that they just have no emotional problems, they're going to handle it well. Other patients, you can detect early on that they are emotionally labile, and they really need psychological support. I think a positive attitude is important in the treatment of any disease, whether it be cancer, pneumonia, or anything. Patients have also asked me about the importance of prayer in cancer, and I think it is important. Personally, I think having faith and having a belief in God can be helpful.

Understanding the Treatments

For us as physicians, learning more about our patients is important — and not just the physical or medical background but some of the social issues, economic issues. We need to ask: How do you react to this? What is your reaction to this diagnosis? Are you very afraid? Have you always dealt with adversity before, and won't have trouble dealing with this? What's your attitude toward this? I think it is good to know how they feel about it up front.

CHAPTER 8

Radiation Therapy for Breast Cancer

Abram Recht, M.D.

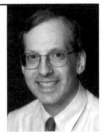

R adiation therapy has been used since the early part of the twentieth century to optimize the postsurgical treatment of women
with breast cancer. Radiation therapy improves the chances of
cure by destroying tumor cells left after surgery. For patients who cannot undergo surgery, radiation therapy can also be given first, to shrink
tumors and thus make surgery possible.

Radiation therapy has an important place in treating patients with
invasive breast cancer or with ductal carcinoma in situ (DCIS). It is useful to understand not only the treatment process but also the short-term
and long-term side effects; the nature of clinical follow-up after treatment; and how recurrences of cancer in the treated breast are managed.
The very word *radiation* is frightening to some people, though the treatments described in this chapter have saved many lives. Radiation therapy is a powerful force for cure.

A Brief Description of Radiation Therapy Procedures

Before a woman's radiation treatments are started, they are "simulated"
a thirty-to-sixty-minute process that creates a precise map of how the

treatments will be delivered to that particular woman. This simulation is done with the aid of either an X-ray machine designed to move like a treatment machine (a "simulator") or a CT machine. At the end of the simulation, measurements and X-rays are taken.

During the simulation, marks are placed on the patient's skin to help guide the radiation therapists in performing the individual treatments. This can be done either with magic marker (which can fade or wash off) or with small permanent tattoos that look like tiny birthmarks or freckles. Once the planning session is complete, an expert calculates how long the treatment machine should be left on to achieve the physician's prescribed dose of radiation, as well as other technical aspects of treatment.

The patient is treated lying on her back with her arms above her head. Usually, an apparatus is used to help the patient maintain this position. The variation of patient position in daily treatment given by well-trained radiation therapists is rarely more than one-fifth of an inch. Each treatment only takes a few minutes for the machine to deliver (see Figure 8.1).

It also takes a few minutes to properly position patients on the treatment table. Hence, most patients are in and out of the treatment room within ten or fifteen minutes. X-ray films of the areas treated (called *port films*) are usually taken once each week to check that the treatment is being carried out accurately.

Radiation Therapy in Detail

There is little evidence about the "best" way to give radiation therapy after lumpectomy, either for patients with invasive breast cancers or for those with DCIS. Many different approaches are taken by different institutions and physicians. Fortunately, it appears that these different approaches all result in about the same success rates. Some of the issues concerning the details of radiotherapy programs are discussed below. There is considerable controversy among experts about these details.

The Timing of Radiation Therapy

The length of time between surgery and the start of radiotherapy is called the "surgery-radiotherapy interval." Waiting too long can increase the risk of local recurrence because any remaining tumor cells may divide

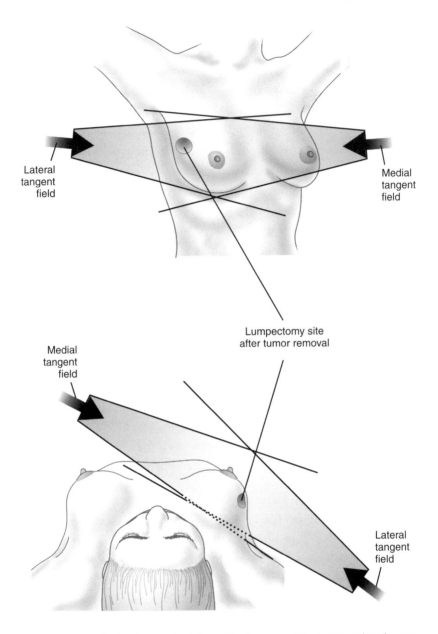

Lateral
tangent
field

Medial
tangent
field

Lumpectomy site
after tumor removal

Medial
tangent
field

Lateral
tangent
field

FIGURE 8.1. Radiation therapy is delivered to the area of the tumor and to the surrounding breast tissue on angles (tangents) that are designed to minimize the effect of the radiation on normal tissues in the lung and the heart. A patient is positioned precisely on the table, and the radiation beam is aimed precisely during each treatment.

and increase in number during this time. There is no evidence that starting early after surgery will improve the cure rates, however, and it is therefore reasonable to wait at least three to four weeks after surgery, to allow for healing, before starting radiation treatments. It seems prudent to begin radiotherapy within about two months of the last breast surgery when chemotherapy is not given, but starting treatment up to three or even four months after surgery may not harm patients with negative margins.

Usually, chemotherapy and radiation therapy are given sequentially rather than at the same time. The first is completed before the second is begun. While it may seem expeditious to give chemotherapy and radiation therapy within a few hours or within a day or two of each other, this approach increases the risk of side effects. Another option is to give part of the chemotherapy program for several months, then do radiation therapy, then complete the chemotherapy program. This "sandwich approach" has had excellent results in several studies, but there has

---

TABLE 8.1. INTEGRATION OF CHEMOTHERAPY AND RADIOTHERAPY GUIDELINES

All Patients:
Chemotherapy and radiotherapy sequentially, not simultaneously, unless patient is enrolled in a study.

BCT Patients:
- For patients with microscopically negative margins at least 1 mm in width: Chemotherapy, then radiation therapy.
- For patients with microscopically negative margins, but less than 1 mm in width ("close"):
An 8- to 16-week course of chemotherapy, then start radiation therapy within 4 months of the last breast surgery; more chemotherapy after radiotherapy is completed if desired.
- For patients with positive margins:
An 8- to 16-week course of chemotherapy, then start radiation therapy within 4 months of the last breast surgery; more chemotherapy after radiotherapy is completed if desired, or simultaneous chemotherapy and radiation therapy, or change the treatment plan to mastectomy.

Mastectomy Patients:
Radiation following chemotherapy.

---

been concern that breaking up the chemotherapy program reduces its effectiveness.

Areas Treated

Traditionally, the entire breast or chest wall has been treated with radiation in all patients. Treatment of the entire breast is done using high-energy X-rays produced either by a machine called a *linear accelerator* or by the X-rays released by a radioactive metal, cobalt-60. The treatment fields are called *tangents,* since they are directed at an angle to the body designed to treat the entire extent of the breast, from the side to the midline, while minimizing radiation exposure of healthy tissues. When the supraclavicular and/or axillary lymph nodes above the breast need to receive radiation, it is necessary to use an additional radiation field (or fields) aimed at these areas.

Many patients receive an extra "boost" dose of radiation to the area of the lumpectomy. This can be done using external treatments with either X-rays or high-energy beams of electrons. Another method, called *interstitial radiation implantation* (or an *implant*), involves placing needles through the tissues in this area to deposit radioactive material temporarily. Results are similar with each of these techniques.

If the internal mammary lymph nodes are to be treated, they can either be included in the same fields used to treat the breast or in a separate field directed straight down at the sternum.

Some studies of BCT have examined the results of treatment when radiation is given only to a more limited volume surrounding the tumor (called partial-breast irradiation). Such treatment can be done using either a radioactive implant, a "balloon" device that contains a radioactive source, or external radiation treatments. This seems to be a promising approach for some patients, but at present it is not yet standard practice outside of a research study.

Axillary node (armpit) recurrences occur in only 1 to 2 percent of patients treated with a standard axillary dissection, whether the lymph nodes are positive or negative. Axillary recurrences are also rare after a negative sentinel node biopsy. Because giving radiation treatments to the axilla after dissection can increase the risk of surgical side effects, it is generally not recommended. However, some patients may be at a much higher than average risk of axillary recurrence (for example, those with many positive axillary nodes). Axillary radiation therapy may be warranted in such individuals, despite the potential side effects. It is controversial whether patients with a positive sentinel node biopsy should go ahead with a "completion" axillary dissection or whether they can instead be treated with axillary radiation therapy with equal results.

Relapses in the internal mammary and supraclavicular nodal areas are also rare. It is controversial whether there are benefits to treating these lymph nodes, especially since giving radiation therapy to these areas can cause complications. At present it is considered acceptable either to give or not to give radiation therapy to the internal mammary lymph nodes for patients with positive axillary nodes. The supraclavicular nodes are treated with radiotherapy routinely when four or more axillary nodes are positive. Treating them is optional when only one to three axillary nodes are positive.

Radiation Doses

Three critical factors influence the effectiveness and side effects of radiation therapy: the areas of the body treated, the total amount of radiation given (the "dose"), and the amount of radiation given during any single treatment (the "fraction size"). Most centers in the United States and Western Europe give radiation doses to the entire breast of 44 to 50 Gray in twenty-two to twenty-five treatments ("fractions") of 1.8 to 2 Gray, with one treatment given daily five times per week. (One Gray, abbreviated as "Gy," equals one hundred rads, the old unit for measuring radiation dose.) However, other schemes are frequently used in Canada and the United Kingdom.

For patients treated with breast-conserving surgery, doses of approximately 50 Gy given to the entire breast have provided excellent results in a number of studies in which all patients had negative resection margins. Many institutions and physicians (including myself) combine treatment of the entire breast, usually to a dose of 45 to 50 Gy, with a "boost," or extra treatment, restricted just to the lumpectomy site with some surrounding margin. There is little proof that this extra treatment adds much to the outcome for women with negative margins, especially those older than age 50. However, doses higher than 50 Gy may be of greater benefit for patients whose specimen resection margins are positive or not evaluated, because these patients may have many more tumor cells left in this area after a lumpectomy than do patients with negative margins. Total doses of 60 to 66 Gy are usually given in this situation.

Must Radiation Therapy Follow Lumpectomy in Patients with Invasive Breast Cancer?

Today, patients with invasive cancers who are considered candidates for breast conserving therapy have a very low risk that cancer will reappear in the treated breast in the ten years following treatment with radiation therapy. The risk is most closely related to the margin status. When negative margins are achieved by the surgery, then the risk of local recurrence is less than 5 to 10 percent. Patients with "close" margins (where the tumor is not at the edge of the tissue removed, but within one to two millimeters of the edge) have about the same risk as patients with wider margins. When the margins are positive, the risk depends on how many tumor cells are at the edge of the excised tissue. When there are relatively few cells at the edge of the specimen, then the risk may be 10 to 20 percent. This risk may be reduced below 10 percent when patients receive chemotherapy or tamoxifen as well as radiation therapy. When many tumor cells are present at the edge of the specimen (called an "extensively positive" margin), the risk of relapse in the breast may be 20 to 40 percent, even with the addition of chemotherapy or tamoxifen.

One question often asked by patients is whether it is necessary to give radiation therapy after lumpectomy for invasive cancers if the margins of the removed tissue are negative. Many studies have looked at this question, and nearly all of them show that the risk of relapse in the breast is much higher when radiation is not used (20 to 40 percent) than when it is (5 to 10 percent). With local recurrence, mastectomy is usually necessary. Because relapse is a traumatic experience with its own impact on survival rates, the standard treatment around the world is to follow lumpectomy with radiation therapy, thus reducing the chance of recurrence.

Some patients, particularly women over the age of 70, with certain specific kinds of breast cancer who take hormonal therapy such as tamoxifen or aromatase inhibitors, may be exceptions to this rule; they have a very low risk of relapse when radiation therapy is not given after lumpectomy. This approach is becoming more popular, but there is no agreement yet among breast cancer experts as to who these individuals are.

Must Radiation Therapy Follow Lumpectomy in Patients with Ductal Carcinoma in Situ?

Recurrence rates for patients with ductal carcinoma in situ (DCIS) who have been treated with lumpectomy and radiation are similar to those for patients with invasive breast cancers. That is, for patients with negative or close margins, the risk of having the tumor return at or near the lumpectomy site is probably about 5 to 10 percent in the ten years following surgery. The risk is higher for patients with positive margins: 10 to 20 percent or more, depending on how many tumor cells are at the margins.

However, unlike the case with invasive cancer, many patients with DCIS can be treated successfully without radiation or hormonal therapy. Lumpectomy alone for these individuals results in a recurrence rate of 5 to 10 percent. Why this is so for DCIS and not true for invasive cancers is unknown. Radiation therapy will reduce the risk of recurrence even further in such patients, but here the benefits of radiation therapy will certainly be limited.

Breast cancer experts disagree about which patients can be safely treated without radiation therapy. The risk of recurrence seems most closely related to the margin status. Most doctors agree that there is a low risk of recurrence when the tumor is ten millimeters or more from the edge of the excised tissue, or when a patient has undergone a re-excision (second lumpectomy) and no cancer cells were found in the specimen. When the margins are narrower, however, the characteristics of the tumor itself (such as the nuclear grade and the tumor's size) may be important in predicting the risk of recurrence. Again, experts disagree about the risk of recurrence in particular situations. One study completed by the Eastern Cooperative Oncology Group (one of the national cooperative cancer investigation organizations funded by the National Cancer Institute) enrolled patients with tumors less than twenty-five millimeters in greatest diameter, a nuclear grade of 1 or 2, and a tumor-free margin width of more than three millimeters to be treated with lumpectomy without radiotherapy. The chance of a recurrence in the breast was 7 percent at five years after surgery. A number of studies of this issue have also recently been performed by other groups or are currently under way.

There has also been much recent interest in using tamoxifen for patients with DCIS as well as for patients with invasive breast cancer. One study conducted by the National Surgical Adjuvant Breast and Bowel Program (trial "B-24") found that tamoxifen lowered the risk of recurrence in the breast in patients treated with lumpectomy and radiation therapy. The benefits of tamoxifen were greatest in patients younger than 50 years old and in patients whose lumpectomy specimens had positive margins. However, a study performed in the United Kingdom did not show tamoxifen to have any benefits, either for patients treated with lumpectomy and radiation therapy or with lumpectomy alone.

When Is Radiation Therapy Used after Mastectomy?

Enormous controversy exists regarding the question of who benefits enough from postmastectomy radiation therapy to warrant its use. In 1997, the *New England Journal of Medicine* published the results of randomized trials performed in Denmark and British Columbia which showed increased survival rates among mastectomy patients who were subsequently treated with radiation therapy. Since then, the use of postmastectomy radiation has increased and a number of groups, such as the American Society of Clinical Oncology, have promoted guidelines for its use. Nearly all such guidelines agree that patients with tumors larger than five centimeters, those with "locally advanced" (T3–4) cancers, and those with four or more positive axillary nodes should receive radiation treatment. However, there is substantial controversy regarding whether other patients benefit enough to make such treatment routine (for example, those with tumors smaller than five centimeters, those who have only one to three positive axillary nodes, or those receiving preoperative chemotherapy).

Unfortunately, the key information that determines the need for post-operative radiation — the pathologic status of the axillary lymph nodes — is *not* known in most patients until the mastectomy surgery is actually done. This is a problem for women who want reconstructive surgery performed at the same time as their mastectomy because the risk of complications related to reconstruction increases with radiation therapy, particularly when the reconstruction involves a prosthesis. It seems that some (but not all) reconstructions performed using a "pure" muscle flap tolerate radiation therapy well, but these procedures are more complex and have their own potential problems, as discussed in chapter 12.

Side Effects of Radiation Therapy

Cosmetic Results after BCT and Radiation Therapy

Cosmetic results in different centers are difficult to compare, as there is no standard system for describing results. However, 80 to 90 percent of women treated with modern surgery and radiotherapy techniques have good or excellent cosmetic results (that is, little or no change in the treated breast in size, shape, texture, or appearance compared to what it was like before treatment). The details of surgery and radiation therapy affect the appearance and characteristics of the treated breast. Patients with large breasts seem to have greater shrinkage of the breast after radiation therapy than do smaller-breasted patients. This problem usually can be overcome by the use of higher X-ray energies.

Possible Side Effects during Radiation Treatments

There are no immediate side effects from each radiation treatment given to the breast. Patients do not develop nausea when this part of the body is treated. Side effects may build up gradually over the course of multiple treatments, however. So patients usually see their physician and the nurse weekly during the treatment cycle to discuss any side effects that might be developing and to make sure all the patient's questions are answered. It is usually two to three weeks before most patients begin noticing side effects of any kind.

Most patients develop mild fatigue that builds up gradually and that slowly resolves over one to two months following the end of radiotherapy. Blood counts go down very little, if at all. It is not necessary to measure them, even in patients who have previously received chemotherapy, except in unusual circumstances. Many patients develop dull aches or sharp shooting pains in the breast that may last for a few seconds or minutes. It is rare for patients to need any medication for this pain.

The most common side effect requiring attention is skin reaction. Most patients develop mild reddening, dryness, and itching after a few weeks. Some develop substantial irritation. Skin care recommendations vary greatly from center to center and have rarely been subjected to comparative testing. Most include broad guidelines such as keeping the skin clean and dry; using warm water and gentle soap; avoiding extreme temperatures while bathing; avoiding trauma to the skin; avoiding sun exposure (use a sun screen of at least SPF 15); avoiding shaving with a razor blade in the treatment field (use an electric razor, if necessary); avoiding use of perfumes, cosmetics, aftershave, or deodorants in the treatment field (use cornstarch, with or without baking soda, in place of deodorant); and using only recommended unscented creams or lotions after daily treatment. Some physicians recommend application of steroid creams for treating reddened skin and inflammation. Skin reactions usually heal by themselves within a few weeks of completing radiotherapy.

Some patients develop a sunburn-like reaction, with blistering and peeling of the skin, called *moist desquamation*. This reaction usually occurs in the fold under the breast or in the fold between the breast and the arm; it can also occur in the area given a radiation boost. Most patients who have only limited areas of moist desquamation can continue treatment without interruption. When treatment must be interrupted due to skin reaction, the skin usually heals sufficiently to allow radiation to be resumed in five to seven days. Healing need not be complete for treatment to begin. Skin care for women with moist desquamation includes using chlorhexadine gluconate or other antibacterial soaps to cleanse the area; alleviating discomfort with medications such as aspirin, ibuprofen, or acetaminophen if needed; and using nonadherent dressings to absorb drainage and maintain moisture.

It is rare for patients to develop skin or breast infections during radiation therapy. When they do occur, such infections can usually be cured with antibiotics without interrupting radiation therapy.

Possible Long-Term Side Effects of Radiation Therapy

MINOR COMPLICATIONS

Many women develop slight swelling of the breast during radiotherapy. This harmless complication usually goes away within six to twelve months, but sometimes it does become permanent.

Skin in the treated area becomes darker during the course of radiotherapy, just as skin tans in the sun. Like breast swelling, this harmless effect also usually fades gradually over six to twelve months but can occasionally become permanent.

Most women will have aches or pains from time to time in the treated breast or in the muscles surrounding the breast, even years after treatment. Usually there is no apparent cause for these episodes, although sometimes they occur after exertion. It is not clear why they occur. Though annoying, these pains are harmless, and they are *not* a sign that the cancer is reappearing.

Rarely, patients may develop a rib fracture in the years following treatment. This complication occurs in fewer than 1 percent of patients treated with modern approaches. Fractured ribs heal slowly by themselves.

SERIOUS COMPLICATIONS

It is very rare for patients to develop breakdown of the skin, fractures of the sternum (breastbone), or such severe pain in the breast that surgery is required.

Radiation therapy given to the axillary lymph nodes can increase the risk of arm swelling (lymphedema) following axillary dissection. However, as discussed above, such treatment is rarely needed. Treating just the supraclavicular lymph nodes does not increase the risk of arm edema.

If the supraclavicular or axillary nodes are treated, nerves that run from the neck to the arm are in the radiation treatment field as well. This treatment can cause numbness or tingling, or even pain and loss of strength, in the hand and arm years after treatment. Fortunately, this is a rare event in patients treated with current radiotherapy techniques (1 to 2 percent of patients at most). Most of these symptoms will be temporary, although they may be permanent in some patients.

A small percentage of patients may develop radiation pneumonitis between three and nine months after completing treatment. This complication is due to a reaction in the lung under the breast. Individuals with radiation pneumonitis may have cough, shortness of breath, and fevers. It is usually mild enough not to need specific treatment and generally resolves on its own within two to four weeks. There are no long-term complications, such as shortness of breath or difficulty exercising, in women who develop this problem.

Radiotherapy may cause damage to the heart. Fortunately, radiation techniques used now treat much less of the heart than those used in the past. Studies from Boston, Denmark, and Stockholm and from cancer registries in the United States have generally found no increased risk of serious heart disease in patients treated with modern techniques even ten to twenty years after radiotherapy was given. But there is still some uncertainty about whether radiation may cause heart problems after ten or twenty years, particularly in patients who receive drugs with known cardiac toxicities, such as doxorubicin (Adriamycin). So far this does not seem to be the case, but many more studies will need to be done to be certain. Nonetheless, it seems that any potential cardiac risk of radiation is more than offset by the benefit this treatment provides in prevention of cancer recurrence.

At the same time as it cures cancer, radiation can cause cancer—but very rarely. Cancers caused by radiation can take ten to thirty years or more to appear, so it is difficult to estimate how often this might happen in patients treated with current methods. Some studies suggest cancers caused by radiation might occur in 1 in 1,000 patients, but estimates range from approximately 1 in 100 to 200 patients to 1 in 2,500 patients. Women age 45 or younger at the time of treatment may have a slightly increased risk of eventually developing cancer of the other breast because of having radiation therapy. However, the increase in this risk at twenty-five years after treatment due to radiotherapy is small (perhaps 3 to 5 percent or less) compared to the risk patients already have just by virtue of having had one breast cancer (15 to 25 percent). Since few patients in this age group (or their physicians) consider preventive mastectomy for the opposite breast, this small additional risk does not usually stop patients from undergoing irradiation.

Follow-up

The major goal of follow-up visits after treatment is early detection and treatment of possible cancer recurrence or of new tumors in the treated or untreated breast. In patients without symptoms, there is no benefit to routinely doing bone scans, chest X-rays, blood tests, or other studies used to detect distant metastases (spread to other organs).

The optimal timing of follow-up visits is not known. Although many different schemes have been suggested, there are no comparative data to use to choose one of these schedules over another. In my practice, patients have a history taken and a physical examination performed by one of their treating physicians every three to six months for the first several years and then every six to twelve months indefinitely.

The optimal interval between mammograms is also not known. Some physicians recommend taking films of the treated breast every six months for several years after treatment. In my institution, we usually obtain mammograms of both breasts approximately six months after completing radiotherapy and then yearly. The value of other breast-imaging tests (MRI, ultrasound) for routine follow-up is not known.

Cancer Recurrence in the Breast after Lumpectomy and Radiation Therapy

Many patients who suffer a local recurrence desire breast reconstruction. Reconstruction can be done at the time of mastectomy, but it must be done using an approach that is compatible with prior radiation treatment. Irradiated tissues do not very well tolerate foreign bodies such as breast prostheses. Hence, patients who desire breast reconstruction need to have a portion of muscle and skin (*myocutaneous flap*) moved from the abdomen, back, or buttock onto the chest. The risk of complications from this reconstruction is slightly greater than in patients who have not had prior radiation, and the overall cosmetic results may not be as favorable. However, the results are usually satisfactory enough that many patients are glad they had the procedure done.

It is not clear whether there is an advantage to giving patients chemotherapy or tamoxifen after a breast cancer recurrence.

Some patients who have had a breast cancer recurrence after lumpectomy have been treated with another lumpectomy (with or without more radiotherapy). The results have not been terribly good with this approach, with 20 to 30 percent of patients developing another cancer in the breast with time. Giving more radiation also causes more scarring, and the cosmetic results of such retreatment are often poor. Therefore, I generally recommend mastectomy instead of another lumpectomy in the case of recurrence.

Conclusion

Radiation therapy has evolved over the past century to become an important tool for treating women with breast cancer. It is remarkably effective and safe. Further research in many areas of breast cancer radiotherapy is required, especially to identify ways of selecting the best form of treatment for an individual patient and to further decrease the risk of complications. Even so, today radiation therapy provides excellent results for the great majority of patients with breast cancer who require such treatment.

CHAPTER 9

Profiles of Two Radiation Oncologists

Interview with Luther Ampey, M.D.

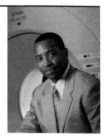

When deciding whether to have lumpectomy with radiation or mastectomy, some patients ask me, "If this were your mother, what would you recommend?" That's a question I would never answer because, as I always tell patients, "I can't answer for my mother." But some physicians might answer that question, "If it were my mother, I would recommend that she have a mastectomy." That's a powerful thing to say to a patient because she is looking to the physician at that time for guidance. So physician bias or preference can play into her decision. But with people becoming more knowledgeable and being able to do research on their own, patients often are a lot better educated when they come in with breast cancer or prostate cancer. They talk to people and discover that their friends and acquaintances have had breast cancer. They research things on the Internet, and they get counseling. Patients now can say, "What about this?" or "I know they had this clinical trial." Or they seek out a second opinion just to make sure that they are getting the counseling that they think they need.

In making the decision about lumpectomy, one question is, "What's the clinical outcome?" When patients understand that mastectomy and lumpectomy with radiation have an equivalent outcome, they feel reassured. Then, another important issue comes in—appearance, and what the breast means to the particular patient—and her decision about mastectomy or lumpectomy with radiation oftentimes will come down to that. I find that this is a more prominent issue for younger women with breast cancer as compared to older women. Finally, the length of radiation treatment can be a factor, but generally the length of treatment involved in six weeks of postoperative radiation doesn't really drive the patients' decision, although some patients opt for mastectomy just to "get it over with." This approach might not be what they really prefer, but their overall life situation dictates such a choice. They might have to take care of a spouse, or they might have another responsibility. Some women really can't take time away.

Radiation is probably the most mysterious of the treatment options. Almost everyone knows something about what happens in surgery—the surgeon goes in and cuts out the tumor. Similarly, almost everyone also knows something about chemotherapy—it can make you throw up or you may lose your hair.

Radiation treatment suffers a bad reputation because of past history— Nagasaki, Hiroshima, nuclear accidents, and what can happen to people who have inappropriate exposures to radiation. I spend a lot of time refuting what the person at the grocery store has told a patient. I try to let patients and their families understand that radiation can be well focused and very effective in the treatment of breast cancer. But just like with any other treatment—chemotherapy or surgery—there are possible side effects, and we go over those in detail. I let them know what their risk of these side effects is, depending on their particular cancer and their anatomy, and we go over what their expectations should be. I try to emphasize, "You're likely to get these, these you may or may not get, and these other side effects are rare." It is helpful for patients to have realistic expectations about side effects so that they aren't shocked when these occur. Some patients want to believe that they are going to have no side effects, and so, when they do, they don't handle it well emotionally. They can have a difficult time getting through their treatment, even if the side effects are minimal. Helping these patients to understand radiation and getting them into the routine of it can be difficult.

Understanding the Treatments

Patients come in Monday through Friday to get external radiation. They come in every single day for six weeks or a little more than that, and their doctors, nurses, and technicians get to know them well. We get to know their personalities, and we can tell when they are having a good day or a bad day, and if it's related to their treatment or not. A lot of patients worry about or get frustrated by their lack of control when they are receiving radiation or chemotherapy. They have to come for treatment at a particular time, they have to get x amount of treatments, and therefore their disease basically is dictating to them how they are going to live their lives for that period of time. So, once they know the routine, they at least feel that they have a bit more control over what is going on. I think this sense of some control helps patients feel that the cancer cannot totally consume their lives.

Interview with Susan Stinson, M.D.

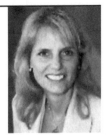

I believe that it is important to emphasize to women with early stage breast cancer that the chance for long-term survival is the same for women who choose mastectomy as for those candidates who undergo lumpectomy and then receive breast radiation therapy. While most women are candidates for mastectomy, not every woman is a candidate for breast conservation (lumpectomy and radiation). Typically, for breast conservation treatment, a lesion should be five centimeters or smaller. There should not be any skin involvement or chest wall involvement. Inflammatory breast cancer is a contraindication to breast conservation. (Inflammatory breast cancer is an unusual and aggressive type of breast cancer.) Margins are an issue also. If a surgeon does a couple of lumpectomies on the same woman and keeps getting positive surgical margins, then there's more cancer there than meets the eye clinically. A woman with this scenario would probably be best served by mastectomy. If a patient has two lesions in two different quadrants of the breast, she may not be an optimal candidate for breast conservation. Aside from these special circumstances, most patients are candidates for lumpectomy and radiation. Again the survival outlook is the same with either procedure.

There are many reasons why women choose one approach or the other. Some women feel strongly about keeping their breast unless there is a compelling reason to undergo a mastectomy, while others feel that they will worry about a recurrence of the cancer in their breast if they do not have a mastectomy. I think some of it may have to do with the bias of the physician who first explains their options. In this area of the country (the northeast), almost all of the physicians favor breast conservation when possible. There are other areas of the country where surgeons don't believe as strongly in this treatment option. Another factor may be availability of services. If a patient doesn't have a radiation center nearby, then she may choose to undergo a mastectomy rather than travel long distances daily to receive radiation treatment. We have excellent doctors in this area who are presenting patients with a full representation of both approaches, so it doesn't bother me when a woman makes an informed choice to undergo a mastectomy.

Treatment of non-invasive breast cancer (DCIS) is becoming a greater part of our practice each year, and the role of radiation in such cases is being investigated and refined. Mammography has greatly improved and mammographers are wonderful at picking up little tiny clusters of calcifications on a mammogram, so we are finding lots of people with non-invasive breast cancer. For these women there is some evidence to suggest that with good margins, lumpectomy alone may be okay if they have low-grade and very low-volume disease. There's a randomized trial (now closed to accrual) that's looking at that option right now for patients with non-invasive disease. I encouraged eligible women to be part of that study and did enroll a few patients. It gave them a fifty-fifty chance of getting radiation versus close follow-up. I discuss the trial with women and go over the risks and benefits of radiation or observation alone.

If a woman with DCIS wants to keep the in-breast recurrence risk as low as she can, then the way to do that is with radiation. If, however, a patient's risk is really low because she has a favorable presentation, the radiation would decrease the recurrence risk but may not decrease it enough to make an impact. If the patient makes an informed decision for close follow-up that is off protocol, I won't strongly disagree, and I will help arrange close follow-up. Some people do opt for close follow-up without radiation because there are a lot of nonrandomized data suggesting that recurrence risks are low in that situation after surgery alone. Many other patients opt for treatment with radiation even if they have had a small non-invasive breast cancer because they do want to reduce the risk of recurrence of what could then be an invasive cancer.

There is growing interest in treating a smaller portion of the breast with radiation, which is known as partial breast irradiation. Partial breast irradiation has never been studied in a prospective randomized phase-III trial. One of these trials started in spring 2004; my hospital-based clinic participates in that. Essentially this is treatment to the lumpectomy site and about a centimeter and a half of the margin around it. There are three ways you can do it. The first uses three-dimensional conformal external beam radiation that is similar to the regular treatment but focuses carefully on the tumor bed with a margin around it. A second technique involves placing hollow needle catheters into the breast and then inserting radiation sources into these needles for a certain amount of time each day.

Finally, a newer technology, called the MammoSite, is becoming available. The MammoSite and the catheters discussed above are brachytherapy (*brachy* means short distance radiation). In both types of brachytherapy, you put your source right at the site, and radiation is given off over a specific time period, depending on the source strength. Beyond a few centimeters, the radiation dose is basically zero. The MammoSite is a little balloon that is inserted into the bed where the tumor was excised and then the balloon is inflated and radioactive material is placed in it for a specified amount of time over a five-to-seven day period. The theory is that potentially the patient can get more even radiation to the area at highest risk of recurrence. One concern with that is that you get a very high dose of radiation right around where the balloon is and then it diminishes beyond that so that other areas of the breast are not treated.

We don't know right now if this type of treatment is as effective as the traditional approach for all women with breast cancer or for certain subgroups. For example, for women who have one to three positive lymph nodes, we need to determine if radiation should be provided to a wider field and be more "local-regional" in nature or not. Some people think that these women need to receive radiation to a standard field that includes the entire breast and some of the areas containing lymph nodes. Some people think that patients with positive nodes who have received state-of-the-art chemotherapy don't need local-regional radiation but need only breast radiation. My partners and I still tend to feel that, in that situation, where there's lymph node positivity, treating the breast and regional lymph nodes may also be sterilizing the micrometastatic disease, which are potentially very small amounts of tumor that may be present in remaining lymph nodes. One trial out of Canada has addressed this issue. The trial is closed to accrual now, so hopefully data analysis will begin in the next year or two. We all will benefit from well-conducted clinical trials to answer this and other important questions.

CHAPTER 10

Beyond Local Therapy

Hormonal Therapy and Chemotherapy

Antonio C. Wolff, M.D. *&* Nancy E. Davidson, M.D.

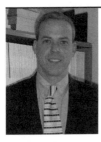
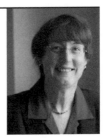

Today, breast cancer is usually diagnosed early and can potentially be cured with local therapy (mastectomy or lumpectomy,
with or without radiation) often followed by adjuvant systemic
therapy. Women diagnosed with ductal carcinoma in situ (DCIS) have
a non-invasive form of breast cancer that is treated with local therapy
(surgery alone or surgery followed by radiation therapy), sometimes followed by tamoxifen; DCIS generally does not spread outside the breast.
Women diagnosed with invasive breast cancer, however, are at a risk for
developing metastatic breast cancer. The degree of risk varies widely.
Jane and Doreen both had breast cancer, but the difference in their risk
of developing metastatic disease is significant.

*Jane is a 40-year-old woman who was found to have a five-centimeter (approx-
imately two-inch) breast cancer that had spread to eleven lymph nodes in her
armpit. Jane has a high risk of developing recurrent breast cancer elsewhere in the
body (metastatic disease).*

Doreen is a 62-year-old woman who was found to have a breast cancer that measured 0.3 centimeters (one-eighth of an inch). No cancer was found in the lymph nodes in her armpit. Doreen is at low risk of developing recurrent breast cancer.

Most women with invasive breast cancer have a level of risk for cancer recurrence elsewhere in the body in the range between Jane's level of risk and Doreen's level of risk. It is important to estimate the risk of recurrence for the individual patient because, while not precise, this information helps the patient and her doctors in their discussions about what treatments to consider. There are several tools that help doctors and women make decisions; these tools use individual characteristics of the patient and her disease to estimate the risk of recurrence and death as well as the potential reduction in risk with specific therapies. Although a major step forward, these web-based programs describe the expected risk and benefit for a *group of women* with those characteristics, not the risk and benefit for a specific individual. Therefore, researchers are increasingly interested in exploring individualized factors that predict outcome and benefit from a specific therapy for a specific patient. Several tissue-based tests that identify the genetic make-up of the patient's tumor are now being evaluated for this purpose.

Understanding the Risk of Recurrence

Non-Invasive Breast Cancer

For a woman with ductal carcinoma in situ (DCIS), the risk of a local recurrence is virtually eliminated by mastectomy or is significantly decreased with breast conservation therapy (lumpectomy usually followed by radiation). Women treated with breast conservation surgery whose cancers express the estrogen receptor often take tamoxifen for up to five years after surgery. Mastectomy and breast conservation therapy offer similar chances of survival. Furthermore, in women who do not have invasive disease, the cancer is not expected to recur elsewhere (systemic recurrence).

Invasive Breast Cancer

For a woman with invasive breast cancer, the risk of local (in the same breast) or systemic recurrence is related to a number of different factors, including:

- the number of involved lymph nodes,
- tumor size,
- tumor grade (how aggressive the tumor appears to be under the microscope), and
- tumor biology (the presence of hormone receptors and levels of expression of the HER-2 gene).

Women with invasive breast cancer are at risk for systemic recurrence — a recurrence of breast cancer elsewhere in the body. This risk is due to clusters of cancer cells that may have left the breast before surgery and spread through the bloodstream to other sites in the body. The two factors with the greatest impact on risk of recurrence and survival are the number of lymph nodes with cancer and the size of the tumor (see Table 10.1), but even women with small tumors that have penetrated through

TABLE 10.1. EFFECT OF TUMOR SIZE AND NODES ON SURVIVAL AT FIVE YEARS

Tumor Size	Survival at Five Years (%)		
	Negative Nodes	One to Three Positive Nodes	Four or More Positive Nodes
‹0.5	99.2	95.3	59.0
0.5–0.9	98.3	94.0	54.2
1.0–1.9	95.8	86.6	67.2
2.0–2.9	92.3	83.4	63.4
3.0–3.9	86.2	79.0	56.9
4.0–4.9	84.6	69.8	52.6
›5.0	82.2	73.0	45.5

Source: Adapted from S. Hellman, M. E. Lippman, M. Morrow, and J. R. Harris, eds., *Diseases of the Breast, Natural History of Breast Cancer* (Philadelphia: Lippincott-Raven, 1996), 12:383.

Understanding the Treatments

Balancing Risks and Benefits

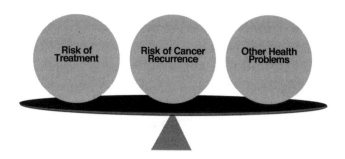

FIGURE 10.1. Decisions about postoperative treatment (adjuvant therapy) must balance the risk of the cancer recurring with the risks and side effects of the therapy, as well as consider the patient's age, general health, and life expectancy.

the inner wall of the duct and lymph nodes that are free of cancer involvement are at risk for recurrence.

Adjuvant Therapy to Reduce the Risk of Recurrence and Death

To help reduce the risk of recurrence, people with cancer often take adjuvant therapy, either as pills or as injections. Endocrine therapy (also called hormonal or anti-estrogen therapy) is often recommended in women with estrogen receptor (ER) positive disease. Endocrine therapy includes tamoxifen by mouth (in premenopausal women and postmenopausal women), aromatase inhibitors by mouth (in postmenopausal women), and LH-RH in monthly subcutaneous injections (in premenopausal women). Chemotherapy regimens are often considered for women with node-positive tumors, large node-negative tumors, and many women with ER-negative disease. Decisions regarding the use of adjuvant therapy (and the type) should balance the risk of recurrence, the potential benefit from treatment, other existing medical problems and life expectancy, and risk of side effects from treatment (see Figure 10.1).

Who Is at Low Risk and Does Not Need Adjuvant Therapy?

A few studies have found that, after surgery, women with breast cancers that are very small and low grade, that have no lymph node involvement, and that express the estrogen receptor may have a five-year survival rate not much different from similar aged women who have never had breast cancer. Women with ER-positive tumors are often treated with endocrine therapy such as tamoxifen (all age groups) or an aromatase inhibitor (if postmenopausal). Endocrine therapy helps reduce the risk of cancer recurrence in the same breast (if the woman was treated with breast conservation surgery), the risk of a new cancer in the other breast, and the risk of developing metastatic disease to other parts of the body. In low-risk women with ER-positive disease treated with endocrine therapy, the added benefit from a few months of chemotherapy given before tamoxifen may be very small. Nonetheless, chemotherapy might offer added benefit, especially for larger tumors, node-positive disease, or in very young women. Still, it is important to remember that endocrine therapy is the most important adjuvant treatment in a patient with ER-positive disease and/or progesterone receptor (PR) positive disease.

Endocrine therapy is not recommended for women whose tumors do not express either the estrogen receptor or the progesterone receptor. Even women with tumors with low levels of expression of hormone receptors can benefit from this therapy, though, which means that the doctor and the patient need to make sure that ER testing was correctly done when making decisions so that women are not incorrectly denied a potentially useful adjuvant treatment.

Options for Reducing the Risk of Recurrence: Endocrine Therapy

Tamoxifen

Breast cancer is often an estrogen-dependent disease. If the tumor depends on an intact ER pathway, the cancer growth is stimulated by the hormone estrogen (see Figure 10.2). Tamoxifen binds to the estrogen receptor differently from the way estrogen binds to the receptor, and that

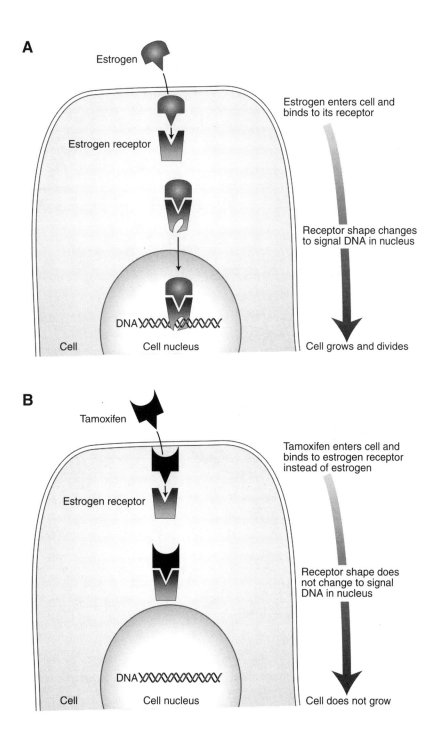

A

Estrogen

Estrogen receptor

DNA

Cell

Cell nucleus

Estrogen enters cell and binds to its receptor

Receptor shape changes to signal DNA in nucleus

Cell grows and divides

B

Tamoxifen

Estrogen receptor

DNA

Cell

Cell nucleus

Tamoxifen enters cell and binds to estrogen receptor instead of estrogen

Receptor shape does not change to signal DNA in nucleus

Cell does not grow

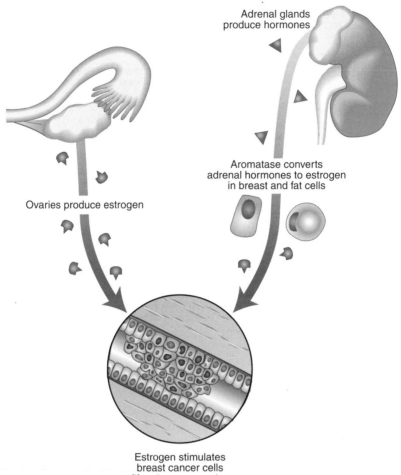

Adrenal glands
produce hormones

Aromatase converts
adrenal hormones to estrogen
in breast and fat cells

Ovaries produce estrogen

Estrogen stimulates
breast cancer cells
with estrogen receptors,
causing cell growth

FIGURE 10.2. The source of estrogen in women prior to menopause is primarily the ovaries. After menopause, the adrenal glands (which sit above the kidneys) produce hormones that can be converted to estrogen by a special enzyme in fat and breast cells called *aromatase.* So even after menopause there is estrogen available to stimulate breast cancer cells to grow if they are receptive to estrogen.

is how tamoxifen modifies the usual function of the estrogen pathway (see Figure 10.3). Tamoxifen often provides the best risk to benefit ratio among adjuvant therapy options, especially in women younger than age 50. Tamoxifen can help both premenopausal and postmenopausal women but is of no use in women with tumors that are completely neg-

ative for the ER and PR. Because the test that measures the estrogen receptor is not standardized across pathology labs, it is important to confirm that a negative ER result is indeed correct — that it is not a false negative, which would cause women to be denied potentially effective therapy.

- Women can benefit from treatment with tamoxifen if the tumor expresses the estrogen receptor and/or the progesterone receptor (ER-positive and/or PR-positive), but if neither receptor is expressed, there is no benefit to tamoxifen treatment.
- Women who receive tamoxifen after radiation therapy have a lower risk of recurrence of the cancer in the breast that was treated with radiation.
- A longer duration of treatment with tamoxifen (up to five years) offers increasing benefit in reducing the risk of recurrence. Treatment with tamoxifen for five years essentially halves the risk of developing a new cancer in the other breast (called contralateral breast cancer). Current evidence suggests that tamoxifen should not be used beyond five years.
- The relative benefit in reducing the risk of recurrence and death offered by tamoxifen is the same among all women with hormone receptor–positive tumors, regardless of age, tumor size, and lymph node involvement.
- In premenopausal women, five years of tamoxifen is the standard treatment. New information in postmenopausal women indicates that most women should receive an aromatase inhibitor alone or in sequence with tamoxifen (see discussion below).

FIGURE 10.3. (A) Many breast cancer cells have a special receptor for estrogen known as the *estrogen receptor*. Estrogen enters the cancer cell and binds to the estrogen receptor, which is custom made to receive it. When the estrogen is received, the protein that binds the estrogen and the estrogen itself send a message to the cancer cell to grow. (B) When tamoxifen is present it modifies the ability of the cancer cell to bind the estrogen, and the message is not generated to the cancer cell to grow. The tamoxifen looks similar to estrogen, so it can fill the space that is normally occupied by estrogen, and yet it is different enough from estrogen to not change the way it stimulates the cancer cell.

- Treatment with tamoxifen can have other benefits, as well, including a reduction in the risk of bone fractures in older women and a lowering of certain types of cholesterol (though without a reduction in the risk of heart disease).

TAMOXIFEN: WEIGHING RISKS AND BENEFITS

Treatment with tamoxifen is associated with an increased incidence of hot flashes, vaginal discharge, and night sweats. Anecdotally, many women and doctors believe that it is associated with weight gain, although well-conducted trials have not demonstrated that weight gain is necessarily related to the tamoxifen. Rather, this weight gain may be associated with the onset of menopause, treatment with chemotherapy, and other poorly understood factors. Tamoxifen may cause menstruation to stop in some women, especially in women over age 45 who may be approaching menopause. Other side effects include a slightly increased risk of problems associated with blood clots, but less than 1 percent of women develop clots. Some eye problems have been reported, and therefore an eye examination during the first year of treatment is sometimes recommended (see Figure 10.4).

THE RISK OF UTERINE CANCER AND OTHER POTENTIAL RISKS

Tamoxifen changes the way estrogen affects breast cancer cells, but it can also stimulate other types of cells in the body, just like estrogen does. Large studies have demonstrated that women being treated with tamoxifen are more likely to develop uterine cancer than women who have not taken the drug. For example, in the NSABP P1 Prevention trial, the risk of endometrial cancer was approximately one-fourth of one percent in the placebo group and one-half of one percent in the tamoxifen group. Although the incidence of endometrial cancer was doubled, the absolute increase was very small. Also, most of the cases of endometrial cancer in women who were taking tamoxifen were diagnosed early and were cured with surgery. However, other studies showed an increase in hysterectomies in women treated with tamoxifen, perhaps reflecting an increased concern about endometrial cancer and use of prophylactic procedures. There may be a slightly higher risk of another type of uterine cancer known as a uterine sarcoma, though this is a rare cancer. Women taking tamoxifen need to alert their doctors if they have any

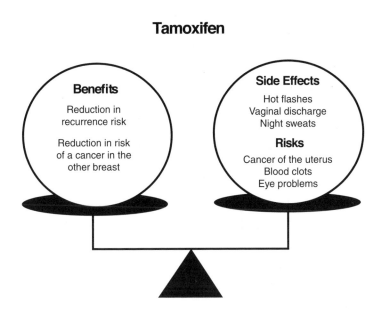

Tamoxifen

Benefits

Reduction in recurrence risk

Reduction in risk of a cancer in the other breast

Side Effects

Hot flashes
Vaginal discharge
Night sweats

Risks

Cancer of the uterus
Blood clots
Eye problems

FIGURE 10.4. Treatment with tamoxifen has benefits as well as certain risks and side effects.

abnormal spotting or bleeding, and they should have regular screening gynecologic evaluations, especially if they are postmenopausal. Many women taking tamoxifen have benign thickening of the lining of the uterus; the benefit of routine use of transvaginal ultrasound or endometrial biopsy in women without symptoms is not clear.

Aromatase Inhibitors in Postmenopausal Women

Estrogen is primarily produced by the ovaries. After menopause, the ovaries stop producing estrogen, and postmenopausal women produce less than 20 percent of the estrogen they produced before menopause. The estrogen in a woman's body after menopause is produced by conversion of hormones from the adrenal glands in some other tissues in the body and also locally in the breast. These sources of estrogen production can be blocked with a newer type of anti-estrogen drugs called *aromatase inhibitors* (see Figure 10.5): anastrozole (brand name Arimidex), letrozole (Femara), and exemestane (Aromasin). Important facts about these drugs are:

- They should only be given to women who are beyond menopause.
- They help reduce the risk of systemic recurrence (outside the breast).
- They help reduce the risk of a new breast cancer in the other breast.
- They are being tested as preventive in women at high risk for developing breast cancer and in women diagnosed with ductal carcinoma in situ (non-invasive cancer) of the breast.

Recent studies have shown a benefit of aromatase inhibitors after initial surgical treatment for invasive breast cancer in the following three situations:

- when taken for five years instead of tamoxifen (that is, taken in years 1 to 5),
- when started after three to five years of tamoxifen therapy, or
- when taken for two to three years after initial use of tamoxifen for two to three years.

These studies confirm the value of using aromatase inhibitors in post-menopausal women diagnosed with hormone receptor–positive invasive breast cancer. However, determining their optimal schedule and duration of use (up to five years or longer) is the objective of intensive ongoing studies, and we expect more information will become available in the next few years.

Aromatase inhibitors are generally as well tolerated as tamoxifen. They are less likely to cause vaginal bleeding or vaginal discharge, blood clot-

---

FIGURE 10.5. The source of estrogen in women prior to menopause is primarily the ovaries. After menopause, the adrenal glands (which sit above the kidneys) produce hormones that can be converted to estrogen by a special enzyme in fat and breast cells called *aromatase*. So even after menopause there is estrogen available to stimulate breast cancer cells to grow if they are receptive to estrogen. Treatment with the aromatase inhibitors reduces the conversion to estrogen of other hormones produced by the adrenal glands. The aromatase inhibitors have risks and side effects as well as benefits.

Understanding the Treatments

ting problems, and cancer of the uterus. However, they have a similar risk of causing hot flashes and a greater risk of causing osteoporosis, joint achiness, and vaginal dryness.

Aromatase inhibitors should not be taken by women who are still having menstrual periods, and they should be taken with caution by women with chemotherapy- or tamoxifen-induced cessation of menstrual cycles, because ovarian function may resume even years after these other drugs are stopped. The safety and effectiveness of using aromatase inhibitors with a drug that suppresses ovarian function (LH-RH analogues) in premenopausal women is the subject of ongoing research.

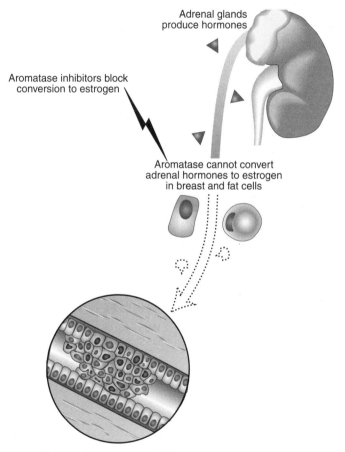

Adrenal glands produce hormones

Aromatase inhibitors block conversion to estrogen

Aromatase cannot convert adrenal hormones to estrogen in breast and fat cells

Estrogen is no longer available to estrogen receptor–positive breast cancer cells

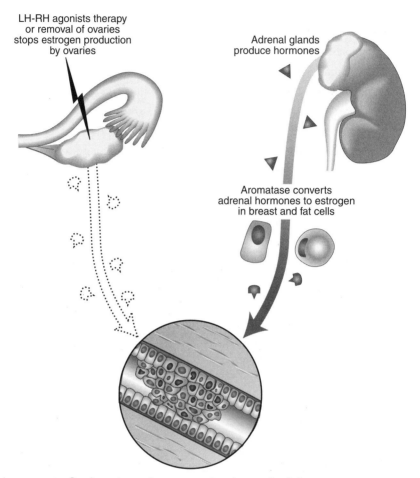

LH-RH agonists therapy
or removal of ovaries
stops estrogen production
by ovaries

Adrenal glands
produce hormones

Aromatase converts
adrenal hormones to estrogen
in breast and fat cells

Ovarian estrogen is suppressed, no longer stimulating
estrogen receptor–positive breast cancer cells

FIGURE 10.6. In women who are still having their menstrual periods, estrogen levels are typically high. This estrogen can stimulate the growth of cancer cells that have the ability to receive estrogen (they have the estrogen receptor). In these premenopausal women, the levels of estrogen can be reduced either by removing the ovaries (oophorectomy) or by administering medications called LH-RH antagonists, which reduce the stimulation of the ovaries to produce estrogen. Woman who undergo oophorectomy or are treated with LH-RH antagonists are similar to postmenopausal women and can also be treated with the aromatase inhibitors.

Ovarian Suppression

Suppressing the functioning of the ovaries, either surgically or nonsurgically, is called oophorectomy. Oophorectomy has long been studied as an effective form of breast cancer therapy in premenopausal women with metastatic disease. Effective forms of ovarian suppression include potentially reversible ones (such as LH-RH agonists taken as a monthly skin injection) and permanent ones (such as ovarian irradiation and surgical oophorectomy) (see Figure 10.6). Many studies showed that ovarian suppression as adjuvant treatment and chemotherapy as adjuvant treatment bestowed similar benefits. However, most of the available information comes from studies that did not compare oophorectomy with modern chemotherapy regimens containing a class of drugs called anthracyclines or oophorectomy followed by tamoxifen. The potential benefits of adding ovarian suppression to oral anti-estrogens (such as tamoxifen) in premenopausal women who did not take chemotherapy or who continued to menstruate after chemotherapy is the subject of current research.

Options for Reducing the Risk of Recurrence: Chemotherapy

Chemotherapy drugs are medications that help to destroy cancer cells in many different ways. Some prevent the cancer cells from dividing, while others interfere with the cancer cells' metabolism or repair process. They may also benefit young women with hormone receptor–positive disease by interfering with the production of ovarian hormones (see Figure 10.7).

Many important research studies have helped to shape treatment recommendations. Landmark trials on breast cancer have revealed that women who receive several months of a combination of multiple chemotherapy drugs following surgery for breast cancer have a lower risk of recurrence and of death from breast cancer than women who receive no postoperative therapy. Numerous combinations of chemotherapy drugs have been developed and studied. Examples of commonly used regimens include those shown in Table 10.2.

A large overview (metaanalysis) of dozens of clinical trials reported that treatment with chemotherapy was associated with a reduction in breast cancer recurrence and mortality. This relative benefit was seen in women of most ages, especially women younger than age 50. Unfortunately, little information on the benefit of chemotherapy is available for women over age 70. Chemotherapy treatment offers a similar relative

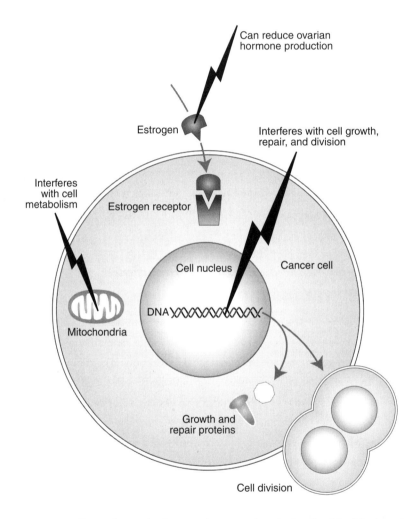

FIGURE 10.7. Chemotherapy is often very important in reducing the risk of the breast cancer recurring. The chemotherapy drugs work by many different mechanisms, including interfering with cell metabolism, preventing the cells' genes (DNA) from duplicating or from repairing themselves, or preventing the cancer cells from dividing. Chemotherapy has risks and side effects as well as benefits.

Understanding the Treatments

TABLE 10.2. ADJUVANT CHEMOTHERAPY

FAC/CAF (cyclophosphamide, doxorubicin, and 5 fluorouracil)
FEC/CEF (cyclophosphamide, epirubicin, 5 fluorouracil)
AC (doxorubicin, cyclophosphamide) ± paclitaxel
EC (epirubicin and cyclophosphamide)
TAC (docetaxel, doxorubicin, and cyclophosphamide)
A followed by CMF
E followed by CMF
CMF
AC followed by paclitaxel or A → T → C, every two weeks with colony
   stimulating factor
TC (docetaxel and cyclophosphamide)

Source: Adapted from 2005 NCCN Guidelines.

risk reduction in women with or without lymph node involvement, although women with ER/PR-negative disease appear to benefit more from chemotherapy than women with hormone receptor–positive disease also being treated with endocrine therapy.

In women with hormone receptor–positive disease, endocrine therapy should be seen as the most important systemic treatment, though chemotherapy offers some additional benefit, especially if there is evidence of lymph node involvement. In women with hormone receptor–negative disease, chemotherapy is the only option and often considered even for those with small tumors and lymph nodes free of disease. Younger women also appear to benefit more from chemotherapy, perhaps due to its indirect effect on suppressing ovarian function, at least temporarily, in women with hormone receptor–positive disease. Women being treated with chemotherapy and endocrine therapy generally receive them in a sequential fashion, with all chemotherapy given first.

During 2005, several clinical trials showed an improvement in survival for certain groups of patients with HER-2 positive breast cancer treated with chemotherapy and up to one year of the monoclonal antibody trastuzumab versus chemotherapy alone.

These clinical trials included patients with node-positive breast cancer and a smaller number of patients with high-risk node-negative breast cancer (for example, tumors greater than one centimeter and ER/PR

Hormonal Therapy and Chemotherapy   147

negative). At present, there is less information on the benefit of using trastuzumab in node-negative patients with smaller tumors.

HER-2, or human epidermal growth factor receptor 2, is over-expressed in approximately 20 percent of invasive breast cancers. Tests commonly used to identify these tumors include immunohistochemistry (3+ is considered positive) and fluorescent in situ hybridization (a FISH gene amplification ratio of 2.2 or greater is considered positive).

Because of an increased risk of heart damage when combined with doxorubicin or epirubicin, trastuzumab is started at the beginning of taxane therapy or following the completion of all chemotherapy. There-fore, patients often receive it during radiation and anti-estrogen therapy.

Several important chemotherapy principles have been established based on a long series of large studies.

- Treatments that include anthracycline drugs (for example, dox-orubicin [Adriamycin] or epirubicin [Ellence]) may offer a greater benefit than those without them, especially in women treated with six cycles of therapy.
- The addition of a taxane drug (paclitaxel [Taxol] or docetaxel [Taxotere]) seems to further reduce the risk of recurrence in women with lymph node–positive disease.
- The use of the chemotherapy regimen AC followed by Taxol given every two weeks instead of every three weeks further decreases the risk of recurrence and death from breast cancer.
- The use of high doses of chemotherapy with bone marrow trans-plant support has not shown any meaningful benefit and should not be used outside of clinical trials.
- Trastuzumab should be considered in addition to chemotherapy in women with HER-2-positive high-risk node-negative disease.

Risks and Side Effects with Chemotherapy

Most chemotherapy regimens have the potential to produce side effects and pose risks. The side effects and risks are different in type and inten-sity depending on the drugs used. Common acute side effects include reversible hair loss, nausea and vomiting (controlled in most patients), low red blood count (anemia) and low white blood count (greater risk of infection), changes in taste and sensation, and joint achiness. Some regimens include the use of white blood cell growth factors to reduce the risk of infectious complications. Side effects are rarely life-threatening or fatal. Other common side effects include fatigue, weight gain, possible cognitive dysfunction (for example, memory problems), and the onset of early menopause. Anthracycline drugs have a small risk of causing cardiac weakness, and taxane drugs have a small risk of causing peripheral neuropathy (numbness or tingling in hands and feet). Some of these drugs are associated with a higher risk of leukemia. Hot flashes often occur in postmenopausal women who stop taking hormone replacement therapy after being diagnosed with breast cancer or in premenopausal women who stop menstruating with chemotherapy. Trastuzumab is associated with a small risk of potentially life-threatening heart failure.

How Significant Is the Reduction in Risk Offered by Systemic Therapy?

As noted above, the risk of recurrence is smaller in women with small tumors and uninvolved lymph nodes. If the tumor is hormone receptor positive, most of the benefit will be from endocrine therapy. If the tumor is hormone receptor negative, only chemotherapy should be considered. There are a few online tools available for health care professionals to use, often while the patient is in the office with the physician. The patient's specific characteristics are entered into the program, and it calculates statistics for outcomes. These programs are useful in describing the risk of death from non-breast-cancer-related causes associated with age and other comorbid conditions; the most commonly used program is Adjuvant! (www.adjuvantonline.com). Here are two examples of how this program works.

Patient A is a 60-year-old woman with a breast cancer smaller than one centimeter with negative nodes and positive estrogen receptor. At ten years, 15 out of 100 women like her will have had a systemic relapse if given no systemic therapy.

With tamoxifen alone this would be reduced to 10 out of 100 women; and with chemotherapy and tamoxifen it would be reduced to 9 out of 100.

The risk of recurrence is greater in women with larger tumors or involved lymph nodes. The risk/benefit ratio of adding chemotherapy may favor its addition to the treatment plan.

Patient B is a 40-year-old woman with a breast cancer larger than one centimeter with one to three positive nodes and a positive estrogen receptor. At ten years, 52 out of 100 women like her will have a systemic relapse without systemic therapy. With tamoxifen alone this would be reduced to 34 out of 100; with chemotherapy alone this would be reduced to 33 out of 100; and with chemotherapy and tamoxifen this would be reduced to 20 out of 100.

Predictive Markers

The available tools describe risk for a group of patients without providing a yes or no answer for an individual patient, and therefore many women are excessively and unnecessarily treated with chemotherapy because we do not know which women will be helped by the treatment. Thus, there is major interest in developing tools to predict the individual future behavior of the disease in a particular patient with or without adjuvant systemic therapy. Predictive factors could make it possible to predict the response or resistance to a specific therapy in a specific individual. New technologies based on the genetic analysis of tumor tissue are being gradually tested and introduced in clinical practice. One example is a twenty-one-gene tissue assay that can be performed in pathology tissue blocks available in most cases. In late 2004, retrospective results from the Oncotype DX assay showed that it is possible to divide a group of patients with node-negative, ER-positive disease into three groups: low risk (approximately 50 percent of women), intermediate risk (25 percent) and high risk (25 percent). Subsequent retrospective validation of these findings using tissue specimens from mature studies conducted by the National Surgical Adjuvant Bowel and Breast Project (NSABP) showed that the average low-risk patient gained all the risk-reduction benefit from tamoxifen and none from chemotherapy, while the exact opposite was seen in the average high-risk patient. This assay appears to help identify the women with ER-positive, node-negative disease who are most likely to benefit from specific therapies, thereby reducing the number of women unnecessarily exposed to potentially toxic therapies of minimal or no utility for them. This assay is already commercially available and is now undergoing further study to examine the intermediate risk group. New methods using breast tissue, peripheral blood, and imaging studies are exploring the usefulness of other markers in women treated with adjuvant therapy before or after surgery.

Preoperative Chemotherapy or Hormonal Therapy

Chemotherapy was initially used for a period of time before surgery in women who had locally advanced disease and inoperable tumors, and more recently it has been used in women with smaller tumors and operable disease. This approach is also called neoadjuvant, preoperative, or primary systemic therapy. Available evidence shows that giving the same chemotherapy before or after surgery offers the same chance of survival and a small increase in the rate of breast conservation. More important, preoperative systemic therapy offers the opportunity to examine upfront the response of the cancer to systemic therapy, while allowing a small increase in the number of women treated with breast conservation. This approach is viewed as an important research avenue to study new techniques for early identification of antitumor activity and new therapies. This is important because women who achieve a complete pathologic response (no residual cancer at surgery) in the breast and axilla after preoperative systemic therapy appear to be the women most likely to do well in the future.

Future Directions

Ongoing studies are examining the role of efforts to enhance the immune system against breast cancer using approaches based on vaccines. Several new drugs against specific molecular pathways that might be important for breast cancer survival are also being tested in the adjuvant setting. In addition, trials examining the value of agents targeting new blood vessel formation are also in progress.

Questions to Review with Your Breast Cancer Specialist

At times it may seem overwhelming to absorb so much medical information. The following list of questions is intended to help you gather important, personalized facts from your own doctor which will help guide your treatment decisions. These questions do not address the emotional side of your experience right now, but that, too, is critical. Many women find that focusing on concrete facts can help bring step-by-step coherence to the frightening and often disorienting task of treatment planning. Here are some fundamental questions to review with your breast cancer doctor.

What type of breast cancer do I have?

If the cancer is non-invasive (DCIS), then what are my options for local control of the tumor (lumpectomy alone, lumpectomy with radiation, or mastectomy)?

Am I a candidate for endocrine therapy? (Does my tumor express the estrogen receptor?)

If I take endocrine therapy, how much benefit can I expect in reducing the risk of another breast cancer in the same breast or the other breast?

If the tumor is invasive, how large is it, what grade is it, and were the lymph nodes involved?

What stage cancer is this?

What did you learn about the biology of the tumor? Does it have the receptor for estrogen or progesterone? Does it overexpress HER-2?

What is the risk of a recurrence elsewhere in my body in the next several years? How can I best reduce this risk?

Will hormonal therapy, chemotherapy, or both help reduce my risk of recurrence? By how much in absolute terms?

If the tumor is HER-2 positive, am I a candidate for therapy with trastuzumab with or following chemotherapy?

What are the side effects and risks of treatment, both short and long term? How do the risks compare with the possible benefit?

Am I eligible for any research clinical trials that may benefit me or other women with breast cancer?

Understanding the Treatments

CHAPTER 11

Profiles of Three Medical Oncologists

Interview with Claudine Isaacs, M.D.

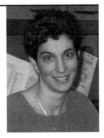

A s medical oncologists, our main role is to make recommendations regarding the use of systemic therapy. The aim of systemic treatment is to decrease the risk of breast cancer recurrence and to improve survival. When I meet with a patient, we have a
detailed discussion about whether treatment with chemotherapy, hormone therapy, or, more recently, antibody treatment such as Herceptin
is indicated. These discussions take into account a woman's age and
other medical conditions, as well as the features of the tumor, such as
whether there are any involved lymph nodes, the size of the tumor, and
whether it is hormone receptor positive or HER-2 positive.

As a doctor, it's generally harder not to do something than to do something, particularly in American medicine, where the tendency is to do
more rather than less. I review with women the results of clinical trials
and what they show us about the potential benefit of these treatment
options. For some women the benefit of chemotherapy is considerable,
but for others there is only a small benefit. I don't necessarily use specific numbers, but I share the range of benefit one might expect from
chemotherapy, explaining that we can't individualize who precisely will

benefit or suffer a significant side effect from this treatment. I also make it clear that none of our therapies reduce the risk of recurrence to zero. In some cases, there may only be a 1 to 2 percent improvement in long-term survival, whereas in others the benefit is more marked. Different people have different takes on whether that 1 to 2 percent benefit is worth it, and I think it is important that women are informed of the magnitude of benefit.

There are situations where I do not recommend chemotherapy. I'll say, "Medically, I'm leaning more against it because there are some rare and unusual side effects of chemotherapy and . . . " While these side effects don't happen very often, if they happen to somebody for whom chemotherapy only provides a 1 to 2 percent reduction of the risk of recurrence, that ends up being a pretty high price to pay. I'll say, "This is a personal decision, and you might feel this is worth it." "But you need to know that there are potential serious risks, and these risks start to add up and, in your case, equal the potential benefits. You're balancing the risks and benefits."

As we spend more years in practice, I think we feel increasingly comfortable with the recognition that there is often no single right answer. In breast cancer care, there are many controversial areas, where different clinicians may disagree and where nobody is right and nobody is wrong. I'll usually make it a point to tell patients that this is a controversial area and that there is not one right way to proceed. I think it helps them to understand why they may be getting two or three seemingly different opinions if they see several oncologists. In the breast cancer field, we are fortunate that so many women have agreed to participate in clinical trials and have allowed us to make all of the advances that have occurred in the treatment of this disease. These trials answer important questions and also raise questions for today and tomorrow. As a result, there is not a single way to treat women with breast cancer, and I think there are many situations where there are a number of perfectly reasonable options.

A critical component of decision making is the patient's own perception of how the risks and benefits of any therapy weigh out. It is important for clinicians to make recommendations for or against a treatment but also to involve individuals in the decision making. For people to make that type of decision, I think it is important that they have a clear understanding of the choices and their associated benefits and risks. I end up having a dialogue with patients and getting a feel for what type of information they want. I tend to start out speaking in general ways about the benefits of therapy, and then, depending on a particular person, I talk to them about numbers or the anticipated magnitude of a therapy's benefit. I tell patients that numbers don't apply to individuals but that they apply to populations. Computer algorithms now exist to help us figure out the benefits of different therapies, but it is important to tell people that those numbers are not as hard and fast as they appear. If somebody wants to know numbers, I will tell them numbers. But many people don't want to know numbers; they want to get a general sense of benefit.

If a woman is making a decision that is very counter to the standard of care, I'll explore with her what her issues and concerns are. In such a case I tend to make sure that people understand the magnitude of the benefit of the recommended therapy. I want to make sure they're really making an informed decision and that they know what they are choosing and what the potential benefit or risks might be.

For women for whom chemotherapy is recommended, I start off by talking to them about how women generally feel on chemotherapy and then discuss the common side effects. Most women fear chemotherapy, but what we see on TV or read about is generally worse than the real thing. With the chemotherapy we give for breast cancer, women usually do better than they thought they would. I first discuss the common things that people worry about: the fear of nausea and vomiting with chemotherapy. I'll then explain to them that the newer anti-nausea medications work very well. I tell them, "We work with you, and we aim for little or no nausea. Although the first cycle might not be perfect, the second time we often modify things to reduce either residual nausea or side effects from the medications." We discuss hair loss, and I am clear with them about what to anticipate and that we recognize that this is a psychologically unpleasant side effect of chemotherapy. We also discuss the impact on the white blood cell count and the risks of infection associated with that and what we need to watch for. Then we'll talk about other side effects like menopause, and other less common but potentially serious side effects, and try and put them in some perspective. As I mentioned

Interview with Sandra Swain, M.D.

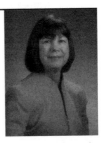

M y work is at the National Cancer Institute and the Naval Medical Center. We have a multidisciplinary breast cancer clinic, and the patients usually have a diagnosis of cancer when they come to the clinic, or they have had just a biopsy. Our patients are seen by a radiation oncologist, and they are seen by one of our medical oncology fellows. Then the cases are all presented at 11 o'clock at our conference. We look at the mammogram or any other imaging, and we look at the pathology. We have the surgeons, the radiation oncologist, the rehab doctors, the pathologists, radiologists, medical oncologists, and we make initial recommendations for the patients regarding the treatment of the breast cancer with surgery and/or radiation. Later on, after surgery, the results will be brought back to the conference, the patient discussed, and then the systemic treatment recommendations will be made.

We put all the information into a computer program and print out information about the risk of recurrence and survival, the expected benefit of treatment with hormonal therapy and chemotherapy, or the combination, and then we go talk with the patients. So then, with the recurrence rates and the changes in rates with treatment clearly defined, we make our recommendations. We share these numbers with the patients and get to know what the patients' issues are and have dialogue about it. And usually they don't make a decision right then. Usually, they'll think about it and come back the next week.

Some women get other opinions, which can be harder for patients in a way. A lot of patients don't like to have to be involved in treatment decision making. They say, "Well, I want to come to a doctor and have him or her tell me exactly what I should do." It's not where the field is yet, though. We don't know exactly what each woman sitting in front of us should do. She wants numbers, but that patient is not a number. She is a person who has thoughts and feelings about what she wants to do.

If you look at the studies, you see that some women will say a 1 percent difference would convince them to get chemotherapy—about 50 percent will say that—and there is another group of women who will say "I need 5 or 10 percent benefit before I will undergo chemotherapy," so it's very individual. I think people who have a good support system tend to want to get chemotherapy. This has been shown in a study. Most people are scared. A lot of fear comes with that first visit or two. It usually takes a couple of times to make a decision. One thing that's very hard for patients to understand, and I have explained this probably to two thousand or more patients, is the difference between getting radiation and getting chemotherapy. They think, "Okay, I'm getting radiation, I don't need chemotherapy." So I try to explain to them that radiation (or mastectomy) provides local treatment, and chemotherapy is for the systemic treatment.

During a typical consultation with a newly diagnosed woman, I often start out with saying, "Your tumor has a lot of very good features." "Your tumor is small." "It's less than an inch," or whatever the size is. "It doesn't have the oncogene, the cancer gene, HER-2 which gives you a higher incidence of recurrence. You don't have that." "You do have estrogen receptor present, which just gives you a better prognosis or less of a chance of recurrence because it shows that the cancer cells are able to make the protein." "You don't have nodes involved, so you have very good features to your tumor, and you're in very good health, so most likely you could be cured with local treatment." This is the most common scenario. "Over 50 percent of patients now fall in this category, that is, with negative nodes, but there are still probably 20 to 30 percent of women in your situation who might have a recurrence. We're not smart enough right now to figure out if you're one of those patients or not."

We're trying to learn more by looking at genes and have a new test that helps, the Oncotype DX, which is based on genes in a patient's individual tumor. If this is not done, we have recommendations of past experience of thousands of women in clinical trials. I might say, "So what these data show for you is that if you get hormone therapy, you're going to have a 3 percent or 4 percent benefit, and if we add chemotherapy, it only increases it by about 1 percent more, so the combination will give you about a 5 percent benefit. Now that certainly is up to you as to what you'd like to do and how you feel about that. If you think that 1 percent is important, then we can give you chemotherapy. I would probably not recommend chemotherapy in that situation because most likely you are cured of your breast cancer, but you know it is an option that we can talk about." A large component of a woman's decision can come from fear. When I do talk about it, I try to be positive. Even though I am recommending chemotherapy, I balance it with saying, "Well, this may actually help you and decrease the recurrence rate." It is best when women can make informed choices in a careful manner without an overwhelming sense of fear.

We carefully review the side effects of chemotherapy with our patients. We talk about the psychological aspects of possibly going through menopause, which is a big thing for a lot of patients because they're young. I think one of the biggest side effects, to me, that I see, that affects people is going through premature menopause because they can have the hot flashes and some mood changes. It's already hard having the cancer and going through chemotherapy and then having menopause start on top of it can be really difficult. So I always try to tell women about that so they're not surprised. Some women diagnosed at a young age want to have children, and it just depends on their age at diagnosis and if they are getting chemotherapy whether they will be able to do that. That's probably a big struggle with a lot of our patients. I also tell women that they may have some fatigue, which is pretty common, not only from the chemotherapy but from the drugs that prevent nausea. Usually, we treat patients on Thursday so that if patients are working and want to take off Friday, they have the weekend to rest and feel better.

A positive outlook is extremely important, especially with breast cancer. Everyone knows someone who has had cancer and has died—for example, a patient had an aunt who had pancreatic cancer and died, and

Interview with Chitra Rajagopal, M.D.

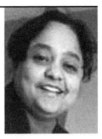

As a medical oncologist I see women after the diagnosis of breast cancer has been made. In some ways women fear chemotherapy more than cancer. It's not the diagnosis of cancer that most people worry about, it's the consequences of treatment that people are really worried about, and so we'll often sit down and talk about the bad news. Some of the most difficult discussions are for women in the adjuvant group because they're now asymptomatic from the disease and it becomes hard, for most of us I would think, to voluntarily subject ourselves to therapy that could deliberately make us sick and disfigure us. That's one of the hardest parts of talking to patients and explaining to them why it is that we think that short period of discomfort will ultimately help them in the long run.

I talk to a woman about the projected risk of recurrence and about her options in helping reduce her risk. Is she a candidate for systemic hormonal therapy or not? Is she a candidate for adjuvant therapy or not? And what is the relative benefit of each one? I almost never, ever tell a patient, "You have to do this," except perhaps for when they balk at hormonal therapy. I tell them it's really not a good option to refuse hormonal therapy if they can benefit from it. I share my view of where the data are, and I end by saying, "This is my recommendation with respect to how much hormonal therapy will help you, how much chemotherapy will help you, how much the combination is going to help you, and what I would recommend based on this."

I used to be a stickler on educating women about the normal breast anatomy and development, but I've become a little less obsessive about it. I have tempered that talk a lot more. I had this lovely and intelligent patient who worked for the Justice Department. After I talked to her for about forty-five minutes, went through her options exhaustively, she looked at me and said, "I am so sorry, I have not listened to a word of what you said because I'm waiting to hear what your recommendation is for me." So, I always keep that in mind when I think I'm becoming too demographic and they're waiting for the bottom line. Now I often start out by saying, "We're not going to be discussing chemotherapy for you," and that helps their minds relax and focus more on what I'm talking about. Other times I will say initially, "We are going to be talking about chemotherapy," and I will explain why. So I always now, for the most part, start by talking to them a little bit about what I'm going to tell them about at the end.

The decision to offer chemotherapy in the adjuvant setting to reduce the risk of recurrence is sometimes straightforward, while at other times it can be very difficult. So in premenopausal women with lymph node–positive breast cancer, treatment options are fairly clear. This is an aggressive disease. They have a longer life span at this stage, so I give them the option of the most aggressive therapy possible. That, in my view, would include an anthracycline and a taxane, plus hormonal therapy where applicable. Another scenario would be an older postmenopausal woman with receptor-positive, node-negative breast cancer for whom, just based on the age and other medical problems, the treatment would be hormonal therapy. There is not going to be much discussion about chemotherapy because for that woman chemotherapy may actually harm her more than benefit. But more difficult situations are common, such as whether to recommend chemotherapy for a woman who has a breast cancer that is lymph node and hormone receptor negative and who has a tumor that measures less than one centimeter. That woman still has some risk of recurrence, which will not be helped by the use of hormonal therapy. Therefore, is chemotherapy justified if the tumor measures nine millimeters or eight or anything less than the one-centimeter cutoff used conventionally?

I do talk with women about the potential side effects of chemotherapy and hormonal therapy. I broadly divide them into two major classes of side effects. One—what I call the nuisance side effects that everybody has—they have it, they get over it, and life goes on. The other sort have potentially long-term damaging side effects. So when discussing the nuisance side effects, I tell them, it's something like being pregnant—you know, uncomfortable during those months and then life goes on. Nausea and vomiting are almost always preventable, but there is fatigue and maybe some memory changes, hair loss, and major disruption of their lives. Everybody will experience this to some degree or the other. There is no exception to that rule. For the other group of side effects, we have good medications to try to diminish their severity, but we cannot alleviate all of them. Today, therapies are relatively shorter than they used to be. Now they usually last three to four months. So, I think of it as a short investment of time. Compared to the rest of one's whole life, this is a short period of time, and so it may not be such a major issue. But on the other side is the risk of infections, a small risk of heart damage, and risks of other long-term effects of treatment.

There is reason for great optimism for women who are treated for breast cancer. Mental attitude and optimism are important. On the other hand, we have sort of gone overboard, I think, by saying, "If you don't do well, it's because you didn't think positively about this." I think this can put a burden on women. Among family, friends, and the patient there is an emphasis on "You've got to keep positive." This is sometimes an extraordinarily difficult thing. How does one stay "positive" when facing a serious illness? A positive attitude helps, but it doesn't help to beat oneself up if this is not possible. A positive attitude makes one feel better and makes the decision process easier. On the other hand, it's not a crime to be worried about what one has to deal with.

CHAPTER 12

Breast Reconstruction after Mastectomy

What Are My Options?

Roger J. Friedman, M.D.

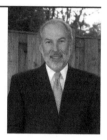

In the treatment of malignant disease, the most important goal is the elimination of the cancer. Breast reconstruction is a different matter—a matter of patient preference. A motivated patient who desires the procedure is the best candidate for breast reconstruction. It can be a positive factor in a stressful situation: reconstruction has been found to improve self-image and self-esteem, as well as help a woman resume her normal routines without being constantly reminded of her cancer.

Breast reconstruction techniques have advanced dramatically over the past fifteen years; today many options are available, and the cosmetic results are impressive. Some reconstructions use breast implants and tissue expanders; others use the woman's own tissues, in the form of muscle and skin flaps (called *myocutaneous flaps*), with implants; and still others use the patient's own tissues without implants. This last form of breast reconstruction is called *autologous reconstruction*; the tissue for autologous reconstruction usually comes from the abdomen. The technique is customized to the patient's needs and desires.

The vast majority of women who have had reconstruction surgery are pleased with their results, but there are limitations to what can be accomplished. For example, surgeons can not exactly match the other breast, even though the results of surgery today are coming close. To make the two breasts more closely resemble each other, some women choose to alter the unaffected breast with procedures such as reduction, augmentation (enlargement) and lift (mastopexy). Because a mastectomy interrupts the nerve supply to the skin, all reconstructed breasts will have less sensation in the skin; part of this sensory change will last forever. All reconstructed breasts have scars, though they usually fade over time. Reconstructed nipples look normal, but they do not change with stimulation and appear to be always erect.

Basic Concepts

The Envelope and the Contents

Two concepts in breast reconstruction are, first, that the *skin* is considered an *envelope,* and second, that the *breast tissue* is considered the *contents.* When a patient has a mastectomy, the general surgeon removes the nipple, the biopsy site, and the contents of the breast. The usual desired goal when a woman has chosen to have breast reconstruction is a *skin sparing mastectomy.* This technique involves removing the contents but attempting to limit the skin excision to the nipple.

All women having reconstructive surgery must have the contents restored after a mastectomy. A physical examination before the mastectomy determines whether there will be enough envelope remaining to hold the restored contents; if not, the patient will need additional skin for the reconstruction procedure. Measurements are taken during the examination to compare the normal breast to the breast with cancer. Because the nipple will be removed, the diameter of the nipple is subtracted from the vertical measurement. (If the cancer involves the skin, this skin — or envelope — is subtracted from the measurement as well; see Figure 12.1.)

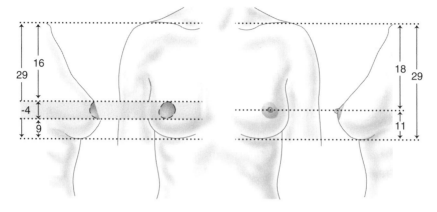

Rt. breast vertical measurement = 25 cm   Lt. breast vertical measurement = 29 cm

FIGURE 12.1. In planning a reconstruction, the reconstructive surgeon needs to consider not only the volume of the breast but also the amount of skin envelope to be removed at the time of the mastectomy. In this example of a skin sparing mastectomy, the deficiency is four centimeters, which is consistent with the diameter of the nipple that has been removed.

Whether a patient will require additional skin (and how much) is determined by the difference between the size of the vertical skin envelope of the normal side and the anticipated vertical skin envelope after the mastectomy. The amount of skin required will play a major role in the choice of reconstruction procedure. Table 12.1 is an algorithm showing the options available to a woman needing between one and seven (or more) centimeters of additional envelope. (These procedures are described in this chapter.)

As noted earlier, for some women the best result is obtained when the opposite breast is modified, as well. If the cancer-free breast is noticeably larger than the reconstructed breast, then the reduction of the healthy breast may be desired. If the healthy breast droops in comparison to the reconstructed breast, then a breast lift may be a consideration. Both of these procedures reduce the skin envelope and may eliminate the need for additional skin on the mastectomy side to attain symmetry.

Timing

The next issue to be considered is timing. Breast reconstruction is classified as either *immediate* or *delayed*. In immediate reconstruction, the new breast is reconstructed at the time of the mastectomy. Once the general surgeon has completed the mastectomy, the plastic surgeon begins the reconstruction as part of the same operative experience. In delayed reconstruction, the operation may take place months or years after the mastectomy. Delayed reconstruction and immediate reconstruction use the same techniques and have similar cosmetic results. Timing, then, is an issue of personal preference with no wrong answer.

Stages in Breast Reconstruction

Breast reconstruction typically requires three steps or stages.

The *initial reconstruction* with mastectomy (if immediate) or without mastectomy (if delayed) requires a general anesthetic and a one- to three-day hospital stay followed by a three- to four-week recovery. The other breast may be altered for symmetry at this time, or that may happen during the second stage.

The *second stage* is a fine-tuning or adjustment and is an outpatient procedure with a weekend recovery in most cases. The second stage takes place when two criteria are met: first, the patient is back to her normal routine, and second, she has completed any adjuvant chemotherapy or

TABLE 12.1. DECISIONS IN RECONSTRUCTIVE SURGERY: WHAT ARE THE OPTIONS?

Amount of Additional Envelope Needed	Options
1–2 cm	Tissue expander
2–7 cm	Latissimus dorsi myocutaneous flap Skin (envelope) + implant (contents)
› 7 cm and/or you do not want an implant	TRAM flap (envelope and contents) Free flap Deep inferior epigastric perforator flap Gluteal free flap

radiation therapy. If chemotherapy is to be followed by radiation therapy, the second stage is delayed six months to a year to enable the tissues to recover from radiation. After radiation the blood supply to the tissues is diminished, and the actual texture of the skin may be affected. The tissues are evaluated, and the timing is set on an individual basis.

The second stage includes revision of the unaffected breast for symmetry. If one side is larger than the other or one breast sits lower than the other, the asymmetry can be corrected. If a tissue expander, a temporary implant, was placed at the initial procedure, it is exchanged for the more permanent implant at the second stage. Finally, if a patient elects to have a nipple reconstruction, it is started at this time. The nipple has two components, the raised part, or *papule,* and the pigmented area surrounding it, called the *areola.* The papule is created at the fine-tuning.

The *third stage* is the tattooing of the nipple to create the areola. This takes place eight to ten weeks after the second stage. The areola tattoo is an office procedure often requiring no anesthesia. In the past, grafts were harvested from the groin region to construct the areola, but today we use tattooing because it provides better symmetry and color match.

Implant Reconstruction

One form of breast reconstruction uses a breast implant. This implant is placed in a pocket that is developed under the muscles of the chest: the pectoralis major, the serratus anterior, and the rectus abdominis. These muscles make up the layer just beneath the breast tissue. A new addition to implant/expander reconstruction is Alloderm (see Figure 12.2). This is a sheet of cadaveric dermis which is placed between the pectoralis major and the fold beneath the breast, eliminating the need to lift the serratus anterior and rectus abdominis muscles. This allows for easier expansion and in some cases the opportunity to place the actual implant at the time of the mastectomy. Alloderm is quite exciting as it allows for the ingrowth of blood vessels and actually becomes a part of the patient's tissues. If the tissues are tight, an expander is placed. In smaller-breasted women, the pocket may be sufficient to accommodate the implant at the initial procedure, although this approach is less common. Moderate- to

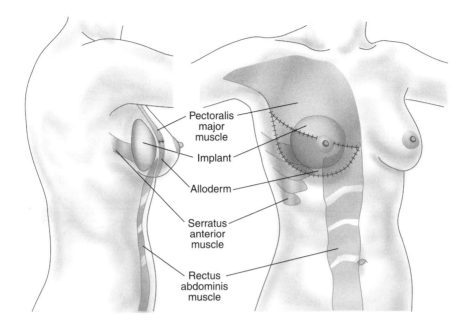

Pectoralis major muscle

Implant

Alloderm

Serratus anterior muscle

Rectus abdominis muscle

FIGURE 12.2. In the case of implant or expander reconstruction, a layer of Alloderm is attached to the lower edge of the pectoralis major muscle and the lower edge is attached to the fold beneath the breast. Together they cover the implant or expander, providing a layer of separation from the overlying skin.

large-breasted women require a tissue expander to stretch the muscle and/or skin to make room for the actual implant.

The tissue expander is a deflated balloon made of silicone with a built-in injection port. During the months following this reconstruction, the patient visits her plastic surgeon every one to two weeks, and the expander is inflated by injecting saline through the skin into the port, gradually inflating the expander. This process causes little or no discomfort. The expander is inflated for several months and then removed. The permanent implant is placed as part of the second stage, the fine-tuning. An alternative to this approach is an expander/implant referred to as a Becker implant. This implant has a remote valve and can be used as an expander; then, at the time of nipple reconstruction, the valve is removed and the implant is left in place.

There are advantages of a tissue expander/implant approach over a flap approach (see below). The advantages include shorter operating time and a less involved procedure, limited to the breast area. This decreases the postoperative discomfort and recovery time. The limiting factor with tissue expansion is that only two to three centimeters of additional skin can be obtained through this technique. If more skin is required, the use of flaps must be considered.

There are some disadvantages associated with the tissue expander/implant option. These include infection, rupture, or leakage of the expander or implant; contour irregularities; frequent visits to the plastic surgeon in the postoperative period for expansion; formation of a capsule or scar tissue around the implant, which may cause discomfort or distortion; and lack of change of implant size with weight loss or gain. Whenever a foreign object is placed in the body (in this case, the expander or implant), the body perceives the object as foreign and forms a wall of scar tissue around it. This scar tissue is termed a capsule. In approximately 20 percent of patients with implants, this scar tissue may tighten around the implant, causing discomfort and possibly a change in shape, which is termed a capsular contracture. Additional surgery may be necessary to interrupt or remove this scar tissue and possibly replace the implant. Capsular contracture may develop at any time from several months to several years following implant placement.

Saline or Silicone?

As a reconstruction patient, women have the option of a silicone gel or saline implant. In the 1990s there was concern about a possible association between silicone implants and symptoms such as muscle aches, joint aches, and fatigue, as well as disease processes such as lupus and scleroderma. The studies to date show that these symptoms do not appear to be related to implants. These include studies from the Institute of Medicine (Safety of Breast Implants, 1999), Brinton study of 7,234 patients and a Danish study with nineteen-year patient follow-up. It is possible that there may be people with sensitivity to silicone, but they would be a rarity.

The silicone gel has the consistency of molasses, and saline has the consistency of water. The gel feels more natural to many, while others prefer the saline. Saline implants have a 3.7 percent deflation rate. This

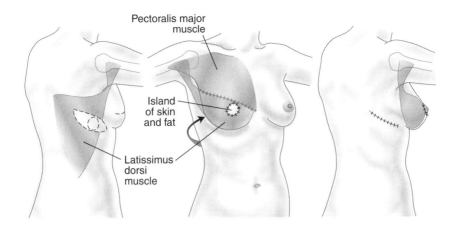

FIGURE 12.3. In this example of a latissimus dorsi myocutaneous flap, the skin and the muscle that provides blood supply to the skin are passed through a tunnel from the back to the breast area to replace the skin island that has been removed and thus enable the surgeon to match the opposite side. The excess skin is removed. The back scar will be hidden by the patient's bra or bathing suit.

means that at some point, this implant may fail, and the patient will call and say she has a "flat tire." Silicone gel implants can also fail. Cohesive gel implants are being studied as an alternative to currently used silicone gel implants. If an implant fails, the pocket is already in place, so only the contents have to be replaced. This can be done in a minimal outpatient procedure with no significant recovery time.

Myocutaneous Flaps

Another approach to breast reconstruction utilizes the patient's own tissues, either with or without an implant. One surgical approach uses a latissimus dorsi myocutaneous flap. This is a muscle from the back which is taken, along with an overlying island of skin and fat, and rotated beneath the armpit to provide the necessary skin in women requiring as much as seven to nine centimeters of skin in a vertical dimension. Depending on the size of the breast to be reconstructed, an implant may or may not be required. There are at least two additional muscles that provide each of the functions provided by the latissimus dorsi, and therefore the woman usually does not notice any loss of function when this muscle is used in a flap (see Figure 12.3).

Breast Reconstruction after Mastectomy   171

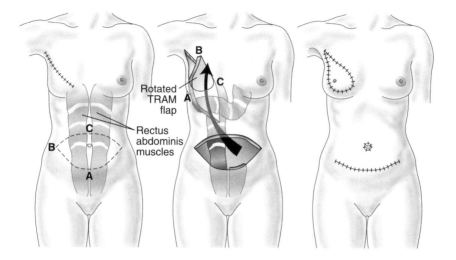

FIGURE 12.4. The TRAM flap provides skin, fat, and muscle. This myocutaneous flap is tunneled under the skin of the abdomen, left attached to its blood supply (traveling through the muscle), and employed to reconstruct the breast without the need of an implant, as the fat typically provides the necessary volume. This flap is rotated ninety degrees, as is shown by the change in position of A, B, C.

Another approach using a woman's own tissues is the transverse rectus abdominis myocutaneous flap, or TRAM flap (see Figure 12.4). This flap employs the lower abdominal tissues that would normally be discarded if a tummy tuck were performed. These tissues are left attached to either one or both of the rectus abdominis muscles, which run from the center of the rib cage toward the pubic bone and are the width of a man's tie. The tissues form an ellipse of skin, which includes fat and muscle. This ellipse is then rotated and placed into the mastectomy defect and the skin and fat are then contoured to match the opposite breast. The donor site is closed, leaving a scar that extends across the lower abdomen from one hip to the other with an additional scar around the navel as would be seen in a tummy tuck.

A variation of this procedure takes the same island of skin and part of one muscle, detaching it from the body and then reconnecting the artery and vein to other vessels in the armpit area using the operating microscope. This variation is called a TRAM free flap.

The TRAM approach has several advantages. First, the TRAM utilizes the patient's own tissues and thus avoids the problems associated with breast implants. In addition, the breast mound is constructed at the initial surgery. This eliminates the need to make frequent trips to the doctor's office. The TRAM flap will shrink approximately 10 percent after surgery. The flap will change somewhat in size with associated changes in body weight gain or loss. As one ages, the breast glandular tissue is replaced with fatty tissue. Thus, the consistency of the reconstructed breast is similar to the breast on the unoperated side.

The TRAM flap also has disadvantages. Approximately 5 to 10 percent of patients will lose a portion of their flap due to circulation problems, which the woman will notice as an area of firmness in the flap. This area is removed at the time of the fine-tuning. There are rare reports of the entire flap being lost due to the same circulatory problems. If this occurs, the flap has to be removed and an alternative method of reconstruction chosen. For women without significant heart, lung, or vascular disease, these procedures are routinely performed without difficulty.

Approximately 2 percent of TRAM flap patients develop a small area of abdominal wall weakness at their donor site. This is more common in cases in which both muscles are utilized. As a preventive measure, a layer of synthetic mesh may be utilized to reinforce the abdominal wall in cases where both muscles are used and in areas that may be exceptionally weak. If this weakness occurs and the woman is uncomfortable despite wearing supportive garments, a surgical procedure is required for repair. Rarely, and more commonly when parts of both muscles are used in a case of bilateral reconstruction, the woman may have difficulty sitting up from a lying-down position. The role of the rectus muscles is to initiate the process of sitting from a lying-down position. When both muscles are used, the abdominal wall may have a temporary or permanent weakness.

Other Flaps

Another option may be to utilize the same abdominal tissues involved in the TRAM flap but leave the underlying muscle alone, avoiding the issues of abdominal wall weakness. This procedure is called a deep inferior epigastric flap or DIEP flap (see Figure 12.5). The blood vessels to

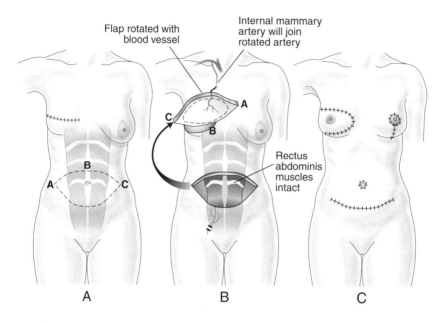

Flap rotated with
blood vessel

Internal mammary
artery will join
rotated artery

A

C

B

Rectus
abdominis
muscles
intact

B

A

C

A

B

C

FIGURE 12.5. The DIEP flap is similar to the TRAM flap except that the muscle is not included. The blood supply is provided by a blood vessel that travels directly into the flap. This free tissue transfer involves taking the flap away from the abdomen and reattaching the blood vessel to a blood vessel in the breast area, which will now provide blood flow to the flap. This flap is typically rotated 180 degrees, as is shown by the change in position of A, B, C.

the flap are dissected through the muscle and preserved, then attached to the island of skin and fat. This is a free flap. A free flap involves cutting the blood vessels to the island of skin and then transferring the island to the chest region and attaching the blood vessel with the assistance of a microscope to local blood vessels in the chest region.

Another form of free flap breast reconstruction, called the inferior gluteal free flap, employs tissues from the lower buttock. This method fully removes an island of skin, fat, and muscle from the lower buttock, centered on the fold; the island is then transferred to the mastectomy site, where the artery and vein are connected to vessels in the armpit using the operating microscope. The advantage of this procedure is that it provides an alternative when the abdominal tissues are not available. The disadvantages include the creation of an asymmetry in the buttock area (unless the procedure is used for bilateral breast reconstruction).

Understanding the Treatments

There is also the potential for *parasthesias*, which are abnormal sensations on the back of the thigh. This procedure takes longer, typically six to eight hours, and technically is more difficult. In rare cases, the entire flap or a portion of the flap does not survive the transfer, and further surgery is required.

Another variation is the superior gluteal free flap, which uses the upper portion of the buttock (see Figure 12.6). Finally, some of the upper abdominal or lower chest wall skin may be moved upward to contribute one to two centimeters of skin to the lower portion of the breast. This procedure is called a lower thoracic advancement flap or Ryan flap.

Nipple Reconstruction

Many patients choose to undergo nipple reconstruction, which is performed at the time of the fine-tuning (see Figure 12.7). As noted above, the nipple has two components: the raised part of the nipple, or papule, and the pigmented area surrounding this raised part, which is called the areola. The papule is developed from the local tissues of the reconstructed

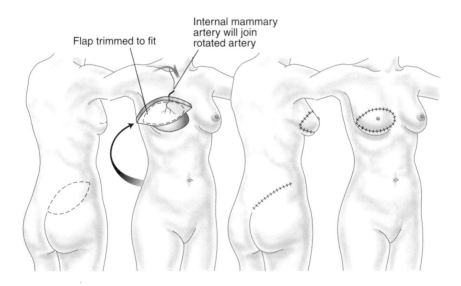

FIGURE 12.6. The superior gluteal free flap uses the upper area of the buttock region as the source for the skin and fat to replace the missing skin of the breast and the necessary volume. This flap also has a single vessel that is reattached to a blood vessel in the breast area which will now provide blood to the flap.

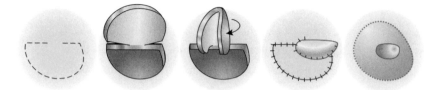

FIGURE 12.7. This form of nipple reconstruction uses the local tissues of the chest area, which are then rolled upon themselves to create the raised part of the nipple, the papule. The area from which these tissues came then is resurfaced by the placement of a skin graft. The papule is always made too long, as it will flatten at least 50 percent over time. The areola, or pigmented portion of the nipple, is created by tattooing at eight to ten weeks after the nipple reconstruction.

breast. It is intentionally made too large, as it will compress approximately 50 percent over the six to eight weeks following nipple reconstruction. A small skin graft may be required to fill the donor site for the papule. This is typically taken from an area of redundancy on the chest wall or the ends of an existing scar. In the past, skin grafts were taken from the groin or labial areas, but this is not done any longer. If a woman has a large papule on the other breast, a portion of that papule may be utilized to create the papule on the side of the reconstruction.

Six to eight weeks following creation of the papule, the areola is created by tattoo and the papule is also tattooed. In the majority of cases, no anesthesia is required for this office procedure. Nipple reconstruction is strictly a matter of patient preference. Although many patients choose to have a nipple reconstruction, some do not. Prior to a nipple reconstruction, women tend to pay attention to the other reconstruction scars. After the nipple reconstruction, her focus is on the nipple, and the scars become less of an issue.

The Other Breast

As noted previously, a woman may decide to alter the cancer-free breast for the purpose of greater symmetry between the two breasts. The alteration may involve prophylactic mastectomy, enlargement, reduction, or lift. For some women, these alternatives represent the most effective means of achieving symmetry. The surgery can be performed at the time

Understanding the Treatments

of the initial reconstruction or at the fine-tuning. Alteration in the opposite side can help limit the amount of skin necessary to achieve symmetry in the reconstruction. A federal law states that for insurance purposes both breast reconstruction and alteration of the opposite side for symmetry purposes are covered procedures.

Lumpectomy and Radiation Therapy

Some patients with a localized small tumor may elect to have a lumpectomy followed by radiation therapy. A lumpectomy involves removal of the tumor and a component of normal breast tissue as well as some of the overlying skin. In most cases, nothing further is required to reconstruct the breast. If, due to the location of the cancer and subsequent skin resection, an asymmetry is created, alteration in the opposite breast may correct this.

A woman with a breast implant may develop a breast cancer and be a candidate for lumpectomy and radiation therapy. As there is a higher incidence of capsular contracture (scar tissue that forms around the implant creating firmness and distortion) associated with radiation, we need to consider removing the implant at the time of the lumpectomy and replacing it with a tissue expander. The expander is then immediately overexpanded until the affected breast is larger than the unaffected breast, prior to the initiation of radiation therapy. At approximately six months after radiation therapy is completed, the expander is removed and the implant is placed.

Sex and Well Being

Some women neither desire nor seek breast reconstruction after mastectomy. They resume their lives and adjust just fine. For some women, however, breast reconstruction provides them the opportunity to feel *whole* after mastectomy. The results are such that the woman is not reminded on a daily basis that she has had a mastectomy or cancer. She feels comfortable wearing any clothes as well as getting undressed in front of her spouse or others. She is able to resume a normal sex life without being self-conscious. (Because the reconstructed breast has less feeling than the other breast, or no feeling, she will need to communicate with her significant other to provide a satisfying sexual experience for both of them.)

BRACA Gene Positive

A woman with a strong family history of breast cancer may elect to undergo gene testing. If she has a positive BRACA gene, she may have up to an 80 percent lifetime chance of developing a breast cancer. Such a woman may feel as if she is walking around with a "time bomb" and may decide to undergo bilateral prophylactic mastectomies with immediate reconstruction. Depending on the amount of envelope, she may have either expander/implant reconstruction or bilateral latissimus dorsi myocutaneous flaps with implant placement.

Conclusion

Breast reconstruction can be an important component of breast cancer recovery for women who choose to pursue it. New surgical techniques have greatly improved the cosmetic results of breast reconstruction, and a woman's decision to consult with a plastic surgeon at the time of her diagnosis makes her better informed when it comes to overall treatment planning. Whether a woman elects to have immediate reconstruction, delayed reconstruction, or no reconstruction at all, it is empowering for her to have options and to play an informed role in choosing the most comfortable path to full recovery.

CHAPTER 13

Profiles of Two Reconstructive Surgeons

Interview with Gregory O. Dick, M.D.

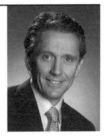

B eing able to create a breast was the reason I switched from general surgery to plastic surgery early in my training. It is rewarding for me to correct a deformity and help a woman to again achieve balance and wholeness.

When I first meet a woman who has breast cancer, I walk into the room knowing that she may be scared of dying and that she may only hear 25 percent of what I am about to say. I describe what I do as the light at the end of the tunnel and say that it is my job to make her feel comfortable looking in the mirror wearing all types of clothing, including swimwear. I need to provide the woman with a lot of information, but most of our conversation is directed toward lifting her spirits and providing her with a ladder to grab on to. The detailed questions can come later. I invite patients to call me at home over the next few days. I also encourage women to talk to other women who have gone through the various types of procedures, and I tell them that those women are doing well and that they were just as scared and confused when they were sitting here trying to decide on their surgery and listening to reconstructive options.

Women often feel that they are given little time to take in all this information and process it, and that their lives are upside down and in complete chaos. I reassure women that no reconstruction has to be done at the time of a mastectomy if they are undecided. They may decide to only undergo the mastectomy first, with no reconstructive surgery. Or I could merely place an expander and begin to stretch the skin, giving them time to decide if they would like to finish the job by replacing the expander with a permanent implant or with a muscle-fat-skin flap. This flap is called a TRAM (transverse rectus abdominus myocutaneous) flap, or, more commonly, the tummy-tuck flap. This procedure is increasingly being done with a microscope to conserve abdominal muscle. For many women, this is wonderful news, because they can quickly recover from their first operation and then take their time and schedule a second operation when it is more convenient for them in terms of their life, their family, their job, and so on.

I show lots of pictures to reassure them that there is a good chance that we will make them feel close to normal or balanced once again. If nothing else, the number of women who've been through the experience of having breast cancer and the variety of options for treatment and reconstruction shows them that they are not alone and that other women, for the most part, have done well. I also encourage women to see and feel some of the implants and the expanders that we have for demonstration purposes in the office. There is now an Internet site where a patient can go and view a tummy-tuck operation from start to finish, if that will help her make a decision. I don't necessarily think this is a great idea because it may provide much more information than the patient may want or need to have at this time. Watching someone else's tape does not allow you to ask questions, and it may produce anxiety.

I take note of who accompanies the patient to my office, and I like to get a picture of the support systems that are available to the patient. This is absolutely critical to the success of the operation. Some women have a great support network, while others may have a spouse or partner who does not have the capacity to provide support, for a variety of reasons. If I see a lack of support, I immediately start thinking of options that carry the least risk of complication, that allow the woman to recover the

Understanding the Treatments

quickest and resume her responsibilities (such as being a single head of household). Similarly, some women might have greater difficulty coping with a complication and with possible additional unscheduled surgeries. I consider the surgery a failure if the breast looks absolutely perfect but the patient is an emotional wreck.

Fewer women are coming in for reconstruction, mainly due to the increasing number of lumpectomies performed. After mastectomy, women make different choices regarding reconstructive surgery. If the patient is devastated by the diagnosis, is in a mild state of shock and disbelief, and has been told that she must undergo a mastectomy, she may not be able to make a decision at all initially. Many of these women eventually opt for reconstruction, and the majority of them choose to have the simplest procedure possible, which is placement of a tissue expander. The idea of a muscle-fat-skin or TRAM flap is overwhelming to some women at first, and their absolute number one goal is to get rid of the cancer. In this case, the husband or relative may be the driving force who helps convince the woman to undergo first-stage reconstruction when she is paralyzed in her decision-making ability. Occasionally, I see a woman who has been thinking about undergoing a tummy tuck but has hesitated due to finances or guilt stemming from vanity issues. These women may be very comfortable with undergoing TRAM flap surgery, getting a free tummy tuck in the process — it is both financially free and guilt-free.

A woman with great personal responsibilities — for example, a single parent with small children, a patient who has her hands full taking care of an elderly parent, a patient with extensive responsibilities at work — or a patient with little support may opt for the surgery that will allow her to recover the quickest. In some cases the choice of reconstructive surgery is limited because the patient has had a previous abdominoplasty or she is morbidly obese (in which case TRAM flap is not recommended because of increased complications and increased risk of vascular compromise to the flap).

If a woman is a smoker, she must not smoke for six weeks before any flap procedure. In smokers, I offer to place the expander, and if she is able to stay off the cigarettes during the time of expansion, about two to three months, then we can consider performing a TRAM flap as a second stage. If she is not able to quit smoking, then the expander is replaced with an implant.

Seventy-five percent of patients at the first visit are not interested in nipple reconstruction, probably because they are worried mostly about their lives. After mastectomy and first-stage reconstruction, 90 percent of patients are open to the idea or themselves broach the subject of nipple reconstruction. Two of my patients have asked me, rather than do a nipple reconstruction, to tattoo a heart on the breast with their husband's initials inside the heart. Both women have an incredible attitude toward life and toward their diagnoses.

No reconstructed breast ever feels like the preexisting one or the remaining one. Men and many women are not forthcoming as to how the reconstructed breast affects their sexual relationships, and it may be that the mere diagnosis of cancer has the major impact, regardless of whether or not reconstruction is chosen or what method of reconstruction is chosen. On the other hand, the entire scenario may be life changing in that the patient becomes more motivated and takes a more active interest in her health and in herself.

Interview with Maurice Nahabedian, M.D.

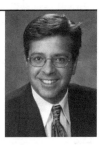

U sually, a woman has seen a number of other physicians before she sees me, so by the time she sees me, she has generally processed the facts that she has breast cancer and that she might lose her breast. She has dealt with these facts for a few weeks or a few months before she comes to see me. In some cases it has been a few years after she has had a mastectomy. But some women come to see me two days after they have been diagnosed with breast cancer. It's probably too early for them to visit me because they have a mental image of their own breasts, and I am going to show them photographs of other breasts that have scars around them, and seeing these photographs is difficult for them. I think it's probably better to wait a couple of weeks or a month or so after the initial diagnosis before meeting with a reconstructive surgeon.

The decision between mastectomy and breast conservation is often made by a woman with her general surgeon and oncologist. If a woman decides on having a mastectomy, then I normally discuss what the various options are and what I can do for her. I tell women there are two ways to reconstruct the breast. One is using your own tissue. The other is using an implant. I describe the pros and cons. I'll say: "The advantages of using an implant are that it is a quick operation with a relatively speedy recovery with minimal downtime. The disadvantages of implants are that they do not last forever. There is about a 10 to 15 percent chance that by ten years they will have to be either removed or replaced." Then

I discuss what is involved in using "your own tissues," and I tell them, "Using your own tissues takes longer and it has a more difficult recovery and the down time is greater. Generally, it takes six weeks before you can get back to your activities of daily living. The advantages are that it lasts forever, and it gets better with time." Weight will cause the tissues to kind of remodel and assume a more natural curve. It remains soft. The scars fade. It just has a much more natural look and feel in the long run.

Some women can go either way. They would be good candidates for using implants or their own tissues. So I have to find out from them what they're interested in. Some women absolutely do not want a foreign object within their body. They don't want me to put an implant in. Some women have heard about the myths associated with silicone implants and are afraid of them, fearing them for one reason or another. They just don't want to have anything to do with implants. Some women come in who are moderately heavy, have a bit of a tummy that they don't like, and they love the idea of taking that abdominal skin and fat and making a breast out of it. That's generally the middle-aged woman, maybe in her mid-forties to early sixties. I'd say probably among younger women it would be fifty-fifty in terms of whether I do an implant or a flap.

I can show women photographs of women who have had reconstructions so they have an idea of what they will look like should they choose to have a mastectomy with reconstruction. And I also show pictures of mastectomy without reconstruction so they can see that, as well. I think it's extremely important for women to have realistic expectations of what a reconstruction is going to look like. Some patients look at the scars and think they are totally unacceptable, even though it was a normal, nice scar from my perspective. Women have to have that visual picture of what things are going to look like; otherwise it's going to be a bit of a shock for them. I think pictures are beneficial in that they give someone a realistic expectation of what she's going to look like.

I show good results, average results, and I show my worst results. I show failures and complications; these all go with the whole package, because not everyone is going to turn out great. Some women are going to have complications. Some implants are going to come out; some flaps are going to fail. I tell women that the risk of flap failure is 2 to 3 percent. If a flap fails, then we try to save it. We go back to the operating room, but if we are unsuccessful, then we have to take the flap away and consider other options, like using an implant. The risk of abdominal bulge or hernia is somewhere between 2 and 4 percent and perhaps with a bilateral reconstruction it is up to 5 to 6 percent—that is, if you use your own tissues. I tell them about wound healing complications, and I tell them about implant complications like rupture, capsular contracture, pain, migration, distortion, all of those things, so they have an idea of the things that can go wrong. I'll spend a good portion of the discussion on some of the complications. It is not just about the benefits. They have to realize that things can go wrong, so they can decide based on all the information.

I think everyone has to get used to a new body image after mastectomy and reconstructive surgery. The breast is generally asensate (lacking sensation) after reconstruction, especially when using your own tissues. With implants you still have sensation, but it's not a lot of sensation, just normal skin sensation.

If you talk to different surgeons, they're going to give different responses. I can say in my practice, patients seem to be more satisfied and better adjusted after having breasts reconstructed with their own tissue rather than implants. Now there are other studies that will tell you that there really isn't a difference and that patients are happy no matter what they have because they accept what's been given to them and then live with it.

CHAPTER 14

Treatment Options for Metastatic Breast Cancer

Daniel F. Hayes, M.D.

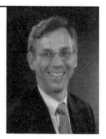

Metastasis means that a cancer that started in one part of the body, like the breast, has spread to other organs, such as the liver, bone, or lung. The cancer is detected through a medical history (a patient's description of symptoms), physical examination, or radiographic tests such as X-rays, CT scans, bone scans, or MRI scans. When breast cancer spreads to other organs, it is still breast cancer, and it still behaves like breast cancer. It does not become bone cancer or liver cancer.

Usually when metastasis occurs, the primary cancer has already been treated with surgery, radiation, chemotherapy, and/or endocrine therapy, all with the goal of curing the cancer. People often refer to metastasis as *recurrence*, since most (but not all) patients have previously had a primary cancer that was presumed to be confined to their breast. It is important to distinguish recurrences in the breast or chest wall (called *local recurrences*) from recurrences outside the breast or chest wall, which are considered true metastases or distant recurrences.

Today, there are more effective therapies for breast cancer than for any of the other common cancers that affect women, such as those that begin in the lung, colon, or ovary. Many of these therapies produce only mild side effects. Unfortunately, when a patient develops detectable breast cancer metastasis, no treatment is likely to eliminate the cancer completely and permanently. But breast cancer, even when it has metastasized, is still very treatable.

Many women with metastatic breast cancer wonder why they should go through treatment if they can't be cured. There are two good reasons for treatment. First, treatment prolongs life, often substantially. Second, when applied judiciously, treatment enormously improves the quality of life for most women with metastatic breast cancer. Doctors call this beneficial effect *palliation.* Put simply, palliative treatment keeps a patient feeling as good as she can for as long as she can. This goal is often accomplished by choosing a series of therapies, each offering the best chance of working for the individual patient and causing the fewest side effects. In this chapter, I describe the strategies used to accomplish effective palliation.

Treatment of metastatic breast cancer acts in one of two ways: locally or systemically. Local therapy, like surgery or radiation, acts on an isolated area of the body. Systemic therapy, such as endocrine therapy or chemotherapy, works throughout the entire body. New systemic treatments also include therapy directed against specific molecular targets like HER-2. The only currently available "targeted" therapy for breast cancer is called trastuzumab (Herceptin).

Choosing the Best Treatment for Metastatic Breast Cancer

Before treatment begins, three important issues need to be evaluated: diagnosis, prognosis, and prediction.

Diagnosis

Most metastases are detected after the patient experiences a new symptom, after the physician finds a change when examining the patient, or when test results indicate that something has changed. Not every new finding means metastases, however. It is wrong to assume that a suspicious symptom, lump, or radiographic finding is a metastasis, because other diagnoses can mimic recurrent cancer—infectious and inflammatory conditions, benign tumors, and new primary cancers from other sites, for example. A biopsy of any suspicious lesion is safe and practical and is a critical part of treatment planning.

Prognosis

Oncologists generally stage a patient with newly diagnosed metastases to determine a treatment proposal. In this case, *staging* is an inaccurate term, since the presence of a metastasis technically places the patient in stage IV. The term *staging* refers to the oncologist's process of understanding the patient's status prior to treatment.

Staging usually includes taking a careful history and doing a thorough physical examination: blood testing for liver and bone marrow function and for tumor markers; and radiographic evaluation, which may include plain X-rays of the chest and/or bones, a bone scan, a CT scan, an MRI scan, or more recently, PET scanning. Rarely would all of the tests listed here be performed. Different doctors prefer to use different combinations of these tests to determine a patient's prognosis.

Prediction

The oncologist seeks to determine which available therapy is most likely to work for the specific patient. Breast cancer is one of the few malignancies for which individualization can be accomplished reasonably well. Sometimes predictive factors argue for the choice of one therapy over another. The oldest known of all predictive factors is the presence or absence of a molecule called the *estrogen receptor* in the breast cancer tissue. We know that many breast cancers require estrogen for growth, just like an automobile needs gasoline to run. If estrogen is the cancer cell's gas, then the estrogen receptor is the gas tank. If you block the receptor, you've sealed the tank.

Endocrine treatments aim to block the estrogen receptor (see below) and therefore are only likely to work in cancers that rely on these receptors to bind estrogen. (In the process called binding estrogen, estrogen

Understanding the Treatments

attaches to the estrogen receptor within the cancer cells, and this action stimulates the growth of these cells.) The estrogen receptor (ER) and its associated molecule, progesterone receptor (PR), are easily and routinely measured in breast cancer tissue after a biopsy or excision.

A second predictive factor that is now regularly measured in women with breast cancer is a molecule called HER-2. The molecule has also been called erbB-2 and c-neu by various investigators, but most doctors now refer to it as HER-2. There is some evidence that ER-positive tumors that also make HER-2 may not respond as well to any endocrine therapy as ER-positive, HER-2-negative cancers, or perhaps may respond only to specific kinds of endocrine therapy but not to others. However, if other factors suggest that endocrine treatment would be appropriate, most doctors will prescribe endocrine therapy even if HER-2 is positive. More importantly, HER-2 is the target for an established drug called trastuzumab (Herceptin), and a newer drug called lapatanib.

HER-2 sits on the outside cellular lining of approximately 20 percent of all breast cancers. If the estrogen receptor is like a gas tank, then HER-2 is like a solar panel for the cancer cell. In this regard, HER-2 may "transmit energy" from outside the cell to inside the cell, much as a solar panel transmits solar energy into the engine. (This analogy is not meant to imply that sunshine has anything to do with breast cancer.) Continuing with this analogy, we can think of trastuzumab (Herceptin) as effectively throwing a blanket over the solar panel. It blocks the HER-2. Thus, oncologists use HER-2 levels in breast cancer tissue to decide whether or not to recommend trastuzumab: yes, if HER-2 levels are high; no, if they are low or absent.

Presently, there are no good predictive factors for the use of chemotherapy in general or for individual chemotherapeutic agents specifically. However, different chemotherapies work in different ways, so there is promise that further research into cellular mechanisms will someday enable doctors to recommend specific agents for a specific individual.

Monitoring Metastatic Disease

Treating a patient with metastatic disease involves choosing the therapy most likely to work with the fewest side effects, and then carefully monitoring the patient to determine if that was the correct therapy or if an alternate one might be more effective in achieving palliation. When a new therapy is begun, four things can happen:

1. The tumor shrinks, and the patient feels better. This is called a *response* or *remission* — the most desired result.
2. The patient stays the same (a condition called *stable disease*).
3. It is obvious that the therapy is not working because symptoms, physical exam, blood tests, or radiographs demonstrate that the cancer is progressing.
4. The therapy has so many side effects that the patient cannot tolerate it.

Most oncologists would change therapies in the case of unacceptable toxicity or obvious disease progression but would otherwise stay with the chosen therapy. In other words, situations 3 and 4 call for a change, while situations 1 and 2 do not.

The oncologist can monitor for these situations in four ways:

1. Taking a history (that is, asking the patient detailed questions about how she is feeling)
2. Physical examination (Are any palpable tumors the same or smaller?)
3. Blood tests (in particular, tests that measure liver function and so-called tumor markers)
4. Radiographic tests (X-rays or scans)

The most important indication that palliation is being achieved, of course, is that the patient says she feels better. Yet symptoms often vary from day to day and may be due to treatment, disease, or nonmalignant causes such as arthritis. So more objective means are helpful to avoid making inappropriate changes in therapy. Physical examination can help identify lesions in the skin, chest wall, and lymph nodes. Most metastatic lesions are in nonpalpable organs, such as bone, liver, and lung. In these cases, physical examination may be of little value.

Radiographic tests permit evaluation of internal metastases and frequently allow precise measurements of the cancer's size to be taken before and after treatment. But radiographic tests are inconvenient and expensive, and, if they are not carefully read, they can be misleading. Therefore, many clinicians also follow serially performed blood tests at each follow-up period (roughly every three to four weeks). For example, decreased levels of circulating liver enzymes in a patient with documented liver metastases provide a good sign of response. A decline in tumor markers is also a good sign. Tumor markers are proteins made by the cancer and released into the bloodstream. The most commonly used tumor markers in breast cancer are CA15-3 or CA27.29 (which essentially measure the same thing) and carcinoembryonic antigen (CEA). A part of the HER-2 molecule can also be measured and monitored in blood, but it is not yet clear how to best apply information about blood levels of the HER-2 protein to patient care.

The FDA recently approved a new test that measures tumor cells that float in the bloodstream. These are called circulating tumor cells (CTC) because they travel throughout the body. A recently reported large trial suggested that if CTC levels do not drop below a certain level (five CTC per 7.5 milliliters of blood) within three to four weeks of starting a new therapy, it is unlikely that the patient will benefit from that therapy. Other studies are ongoing to confirm these results and to determine how best to use this assay in the clinic.

Taken together, the results of these four measures (history, physical exam, radiographs, and blood tests) help shape the decision of whether a patient with metastatic disease should stay on the therapy she has started or whether she should switch to another therapy in the treatment sequence for better symptom palliation. The results of these tests must be used together with the physician's judgment. Any one of these tests may be falsely positive or negative, and therefore treatment should rarely be changed based on the results of one of the evaluations (for example, based on a rising tumor marker alone), if everything else is equal and the patient is doing well. On the other hand, if the history and physical examination suggest that the patient's condition might be getting worse but they are not definitive, a rising tumor marker might be helpful in confirming the clinician's suspicions that it is time to change therapy.

Treatment Options for Metastatic Breast Cancer

Local Therapies

Women with metastatic disease rely on local therapy such as surgery or radiation only in specific situations. These situations include a tumor that is located in a site (notably the brain) poorly accessed by systemic therapy or that is creating an immediate threat, such as a tumor located in or near the spinal cord or chest wall. Radiation and surgery are also often used to treat vertebral bone metastases, especially if systemic therapy is not helping, since these metastases can be quite painful. Well-designed clinical trials have suggested that for patients who have single, resectable brain or spinal cord metastases, surgery followed by radiation is preferable to either therapy alone. Occasionally, surgery and radiation are used to remove or shrink tumors that are threatening to obstruct important structures such as major blood vessels or the breathing tubes (bronchi).

Local therapy is also useful in treating cancer that has spread to the lining of the lungs or heart. When this happens, the patient can develop what is called a pleural (lung) or pericardial (heart) effusion, meaning that fluid collects in the lining of one or both of these organs, posing a risk of compression. In this case, the fluid is often drained with a catheter or even surgically, and then the lining is filled with material to try to prevent a recurrence of the effusion.

Local therapies are not always straightforward options. Because of toxic interactions, oncologists are usually reluctant to combine them with systemic therapies. This means that delivery of local therapy (such as surgery or radiation) may delay the start of systemic therapy for several days or weeks while the patient is being treated and recovering. Surgery, of course, has its own side effects, including the risks associated with anesthesia, infection, and bleeding. It also requires recovery time. Likewise, radiation usually requires daily treatments for several days or weeks, and it may damage normal tissue, such as tissue in the lung and the gastrointestinal tract. Furthermore, radiation to any bone site permanently damages the bone marrow, where red and white blood cells and platelets are made. Blood levels may decrease to very low or occasionally dangerous levels with the radiation. Perhaps more importantly, widespread radiation to many bone sites may decrease effectiveness of chemotherapy in the future.

Systemic Therapies

Most oncologists recommend that treatments for breast cancer metastases be given in sequence, one or two drugs at time, starting with the least toxic therapies. This approach usually eases symptoms by shrinking the tumor, while also minimizing side effects. Therapies that cause more side effects should only be given if the less toxic therapies no longer work.

If the cancer is growing very quickly (particularly in essential organs such as the liver and lung), however, then the oncologist will skip less toxic therapies like hormone therapy and proceed directly to chemotherapy.

Because metastases are generally located in several places at once, it often makes more sense to use systemic rather than local therapy. Systemic treatments include endocrine treatments, chemotherapy, and trastuzumab (Herceptin). Most oncologists do not combine endocrine treatment with the other two types of treatments, for several reasons. First, the goal of palliation is undermined when chemotherapy is added to endocrine therapy, because the patient will almost always have more side effects from the chemotherapy. Combining them essentially eliminates the main advantage of endocrine therapy. Furthermore, there is some evidence that if they are given together, endocrine therapy may lessen the effect of chemotherapy.

Trastuzumab may be given alone; like endocrine therapy, it often has few if any side effects. Trastuzumab alone may work in 20 to 30 percent of women with HER-2 positive metastatic breast cancer and is an acceptable treatment strategy in some cases. There is some evidence that trastuzumab may enhance the effect of certain chemotherapeutic agents — in particular, paclitaxel (Taxol), docetaxel (Taxotere), vinorelbine (Navelbine), and the platin agents cisplatin (Platinol) or carboplatin (Paraplatin). Thus, for a patient with HER-2 positive breast cancer for whom chemotherapy is indicated, combining the chemotherapy with trastuzumab is appropriate. However, *trastuzumab (Herceptin)* should not be combined with doxorubicin *(Adriamycin)*, because trastuzumab itself can cause heart damage, and when combined with doxorubicin, the risk of heart failure can be as high as 20 percent.

Endocrine Treatment

In 1896, a surgeon in England reported that removing ovaries from three young women with breast cancer improved their condition. Although he did not recognize what he had done (because estrogen had not yet been discovered), he had removed the source of the estrogen that the cancer cells needed to survive. Subsequently, many different strategies have been employed to disrupt the interaction between estrogen and the estrogen receptors on cancer cells.

One approach is to stop production of estrogen. This approach is often called an *ablative* approach, since it ablates or removes the source of estrogen. In a premenopausal woman, most estrogen is produced by the ovaries. In a postmenopausal woman, estrogen is made by fat cells and perhaps even by cancer cells, which convert precursors (building blocks) of estrogen into estrogen. This conversion is performed by enzymes (proteins) called *aromatases*. These precursors come from the adrenal glands, two glands that make many different hormones, including adrenaline and cortisone.

Endocrine organs can be ablated surgically, by removing ovaries in premenopausal women or removing the adrenal glands in postmenopausal women. Surgical ablation has many side effects — especially ablating the adrenal gland, which produces so many other important hormones. But today surgery is not necessary. Modern ablative therapy is principally accomplished by more specific medical treatments that are usually safer, easier, and produce few side effects. For example, premenopausal women can take once a month a shot of goserelin (Zoladex) or leuprolide (Leupron), which work by preventing the normal signal from the brain to the ovary which is required for ovarian function.

Perhaps one of the most exciting advances in endocrine treatment for postmenopausal women is the development of specific drugs that block the last step of estrogen production from its precursors. These drugs inhibit the enzyme aromatase, and so are called aromatase inhibitors

(AIs). They include anastrozole (Arimidex), letrozole (Femara), and exemestane (Aromasin). All of these drugs are as effective as previously available agents for treatment of breast cancer (such as tamoxifen), and may even be slightly better. But at this time there is no evidence that one is preferable to another.

A second endocrine therapy approach is so-called additive therapy. In this therapy, agents are administered that bind to the estrogen receptor. Sticking with our gasoline analogy, these agents essentially put mud into the gas tank. They keep estrogen out of the estrogen receptor and effectively "screw up" the engine. The oldest and most widely used of these agents is tamoxifen (Nolvadex). However, since so many patients have already received adjuvant tamoxifen, this drug currently is rarely prescribed for women who have metastases. However, with increasing use of aromatase inhibitors for adjuvant therapy, tamoxifen may regain a role in the treatment of metastatic disease. Other drugs like tamoxifen, in particular toremifene (Fareston), appear equally effective, but they do not seem to work if tamoxifen is ineffective, and so their role is limited. Although tamoxifen is "anti-estrogenic," it can also act *like* estrogen in other tissues, such as bone, liver, and uterus, and sometimes even in breast cancer itself. Thus, like estrogen, tamoxifen decreases osteoporosis (which is good) but slightly increases risk of blood clotting and endometrial cancer (which is bad).

Fulvestrant (Faslodex) is a relatively new additive therapy. Like tamoxifen, fulvestrant binds to the estrogen receptor and blocks it, but without any potential estrogenic capabilities. Studies have shown that fulvestrant is as effective as anastrozole, and the side effect profile is similar. The major difference is that fulvestrant requires intramuscular injection once a month, while the other agents discussed above can be taken orally. Some patients find this requirement a hindrance; others prefer monthly injection to taking daily pills.

Other additive endocrine therapies include medicines that are similar to progesterone (for example, megestrol acetate, or Megace); medicines that like act like the male hormone, called androgens (such as fluoxymestrone, or Halotestin); and even estrogenic agents such as diethylstilbestrol (DES). However, with the availability of the aromatase inhibitors and fulvestrant, these agents are used less frequently.

For postmenopausal women with newly diagnosed ER-positive metastatic breast cancer, most oncologists would now recommend an aromatase inhibitor (AI) as first-line therapy, although tamoxifen is not a bad choice for patients who have not previously taken it. Depending on circumstances, if the first agent fails, another endocrine treatment is appropriate, especially if the first was particularly effective before it stopped working. Often women take one therapy after another over a prolonged period of time, occasionally years. Indeed, sometimes a woman will "re-respond" to tamoxifen if her cancer progressed while she was on it but then she was treated with other intervening endocrine therapy for some time.

Endocrine treatment for premenopausal women usually begins with medical ablation of the ovaries (usually achieved with goserelin); afterward, endocrine therapy proceeds as it would for postmenopausal women. Endocrine treatment is generally well tolerated. The main side effects of endocrine treatment include symptoms typical of estrogen depletion, such as hot flashes and moodiness. Anti-estrogenic therapy can also cause vaginal dryness with irritation, frequent urinary tract infections, and pain during sexual relations. Because it acts like an estrogen in the liver, tamoxifen stimulates the liver to increase production of clotting proteins, a situation associated with heightened risk of blood clots. Megestrol acetate can do this as well. The AIs can cause joint pain; rarely (less than 5 percent of the time) they cause gastrointestinal problems such as abdominal pain.

Chemotherapy

Chemotherapy kills rapidly dividing cells by interfering with the general functioning of DNA, RNA, and proteins. Therefore, unlike endocrine therapy and trastuzumab (which only damage cells with ER or HER-2 receptors, respectively), chemotherapy tends to have more side effects because it kills normal cells as well as cancer cells. Chemotherapy is usually recommended for women whose tumor does not make ER, for women whose tumors are ER positive but for whom endocrine therapy does not seem to be working, and for women with a particularly poor prognosis.

A remarkable number of chemotherapeutic options are available for treatment of metastatic breast cancer. There are several classes of chemotherapies. They include the so-called alkylating agents, such as cyclophosphamide (Cytoxan), and anti-metabolites, such as methotrexate, 5-fluorouracil, and capecitabine (Xeloda). One of the most active classes of chemotherapeutic agents is the anthracyclines, including doxorubicin (Adriamycin) and epirubicin (Ellence). Because these agents can cause heart damage, doxorubicin has been incorporated into structures called liposomes, which serve to protect the heart but do not decrease the drug's activity. These liposomal doxorubicin agents are known as Doxil and Myocet.

Paclitaxel (Taxol) and docetaxel (Taxotere)—known as taxanes—work by interfering with important structures called microtubules that enable cell division. Vinorelbine (Navelbine) and older drugs such as vinblastine (Velban) also interfere with microtubule function. Another older drug that is usually used after most of the other drugs have been tried is etoposide (Eposin, Etopophos, or Vepesid). More recently, a newer drug, gemcitabine (Gemzar), has also proven to be of use in patients with metastatic breast cancer.

Most of these drugs are given intravenously, although some (such as cyclophosphamide) can be given orally. Others (such as capecitabine) not only can be but should be given by mouth. These agents can be used alone or in combinations. Many years ago, when it was shown that combinations of different chemotherapies led to cures in other malignancies, such as leukemias, lymphomas, and testicular cancer, this strategy gained popularity in the treatment of breast cancer. Various combinations included CMF, CAF, AC, and more recently AT (Adriamycin and a taxane) or DC (docetaxel and capecitabine), also called XT based on the brand names for these drugs (Xeloda and Taxotere). Many more combinations have been reported, but none appears more or less effective than any others.

It is tempting to assume that treatment using many drugs is better, but few if any studies have demonstrated that survival is improved with combination chemotherapy as opposed to using drugs in sequence. Although more patients will respond to a combination initially, the side effects are also greater. Therefore many oncologists prescribe each agent by itself until it is clear that it's not working, and then go on to the next.

This approach is not used for patients with particularly poor prognoses, for whom time is of the essence; in these patients, the added toxicities of combined drugs are often considered worth the hope for disease stabilization or remission. Not all patients can sustain slower, sequential treatment.

Although the proper dose is important for any agent to be effective, there is no evidence that going above standard doses is likely to bring more benefit. To the contrary, toxicities are much worse with higher doses, and well-designed clinical trials have failed to demonstrate any advantage to increasing the dose of any of the available chemotherapeutic agents above standard levels.

SIDE EFFECTS

Side effects of chemotherapeutic agents include nausea, vomiting, hair loss, and transient decrease of bone marrow function. Since the bone marrow makes white blood cells (which fight infection), red blood cells (which carry oxygen), and platelets (which stop bleeding), patients are at risk for infection, anemia (low red cell count), and bleeding while they are on chemotherapy. Not all agents cause all of these symptoms. In fact, several of the agents, especially if given weekly, cause little nausea, vomiting, or hair loss. Furthermore, new anti-nausea medicines work extremely well and have drastically offset this side effect. New medicines that stimulate the bone marrow to make white blood cells and red blood cells faster have also been helpful in alleviating the side effects of chemotherapy.

Each of these agents may also have its own special side effect or toxicity. The risk of heart damage with the anthracyclines like doxorubicin (Adriamycin) has already been noted. The anti-tubule agents all cause damage to peripheral nerves, resulting in numbness and tingling. At times this symptom can be severe enough to make it necessary to stop taking the agent. Several of the agents cause mouth sores and diarrhea, especially the anti-metabolites. If a woman has any symptoms, she should bring the symptoms to the attention of her physician immediately.

Another way to reduce the side effects is to stop the therapy after several cycles, if a good response has resulted in satisfactory palliation. A few studies have shown that once effective palliation has been achieved, taking a "drug holiday" does no harm to patients. However, modern chemotherapy is so well tolerated by so many women that the use of drug holidays has declined.

Targeted Therapies: Trastuzumab

As discussed above, the anti-HER-2 monoclonal antibody, trastuzumab (Herceptin), can be used by itself in selected patients or in combination with non-anthracycline chemotherapies. Whether trastuzumab should be continued from one chemotherapy to the next as a patient's disease progresses is not known and is being investigated in an ongoing study. The standard method of administering trastuzumab is to give it intravenously every week, but a recent study has suggested that every three weeks works equally well. Trastuzumab does not appear to work in women whose tumors do not make the HER-2 protein.

Bevacizumab (Avastin)

Bevacizumab is also a monoclonal antibody, but it is directed against a different molecule called VEGF. VEGF, which is made by the cancer cell and some normal cells, has many functions. One of these is to stimulate new blood vessel growth, which cancers need to expand. Bevacizumab has been found to be active against colon, lung, and, quite recently, breast cancers. It appears that the optimal time to use bevacizumab is during the first chemotherapy regimen for metastatic breast cancer. Bevacizumab is relatively well tolerated, although it does cause high blood pressure and occasionally bleeding, which is usually insignificant but can, at times, be catastrophic. The precise role of bevacizumab for breast cancer treatment is unproven at present.

Bisphosphonates: To Protect Bones

Metastases to bone are a major source of pain and suffering for patients with breast cancer. The main goal of therapy is to decrease the burden of the cancer with anticancer drugs so that pain will be relieved—that is, to shrink the tumors. But over the last decade it has been shown that agents that strengthen bone reduce the incidence of uncontrolled bone pain and of bone fractures. These agents work by interfering with the action of cells that naturally decrease bone density; they are also used to prevent and treat osteoporosis in women without breast cancer. However, oral agents such as alendronate (Fosamax) that are used to treat osteoporosis do not appear to be as effective as intravenous agents like pamidronate (Aredia) and zoledronate (Zometa).

For women with bone metastases, bone-strengthening agents are infused every three to four weeks, and are generally well tolerated. A few patients have muscle and bone aches after injection; sometimes these are severe. Recently, doctors have reported with pamidronate or zoledronate use the occurrence of a very rare syndrome of severe damage to the bone of the lower jaw (mandibular osteonecrosis) which is quite painful and difficult to treat. This risk does not outweigh the substantial benefits of these agents, but it should be kept in mind when they are used.

Conclusion

Although a diagnosis of metastatic breast cancer can be devastating, it is by no means a hopeless condition. The goal of therapy is principally palliation, which generally can be effectively achieved through local and systemic therapies, in sequence, along with careful monitoring to help guide decision making.

PART THREE

Notes on the Experience of Having Breast Cancer

CHAPTER 15

The Shock of Finding Out

Kenneth D. Miller, M.D.

T
he news comes like a jangling telephone call in the middle of the night. "You have cancer." Most women are stunned at the diagnosis. Some women are unable to utter a meaningful sound. One breast cancer survivor remembers that all she could say was,·"'Oh, dear.' That was all. 'Oh, dear' didn't seem sufficient, but it was all I could muster."

Different Discoveries

A woman finds out that she has breast cancer through a routine mammogram, during monthly self-exam, when her doctor palpates a lump during a routine checkup, or when she notices something unusual about her breast. Many women, fortunately, take an active course rather than postponing a visit to the doctor because they are in denial.

One of the frustrating things about breast cancer is that it takes different forms. Some masses are palpable; some are not. Some feel pebbly and hard; others simply feel like thickened tissue. And while some are almost microscopically small, others seem to grow large overnight.

If a lump or other abnormality is felt on a breast exam, it usually needs to be biopsied, even if the mammogram is negative. In addition, whether it's a lump, a bump, a squiggle, or a thickened spot of breast tissue, anything that looks unusual on a mammogram is normally followed up with a sonogram. What are the differences between these two tests? A mammogram uses a very low-energy X-ray that records an image on film to show anatomical detail. While it can be uncomfortable to have one's breast squeezed between the plates of the machine, mammography is an effective tool for detecting breast cancer in its very early stages. Mammography works less well when breast tissue is dense. Young women generally have denser breast tissue than older women, which is why regular mammography is not routinely recommended for most women in their twenties and thirties.

A sonogram uses sound waves to analyze body tissue. The technology is the same as that used during pregnancy to assess the fetus. It is non-invasive, harmless, and not painful. The sonogram can clarify the nature of any nodules that appeared on a mammogram; for example, it can show whether the lesion is just a fluid-filled cyst or whether it has features suggestive of something else. MRI scans are taking a more prominent role in breast imaging as well.

Follow-Up Tests

If these initial tests indicate a potential malignancy, or if the results are inconclusive, a doctor usually orders follow-up tests. The results of the mammogram, MRI, or sonogram may indicate that a biopsy is the appropriate next step. A biopsy involves taking sample tissue from the suspicious area to determine whether it contains cancerous or precancerous cells. Examining the cells under a microscope is the only way to confirm a diagnosis.

If cancer is found, the first priority is to determine what kind of cancer it is and to identify its stage. (For more information about types of breast cancer and the process of staging, see chapter 2.) Another part of the diagnostic process is to determine whether the cancer has reached any lymph nodes. When lymph nodes are affected, more aggressive surgery and treatment are usually required.

Knowing Your Own Body

Despite modern medical advances, sometimes the best diagnostic tool is a woman's familiarity with her own breasts. Many women say that their breast cancer was almost missed, but that they themselves insisted on follow-up tests, based on a hunch from their knowledge of their own bodies.

Sometimes it takes more than a little persistence to be heard in the medical world. When one woman felt a lump in her right breast, her doctor told her he was not sure about it and suggested she come back in six weeks. She decided to see him again in four weeks because she still felt the lump. Her doctor dismissed her concerns, saying he did not feel anything, but advised her to go for an early mammogram to ease her anxiety. She went, and it showed nothing. All the while, she felt the lump. She consulted another doctor, who recommended that the lump be surgically removed. And the lumpectomy showed that the lump was indeed malignant. It is important to *follow up on any feeling that something has changed in your body.*

Dealing with Diagnosis

After the immediate shock of learning that one has cancer, five stages of normal emotional response usually follow. Not everyone experiences all of these stages or goes through them in a specific order, however, and no one's emotional responses can be predicted. It can be helpful to know some of the patterns of human response to realize you are not alone.

The first stage of emotional response is characterized by *denial and disbelief.* The person's thought, simply, is: "This can't happen to me. This only happens to other people." The worst kind of denial is the kind that keeps a woman from doing self-exams or from getting routine check-ups, simply because she assumes she will never get cancer.

After a period of intellectual denial, the second stage of emotional response commonly involves *anger.* Women may blame themselves or others. Family and friends often bear the brunt of uncontrollable outbursts. These harsh episodes often give way to a third stage, known as the *bargaining* stage. People may petition God with prayer, for example, promising to offer something up in exchange for release from this trial.

Sometimes people even try to make a deal with their own bodies, promising, for instance, to think only positive thoughts in exchange for recovery. Some women hope that a good deed will have a positive effect on healing.

Internal efforts to bargain with fate or God or one's own body often lead to the fourth emotional stage, *depression*. The symptoms of depression include exhaustion, listlessness, and an overwhelming feeling of emotional fragility. Tears may come easily, and a person may have difficulty finding joy in normal activities. Some people who are depressed wonder if life is even worth living. Depression is common, and it is highly treatable. Therapy and medication can ease the symptoms of depression and can liberate people from that immobilizing state where even the simplest or most straightforward decisions seem too much to contemplate. Family members should not allow their depressed loved ones to postpone or avoid seeking treatment. Suicidal thoughts are not uncommon among people undergoing enormous stress; such thoughts need to be taken seriously and managed with professional care.

The fifth stage of emotional response is *acceptance*. Acceptance helps a person find the calm to consider real options. With breast cancer, this stage is especially important, because the treatment choices are complex. A woman is given information about her particular cancer and is then sent home with many decisions to make regarding surgery, reconstruction, and adjuvant therapies.

The emotional stages of response do not follow a single pattern. Even women who believe that they are prepared to hear that they have breast cancer have trouble accepting it. Other women make the decision to accept that they have cancer within minutes of hearing the news.

Many women describe their experiences with breast cancer as journeys, with each stage characterized by its own challenges. Diagnosis and discovery bring their own emotional burdens, as do the later treatment stages. Again and again, women are astounded at the unexpected depth of their own strength and resilience.

Part 4 of this book relates the stories of breast cancer survivors in their own words. Some of these stories are quoted in the next three chapters to illustrate the issues explored in them.

CHAPTER 16

Neceddary Decidiond

Surgery, Radiation Therapy,

and Breast Reconstruction

Kenneth D. Miller, M.D.

M any women with breast cancer are asked to make a decision about surgery, to choose either lumpectomy with radiation therapy or mastectomy. Women scheduled for mastectomy are usually also asked to decide whether they want to undergo
reconstructive surgery, and whether they want to do it at the time of
mastectomy or later. Other complicated issues often demand their prompt
attention, as well:

- A doctor may recommend neoadjuvant chemotherapy before surgery, with the aim of shrinking the tumor to make it possible to
  do a less-extensive operation (sometimes lumpectomy instead of
  mastectomy).
- If the cancer is invasive, a doctor will make recommendations

based on the results of a surgical sentinel node biopsy (described in chapter 5).

- If medically indicated, the surgeon may offer a skin-sparing mastectomy or a nipple-sparing option.
- Or, a woman may be told she is a candidate for lumpectomy alone, without radiation.

Being asked to make an important decision like this is often shocking, especially because it is not like other experiences we have had. Most women rally quickly after the initial distress of being asked to decide, though, and they are able to make a decision with which they are comfortable. Although about 80 percent of women are now considered good candidates for lumpectomy followed by radiation, many of these women opt for mastectomy instead, feeling that the mastectomy surgery gives them a greater sense of security. Others feel equally confident with lumpectomy and radiation.

Charting a Course

Motivational speaker and author Anthony Robbins believes that our decisions, not the conditions of our lives, determine our destiny. Where do you begin, with such weighty decisions to make? Recognizing and acknowledging your own coping style may help you sort out your options. Most people approach important decisions as "doers," "feelers," or "thinkers." You may have a little of each in you, but one style likely dominates.

Anne, a real "doer," writes of her experience: "The biopsy showed multiple lesions, and out of twelve or so lymph nodes examined, two showed cancer. The doctor came to me with a sad expression. I wasn't surprised at the diagnosis, but I could see how much it bothered him. I tried to cheer him up. I assured him that we would just get going and do what had to be done. I had classes to teach and many shows to put on all over the area." (Anne's story can be found in chapter 21.)

Not all women feel comfortable jumping right in. If you are someone who takes months to decide on a paint color for your den, it will be daunting to wade through the research, physicians' opinions, survivors' advice, and information from sources like the American Cancer Society. If you are an especially intuitive person, your decisions may be guided more by spiritual counsel or gut instinct.

A "feeler" may find that talking with other people, reading spiritual materials, meditating, and praying lead to a sense of acceptance and peace about following a surgeon's recommendation.

If you are a "thinker" by personality, you are probably most compelled by research and study. You believe that knowledge is power. You want clear and accurate information so you can make an informed decision based on credible and up-to-date facts. There are many aspects of the disease and its treatment that are beyond your individual control, but learning as much as you can and making a decision based on what you have learned is very important to your peace of mind.

When a choice is not clear-cut, some women find themselves vacillating between options, afraid that whatever choice they make will be the wrong one. One doctor may recommend a mastectomy, and a different doctor may recommend lumpectomy followed by radiation. It helps to remember that there are no guarantees in life, that even getting in a car to drive to the store entails taking risks. Using your own personal coping style, reaching a decision, and moving forward—while keeping in mind that there are no guarantees in life—is sometimes all we can do.

It's easier to make decisions if you consult doctors in whom you have confidence. If you have time to interview and put together your own team of doctors, and if doing so is important to you, you will more likely respect these doctors' opinions.

Breast Psychology

Lillie Shockney of the Johns Hopkins Avon Foundation Breast Cancer Center (see chapter 25) says it is important to understand that some women base their decisions about surgery on medical fears that may be unwarranted. Some women choose mastectomies simply because they feel that getting rid of the entire breast is safer. Although they would most likely have the same positive outcome with lumpectomy followed by radiation, the decision to undergo more drastic surgery gives them the peace of mind they need.

One breast cancer survivor explains that even though she knew an analysis of the facts showed she would be a good candidate for lumpectomy with radiation, she had to go with what felt best: "Knowing myself, I knew I would be checking my breast, and worrying, so I knew I better go for mastectomy. I discussed it with my husband who stated that he married me because of who I am and not because of my breasts. Mastectomy it was."

These decisions are personal. Counselor Carole Seddon (see chapter 23) emphasizes how critical it is for women to feel validated in their decisions. In other words, if the doctor says "It's your choice," then a woman should be comfortable going with the decision that is right for her. Again, this is true if the doctor provides a choice; decisions should not run counter to credible and consistent medical advice.

Lillie Shockney notes that a woman's "personal relationship with her breasts" is also a major part of the decision-making process. "Some women consider their breasts their 'best feature' and do not want to part with them even if it means losing their life. I've seen this, sadly," she says. "Also, how important are a woman's breasts to her in regard to intimacy with her mate? We should never underestimate the impact of a mate's opinion on a woman's choice. She wants to please him." Conversely, for some women, physical appearance is a comparatively trivial factor in the decision-making process. They do not let anything interfere with their focus on health.

Many breast cancer survivors note that humor, even grim humor, is part of the process. Lillie Shockney remembers her 12-year-old daughter asking whether the surgeon would be moving Lillie's right breast into the middle of her chest after removing her left one. Lillie's first thought was that this would create a new medical condition, the "Una-boob." Her daughter also was intrigued by the pocket in her mother's bra that held her breast prosthesis and suggested it might be a safe place to store money while traveling. "It felt so good to laugh," recalls Lillie. "We made a pact that every day for the rest of our lives, we would find something funny to laugh at or do."

Decisions about Reconstruction

The decision to have reconstructive surgery is perhaps the most individual and personal treatment choice of all. A woman's age and stage of life are important factors in this decision. Some women, when they find out that breast reconstruction can add three or more hours to surgery and can slow recovery, decide against reconstruction. Some women do not want to deal with reconstruction at the time of the mastectomy, but they do not rule it out for the future.

Most women who choose reconstruction surgery are happy with their decision, although rare cases of infection or other problems sometimes cause reconstruction failure. Then there is a decision to be made about whether to try the reconstruction surgery a second time.

A conversation with someone who has had reconstruction surgery— or someone who has not had the surgery and is not entirely happy with the prosthesis—may help with the decision. Whether they credit luck, fate, a guardian angel, or the hand of God, many breast cancer survivors say they are grateful to have had the right people placed in their path at just the right moment in their lives. They found people who helped them wade through information, gave support, listened to their concerns, and provided guidance and direction as they made their surgical choices.

CHAPTER 17

Considering Adjuvant Therapy

Kenneth D. Miller, M.D.

Every day, researchers are finding new ways to attack breast cancer. Chemotherapy and hormonal therapy, the treatment options used in addition to surgery, are termed *adjuvant therapies*. They help save lives, but they also require newly diagnosed women to make additional difficult treatment decisions. Even experts in the field of cancer research don't always agree about specific treatment protocols, so there is no black-and-white answer. If you are a candidate for adjuvant therapy, your doctor might recommend that you seek a second opinion. Sometimes the second doctor will offer the same opinion as the first, but only sometimes.

And then there is the other advice . . . from well-meaning relatives, friends, coworkers, and even the casual "friend of a friend" who has heard about your diagnosis. "Depending on the relationship, the impact of those stories may be very frightening," notes Carole Seddon (see chapter 23). "Things like 'I was so sick; it was awful' can sit in a person's mind. Others are frightened by movies they have seen or stories they have read. Some women fear the side effects they have heard about."

Women's personal experiences reflect the different challenges posed by treatment options related to chemotherapy and hormonal therapy. For a variety of reasons, ranging from personal preference to statistic-driven calculations to general medical condition to spiritual pull, women make different choices about adjuvant therapy. Many women choose to do whatever they have to do to overcome the cancer, but not all women follow this route.

According to Lillie Shockney (see chapter 25), "Women in general who refuse chemo as adjuvant therapy are risk takers by nature. They don't value the 2 to 5 percent increase in survival and would rather take their chances, figuring that the side effects, short and long term, are more horrific in their mind than what they will gain. It is all a matter of attitude. Some women will do anything to gain 1 percent, and others must be shown there is a considerable statistical difference to make it worth their while."

Many women testify to the power of making positive, active decisions. And in the face of all manner of serious diagnoses, many people have been helped by their doctor's upbeat and positive attitude about what can be accomplished through treatment.

Weighing the Options

One cancer survivor compares treatment planning to selecting dishes from a Chinese menu: "You choose one from column A and two from column B." It's helpful to remember that the doctors you see will recommend a treatment plan based on several factors that are unique to your body and diagnosis. The "menu" of decisions you are offered is usually based on the following considerations:

- The type of breast cancer
- The size of the tumor
- The grade of the tumor
- The involvement of lymph nodes
- Whether the cancer is localized or has spread
- Your estrogen/progesterone receptor status and HER-2-Neu status

Adjuvant therapies are administered in two basic ways:

- Systemic therapy affects the entire body, not just the cancer site. Systemic therapy is chemotherapy or hormonal therapy, which usually involves tamoxifen or aromatase inhibitors.
- Localized therapy affects only the site surrounding the cancer. It uses radiation to destroy cancer cells that may have been left behind at the tumor site, or may have spread to surrounding body tissues.

As we have seen, individual attitude is a crucial factor when people are making significant decisions. Carole Seddon says that when she is counseling people, she sometimes sees patterns of thinking that get in the way of clear decision making. "A number of women have been health-focused individuals who do not believe in using a lot of drugs, so this is a very difficult thing for them, especially after being told what can happen as a result of taking the treatments."

Lillie Shockney says, "Women too often look at chemotherapy in a negative way. 'Poison' and 'toxic' are common comments. I tell patients to not look at it as poison. Instead, I provide the analogy of antibiotics. We take antibiotics to kill bacteria and don't consider it a negative drug to take. Look at chemo in the same way, and remember it is carrying you even higher up the survival curve."

Carole Seddon says age sometimes plays a role in a woman's attitude toward cancer treatment. "Younger women, in their thirties or even early forties, may have had mothers who have done well after breast cancer and may or may not have taken additional treatments," she says. "There can be that belief among these women — usually those under age 40 — that they just will not die of this disease."

These younger women, she says, are often upset by the side effects of hormonal adjuvant therapy. Since hormonal treatments may put the body in a menopausal state, childbearing may suddenly become impossible. Carole says it also affects the way younger patients view their sexuality. "They fear losing interest in a sexual relationship with their husbands who are also in their thirties. It's tough. Most do take the recommended treatment but can be very angry or depressed."

Practical circumstances also dictate decisions regarding treatment options. To get a particular treatment, a woman may have to use a different doctor than the one she would have chosen because her preferred doctor is not covered by her insurance plan. Some women suffer other complicating health problems that may make treatment more difficult. Often the practical need to hold on to a job or career may be part of the decision-making process.

Thoughts on Chemotherapy

Having a bad taste in your mouth, losing your hair, or feeling like you have the flu can make it difficult to continue, but most women, once they make the decision to have chemotherapy, continue with it despite the difficulties. The stories in part 4 of this book include many stories from women who have found ways to cope with the side effects and other challenges of chemotherapy.

One breast cancer survivor notes that attitude played a big role in her ability to deal with her chosen course of chemotherapy: "I remember very early on the oncologist said something both true and motivating. He told me that a positive attitude would help me get through this ordeal. I may have taken this to an extreme, but it worked. Even on the days when people stopped to tell me how bad I looked at work or to ask me why I had come in, it was still better than sitting at home feeling sick and sorry for myself. Sure I had side effects—stomach problems and mouth sores so bad I could not talk, eat, or swallow medication—but the people at work were counting on me."

Thoughts on Hormonal Therapy

There are two common types of hormonal therapy. Tamoxifen is considered an excellent choice for women who are pre- or postmenopausal and have tumors that are positive for estrogen or progesterone receptors. Aromatase inhibitors, such as Arimidex, are used in postmenopausal women only (see chapter 10).

Most women who have side effects from hormonal therapy have side effects that are uncomfortable but not life threatening. Hot flashes, nausea, and vaginal dryness are common but can be treated with other medicines. But there are more serious possible side effects, because any hormonal therapy can increase the risk of stroke, blood clots, and some uterine cancers.

For one breast cancer survivor, it was very difficult to look past those small risks. "Where was my biggest struggle? It was whether or not to take tamoxifen. It would seem that after surgery and radiation, this would be an easy decision, but it was not. I believe that given my profile, my chance of being harmed by this drug is equal to my chance of being helped. When my doctor mentioned that I should 'celebrate' that daily pill, I felt lost. How could I celebrate something that could potentially kill me? Isn't there some irony in relying on a cure that has life-threatening possibilities to treat a life-threatening illness?"

For Becky (whose story appears in chapter 21), deciding whether to use adjuvant hormonal therapy was the last treatment decision she faced, following a mastectomy and chemotherapy. "After finishing chemotherapy (and yes, I did lose my hair and wore a wig for about nine months), I decided to take tamoxifen. My tumor was estrogen receptive, so tamoxifen would decrease the likelihood of recurrence for me. Again, this was not a difficult decision to make to stay healthy."

CHAPTER 18

Reflections on the Experience

Kenneth D. Miller, M.D.

A fter the diagnosis has been absorbed, the treatment decisions made, and the treatment carried out, how do people deal with the reality of cancer in their every day lives? In this chapter, cancer survivors reflect not only on the amount of time seemingly stolen from their normal routines but also on the unexpected ways in which the ordeal has brought strength.

The Process

Many women look back on the treatment process as a completely separate season in their lives. Writes one survivor, "As I look back on my experience with breast cancer, I realize that somehow I found myself moving through the whole thing step by step, dealing with the overwhelming reality in little bits that I could handle. At some point, this realization freed me. I actually felt empowered. In some weird way, having cancer made me dig deep inside myself for what I needed to get through each day."

For a woman who is being treated for breast cancer at the same time that she is experiencing divorce, death of a loved one, job loss, or any other life-altering changes, it takes determination to persevere and get through to the other side of the crisis. Handling things as they need to be handled, one thing at a time, is one coping mechanism.

Despite the strength women find in the midst of cancer treatment, most are quick to point out that being strong did not make the day-to-day reality of treatment any more pleasant. Sometimes cancer's cure can feel as bad as the disease. "There were a lot of aspects of my experience that were horrible," writes one survivor. "I am not particularly vain, but losing my hair was very traumatic. I did the best I could. I chose a wig and had my hair cut in the same style. When my hair started to fall out, I figured the transition to the wig would be less obvious. Some people were still quite insensitive or just ignorant, however."

Many women recall that their treatment experiences robbed precious hours from their lives, but in retrospect they see value in the time spent managing the crisis. Barbara writes, "It is so important to make every moment count and recognize all the good things that come our way. Now I see breast cancer as a glitch on the radar screen, and I have put it in perspective. I have so much to be thankful for and to look forward to and great friends and family who helped me get to this point." (See the rest of Barbara's story in chapter 21.)

One of the odd aspects of breast cancer treatment is that the various treatments may cause harsh side effects for one woman and cause no side effects for someone else. Some women suffer with severe nausea from chemotherapy, for example, and others simply don't. Some have very uncomfortable hot flashes after hormonal treatments, while others—especially postmenopausal women—find taking the drugs smooth sailing. And while some women fear radiation treatment and have side effects, others find it is the easiest part of their treatment. The women who tell their stories in part 4 relate various experiences and ways of coping with all of these treatments.

The Importance of Support

When women consider what helped them survive cancer, the word *support* surfaces again and again. "My husband was also very helpful in my decision making," writes Karen. "He kept his thoughts and opinions to himself and clearly supported any decision I would have made. But the gift to me was that he and I arrived at the same decision. His total support gave me that extra boost throughout the process." (Karen's story appears in chapter 20.)

Family and friends create distractions from physical and emotional pain when appropriate, and they can provide appealing food and make it possible for the woman with cancer to get needed rest. In fact, the practical efforts of family and friends help most women keep depression at bay. Supportive friends and family are often named as the key element in keeping one's perspective on the cancer experience—and are often seen as being as important to recovery as watching nutrition, trying to maintain a positive outlook, and getting regular physical exercise.

Many women with cancer join a support group where they can meet women of different ages and at different stages of recovery. Hearing the other women's stories can provide useful information and can make it easier to speak up and relate your own experiences. It can be especially encouraging to meet long-term survivors.

While many cancer survivors recommend support groups, others do not. These women do not like to focus on cancer and would rather give their friends a quick update on health matters before moving on to other topics of conversation.

Having the right support system can literally make a life-or-death difference when hopelessness rears its head. Barbara writes that her husband, Jan, kept insisting that she get psychiatric help until she emerged from a personal time of darkness that engulfed her near the end of her treatment process: "After talking to a therapist, I came to realize that what I was feeling was common. I had spent the last several months in a fight for my life and had the support of the general surgeon, the reconstructive surgeon, and the oncologist to help me. But now, all of this was behind me, and I was alone again with my fears that the cancer might return. My support system was gone, at least in my mind, and I was feeling very alone. I joined two support groups. Jan came with me to one support group and helped me get through the uncertainty and fear that I was feeling. Between these groups, Jan's support and love, along with that of the rest of my family, plus the therapy, I was able to . . . get on with my life."

Reflections on the Experience

Another breast cancer survivor recalls the support she received from her teenaged daughters and her husband. She also was touched by the support that came from a variety of other sources. Her friends and her extended family visited, made meals, pitched in to clean the house, and provided emotional support.

One woman notes that you never know how you will handle a crisis until one falls in your lap. "I have always known that I travel in circles of wonderful people, my family, coworkers and friends," she writes. "It is amazing how much strength you can draw from knowing there are truly wonderful people in this world."

Finding Strength in Faith

For women of faith, spiritual strength can make a tremendous difference. They often express this faith as knowing that God loves them. They and their families and friends pray to God, which helps them maintain hope.

For Kathy, overcoming breast cancer meant placing her trust in two places: her physicians and God. "I have a loving husband, family and friends," she writes, "and I controlled what I could control—my attitude and the choice of physicians. But ultimately, I needed to trust in my physicians, their knowledge and experience. And I must add, trust in God, that regardless of the outcome, I would handle it with as much courage and grace as I could muster. Seventeen years later . . . I am thankful every day."

Many cancer survivors believe a healthy connection of mind, body, and spirit is a vital part of healing. "I reached my sister . . . and she said exactly what I needed to hear," recalls Wanda (chapter 21). "She said, 'God has not given you just the spirit but a power of the blood and a sound mind.' Somehow, that was like water thrown on my face. I was like, 'Oh, you're right!' I was emotionally hysterical for half an hour to forty-five minutes before we connected, and when she said that, I said, 'You know what? You're absolutely right.' If I ever was a Christian, it was at that moment. It was as if I began to heal right then and there. All I knew was that it was a big journey ahead. I didn't really know how big the journey was."

Lessons Learned

Cancer can cause fear and panic, pain and loss, heartbreak and grief. But women who have faced its challenge say cancer is also one of life's great educators. In fact, cancer can change a woman's entire attitude toward life. She may decide to deal with things as they happen rather than worrying or anticipating trouble. She may learn to forgive people when they get angry because she recognizes that anger is how they react to stress. She may become more adventurous, visiting exotic parts of the world or backpacking in the mountains. She may change how she chooses her doctors, even being willing to drive out of her way to reach a well-regarded physician or a physician she can talk with comfortably.

Luba (chapter 21) writes of the lessons she learned: "My advice to anyone embarking on this journey of breast cancer is to inform yourself of exactly what your condition is, talk to others who have walked the walk before you, have real life goals ahead of you, try to maintain as much of your normal schedule as possible, and surround yourself with competent medical people. Make your decision based on all of the information you can get and consult with your closest family and friends. Ultimately, however, the decision must be one that you are comfortable with, since it is your life and your body."

Anne (also in chapter 21) writes that she learned that "the doctor's close supervision of your progress as the years go on can make a big difference. Also, it is important for the patient to recognize and follow up on any doubts they have. Never forget that humor can be seen (if you look) in the most unexpected happenings in one's life."

Moving On

"You are in remission." Every breast cancer patient longs to hear these words. But after fighting the good fight for so long, there is a pause, a hesitation, a transition time, as survivors figure out how to move from this chaotic period back into a normal life rhythm. Life without constant medical appointments, life with more certainty. For many women, moving on to life after cancer is almost as disorienting as struggling with the cancer itself.

They may discover that there is no returning to the previous "normal"; instead, they find a new normal.

Anne writes: "In the end, I learned to see what's important in life. I am spending time with my family and friends and doing the things I enjoy or always wanted to do but did not have the time or opportunity to do before. I take care of myself physically, by doing some kind of exercise almost every day; intellectually, by taking classes at a local college; and emotionally, by playing with my grandchildren and seeing my girlfriends often. And often, I count my blessings."

Another breast cancer survivor has a unique way of explaining how she puts her experience in perspective. "Why in the world would I consider myself a breast cancer 'survivor' any more that I would consider myself a survivor of 'life'? I have survived all of the ups and downs of just living, and these daily life events have taught me my strengths. I have experienced pain and heartbreak, loss of jobs and life dreams, birth and death of children and other significant people, and I have experienced many successes. I am most certainly a survivor, but of much more than breast cancer. This illness does not define me, nor is it even the most important part of my life. It is an event, a blip on the screen that I had to deal with just as I have dealt with so many other life events. Neither more, nor less."

And few stories have the exuberance of Madeleine's, who celebrates every part of moving on. "Today, I don't care if my hair's messed up, and I don't care if my clothes don't match. I am here today. I want to help other people and encourage them through all of this. That's my goal. Living every day with my husband and my kids and my grandkids and my family, playing music — that is my life. I am happy with myself. I am happy with my life. I am happy with my decisions in life. I am happy with the way my family came out. I am happy with the closeness we have with my brothers and my sister. I really don't have any regrets in my life, and if something doesn't make me happy, then I choose another way. I find another way."

Survivors

Tell Their Stories

CHAPTER 19

Stories from Women at High Risk

W *hat would you do if you were told that you had a higher than aver-age risk of developing breast cancer? Higher, that is, than the one-in-eight chance that some studies suggest is the typical risk for a woman living in the United States. Risk factors that can increase the likelihood of breast cancer include, for example, a very strong family history of cancer, being a carrier of the breast cancer related gene known as BRCA, or having had a breast biopsy that revealed either lobular neoplasia or atypical ductal hyperplasia.*

Some women with increased risk choose simply to increase their self-surveillance. Others opt to take the hormonal medication called tamoxifen. Some choose to undergo prophylactic mastectomy. There is a story behind every personal decision.

Debbie has a very strong family history of breast cancer and is positive for the BRCA gene. She chose to undergo bilateral mastectomy.

I was only three years old when my mother discovered a lump in her right breast. She was twenty-nine years old and eight months pregnant with her third child. One month after my sister was born (on my mother's thirtieth birthday), she went in for what she thought would be a lumpectomy. When the doctors told my father that it was indeed cancer with lymph node involvement, he was left with an agonizing decision. As she lay there under anesthesia, he felt there was no choice but a radical mastectomy. My mother awoke from her surgery totally unprepared for the news she would have to deal with.

I was too young to remember this time in her life. My first memory of her cancer is from when I was around four years old. I guess I was at a curious age and started to ask questions about things I had heard my parents discussing. She answered all of my questions very patiently and matter-of-factly. I remember asking to *see* her cancer. I insisted that I wanted to see "the cancer" because my older sister had seen it. She looked confused until I insisted that my sister had "seen it." She hesitated and then showed me her chest. To this day, I shudder at my reaction and wish I could go back in time to change it. I can only imagine how I made her feel when I screamed and ran from the room in tears from the sight of her mastectomy. Yet with all that she had endured, my mother found the strength somehow to comfort me and hold me until I stopped crying. I am still amazed at her courage whenever I think about it.

After time, I grew accustomed to seeing her wounds, and our household grew accustomed to listening to discussions of cancer. My mother even sold gel prosthetic breasts in her quest to help others who, like her, had undergone radical mastectomies. The word *breast* became a topic of conversation around our house, spoken with the same frequency as *homework*. It wasn't unusual for my sisters and me to be seen with silicone breasts on our heads or in our shirts as we played house. We laughed as we watched our friends' eyes grow wide when they saw the suitcase filled with "boobies." We joked with our mom that some people's mothers sold cosmetics, but ours sold breasts. I had a very different outlook on breast cancer because, for my family, it was a way of life. This was reinforced even more so when my maternal grandmother was diagnosed, treated, and cured of breast cancer in her mid-fifties.

As I reached puberty, I never really developed a strong bond with my own breasts once they appeared. It could have been that, in my opinion, a size A was hardly a reason to celebrate. Nonetheless, I never was crazy about them and assumed that eventually, like my mother's, they too would have to go. If they would cause me the same grief that my mother

Survivors Tell Their Stories

had experienced, then what did I really need them for? After all, my mother was still the picture of strength and beauty, no matter what scars lay beneath. She taught me that some things were out of our control, and we couldn't spend our time worrying about them. Likewise, difficult situations were to be met with a positive attitude, determination, and lots of courage. Problems were to be faced head-on and not to be dismissed. My mother had proven that you can come out on top after life throws us curve balls.

> *My mother was still the picture of strength and beauty, no matter what scars lay beneath. She taught me that some things were out of our control, and we couldn't spend our time worrying about them.*

That is why the shocking news in May of 1992 threw us all for a loop. My mother had been complaining of abdominal pain, and the doctors blamed it on gastrointestinal problems. The CT scan revealed a grapefruit-sized tumor on her ovary. The surgery that followed determined that it was, in fact, a malignant tumor. The doctors remained hopeful that it had all been removed and that with chemotherapy she had a decent chance of survival. My mother was positive that, like last time, this cancer could be beat. She was determined to win against this ugly disease, and we knew that if anyone could do it, she could. We were all convinced.

In March of 1993, ten months after the initial diagnosis and despite several surgeries and hospitalizations from the complications of her advancing disease, my mother passed away at the age of 53. She was four months shy of being a grandmother for the first time, as I was five-and-a-half months pregnant with my first child.

From that point on, I tried not to think about my own genetic imperfections, placing them on the back burner until I found a better time to deal with them. I managed to put these thoughts out of my head for five years until I was thirty years old. Then it hit me like a ton of bricks. Why was I sitting around waiting for something bad to happen to my family? I was young and healthy with a loving husband and two beautiful daughters. I should get up and do something about it! After all, I knew I was a strong person because I had made it through the excruciating pain of losing my mother when I was about to become one myself. I knew what it was like to spend countless hours missing her so badly and wanting to ask her all the questions I now had about being a mother. Now was my time to take control and face my challenges head-on, just like she had. It was the time to be proactive and not reactive.

Once I came to that realization, I knew that I had to have some definite answers as to my own genetic predispositions. I made the decision to find out once and for all if I carried the newly understood breast/ovarian cancer gene. More importantly, I prepared myself for how to handle the results. If my results were positive, I knew without a doubt, what I would do. I would not sit around waiting for my world to explode. I had a family to think about. I wasn't going to let breast cancer prevent me from one day seeing my own grandchildren.

My results came quickly, and they confirmed what I already suspected. I was a carrier of the BRCA1 gene. This meant that with my genetics and family history, I was now at an 87 percent risk of developing breast cancer by the time I was 80 years of age. In addition, I also had a 40 to 60 percent chance of getting ovarian cancer.

This information provided me with the strength I needed to potentially change my fate. Together, my husband and I decided that I should proceed with a prophylactic bilateral mastectomy followed by immediate breast reconstruction. We spent the next couple months meeting with several plastic surgeons, a surgical gyn/oncologist, and a medical oncologist. Once a surgeon was chosen, many more difficult decisions had to be made. Would I keep my nipples or have them removed? Should I use prosthetic implants or transabdominal muscular flaps? If implants were chosen, would I choose saline or silicone implants? I was shown pictures of each scenario and became overwhelmed and confused. Everyone had a different opinion! I spoke with and visited several women of all ages who had undergone bilateral mastectomies with different reconstructive techniques. I looked at and felt their breasts, while asking a million questions. I was amazed at how kind and open these women were to me. I was also petrified. The reality of what I was about to do set in. I began to have second thoughts on proceeding with such a radical approach, given the fact that I had yet to be diagnosed with a life-threatening breast cancer. Was I taking an overly aggressive approach for my benign breasts?

I finally became comfortable with my decision to proceed with prophylactic surgery, realizing that by doing so I could possibly avoid the horrible toxicity of chemotherapy and radiation treatments. I stopped asking others' opinions and became more confident that my choice was the right one for me. I also realized that it was important to me to be able to look in the mirror and like what I saw. With that in mind, I made the decision to proceed with a nipple-sparing procedure using saline tissue expanders, allowing for minimal disfigurement. This would also require a second surgery four months later to exchange the tissue expanders for the permanent saline implants. The surgeries and recoveries went better than I had expected. I was able to resume my motherly duties within a short time, and I loved my new size C breasts! I had an incredible amount of support from my husband and family as well as my friends. I knew from the moment I came home from the hospital and saw my children's beautiful faces that I had done a wonderful thing for us all.

> *I was able to resume my motherly duties within a short time, and I loved my new size C breasts!*

Five years have passed since that time, and I have never once looked back. In that time, I was blessed with the birth of our third child, a son. I tell others that this surgery was the best thing I have ever done, and I truly mean that. I have also had the opportunity to speak with many women who are considering this radical approach. I can only share my thoughts and feelings in relation to my own decisions and hope that they too will make the choice that is right for them. I have one last hurdle to tackle with regards to having my ovaries surgically removed. I will face that challenge and proceed with a bilateral oophorectomy in the near future. One step at a time.

I am hopeful that through medical advances, the future of gene therapy may someday alter the risk that my own daughters may have to face. We never know what tomorrow brings, but if we had an opportunity to change our daughters' future, what a wonderful world it could be.

Susan is a 47-year-old woman who was found to have atypical ductal hyperplasia and lobular neoplasia, which puts her at high risk of developing invasive breast cancer. After much deliberation and study she decided to take tamoxifen to reduce her risk.

I believe I had three or four lumpectomies since about 1970 on both sides, and they were just benign fibroids. This type of thing runs in my family. There was never any concern about the tissue whatsoever, it was just apparently something that women in my family tend to grow. In 1997 I had some minor surgery on my left breast, and a normal pathology review was done on the tissue. It came as a surprise that I had atypical hyperplasia and lobular carcinoma in situ in my left breast.

I didn't waste any time. I proceeded immediately to consult with various physicians. My husband is a surgeon, and so he took an active part in this. I went to see two oncologists here. I consulted with my gynecologist. I was getting a lot of different opinions as to how to treat this, everything from doing nothing to doing a prophylactic mastectomy.

One of the local oncologists, who is a very astute man, originally told me to have a double mastectomy. He thought that if you have a double mastectomy you're almost out of the woods — not totally out of the woods, because there is still breast tissue within the chest wall, but that would be the absolute extreme that anyone can go to to safeguard themselves. So being fairly aggressive, I think, in how he treats patients, his feeling was, "If you can do that, why not do it?"

It really was a huge range of opinions and quite confusing at the time. And so I decided that there were too many cooks in the kitchen and that I really had to take matters into my own hands.

It really was a huge range of opinions and quite confusing at the time. And so I decided that there were too many cooks in the kitchen and that I really had to take matters into my own hands.

I made an appointment at Sloan-Kettering, in New York. Before I went to Sloan-Kettering, I all but decided that I was going to follow their advice. They were alarmed that I had been diagnosed with atypical hyperplasia and lobular carcinoma in situ but not to the extent that they would recommend prophylactic mastectomy. They thought that we should treat it by increased vigilance and by taking tamoxifen prophylactically.

Back in 1995, tamoxifen had been used for women who had already had breast cancer, and it had been determined to have a very high rate of success in preventing a second breast cancer. But they were figuring out that it could also be used in women who have never had breast cancer but are at a higher risk, to prevent a first breast cancer. Sloan-

Kettering felt very strongly that that was the road that I should take and that I should be examined professionally by a physician, with breast exams on a very regular basis, three to four times a year; that I should continue with an annual mammogram; and that I should start on a five-year stint of tamoxifen.

I brought that information back here with me and resumed my care with my doctor, a wonderful, intelligent man. He was the one who originally recommended mastectomy. He also has great respect for Sloan-Kettering. I think my doctor saw the merit in both forms of treatment, and he really left the decision up to me. At one point I said to him, "If this were your wife, what would you tell her to do?" and there was no question in his mind that he would have told his wife to have a double mastectomy. However, he also saw the merit in not doing a double mastectomy and just having highly increased vigilance, keeping up with the mammogram and absolutely, without question, taking the tamoxifen.

So taking the tamoxifen, for me, was a big step, believe it or not, because it's very difficult to go from being a totally healthy young woman to having to take what I felt was a very toxic medication. At that time it was an extremely difficult decision because I had to, first of all, admit to myself that I had a problem, and it's very easy to deny the fact that you're a candidate for a problem because hey, there's nothing wrong with me. I'm fine.

What happened then is that I did not take the tamoxifen right away. We really talked about it for quite some time, and emotionally I had a very difficult time, even though I was aggressive in finding out what it was that I had to do. It took me a long time to get myself to take the medication. My husband left the decision mostly up to me. From a professional point of view and the research that he did, he felt very strongly that I should take the tamoxifen. My hesitation with taking the tamoxifen was that to me it seemed like a toxic medication. I believe what it does is put you into a chemically induced menopause, and I wasn't ready for that. You know, I was young, and I felt full of life. I didn't feel sick at all. I also happen to be one of those people who reacts very strongly to medicine, so if I ever take a medication, I usually have to take the children's dose. I was afraid to take the medicine because I didn't know what it would do to me. It turns out my fears were substantiated because I had every reaction in the book.

I had very severe headaches from it. I went from being a very active, energetic person to a person who was exhausted all the time. It causes vaginal dryness, and that just hit me from the blue. I had never experienced anything like that before. I had heard people talk about it but I never knew what it was until it actually happened to me. I also had daily upset stomachs. It causes sleeplessness.

I had to tell myself, "Well, maybe there was an emotional aspect to this also." But over the course of five years, I was able to separate the emotional strain of taking the tamoxifen from the actual physical effects because we started treating the physical effects. I was able to treat the vaginal dryness. I started taking sleeping pills so that I could sleep. I started taking things to help my upset stomach, and it was very difficult to take it.

I also had problems with hot flashes. Only another woman who has had them can truly understand what they are. It's just a flash of heat that begins on the inside of your body and just overtakes you. You never know when it's going to happen, and you just break out into a sweat and your hair gets wet. Even worse were the night sweats because they disrupt your sleep, and you wake up drenching wet. You have to change your nightgown and sometimes the sheets. And then you can't fall back asleep.

So I had just about every side effect in the book. How did I get myself to stay on the tamoxifen? I intellectualized about it. I told myself I was on a greater mission, and I knew that it was for five years, so I always felt that there was a light at the end of the tunnel. If I could survive this for five years, at least I knew that chemically I had done everything that I could to reduce the possibility of developing breast cancer. That's how I got myself to do it, and for five years it was a daily challenge. Now some things did get better over the course of the five years. The upset stomachs were not as severe. I think I just got used to the side effects.

> *How did I get myself to stay on the tamoxifen? I intellectualized about it. I told myself I was on a greater mission, and I knew that it was for five years, so I always felt that there was a light at the end of the tunnel.*

I really felt that I was on a mission. That's how I spoke to myself. That I was on a five-year mission and that there was a purpose for it, and I thought a lot about my children, who now are in their early twenties but were teenagers when this all started. I think the last time I spoke to my doctor about it, he told me that taking the tamoxifen reduces your chance of breast cancer by up to 85 percent, and not only that, but the benefits of it stay with you after you finish taking it.

I've never been tested for the BRCA gene. We've talked about it, and there's a possibility that I will. My first thought is, "Why not?" I know all the pros and cons, all the reasons why it's good to do it and all the negative reasons for doing it.

I think if I were tested for BRCA, my main reason would be for the benefit of my two daughters. If I were tested for BRCA and it was a positive test, then I would opt more seriously for a mastectomy and I would just counsel my children, again, to have increased vigilance. Knowledge is power. The more you know, the better off you are.

Then, of course, I am aware that there are other things that can happen if you test positive for BRCA. You have to decide about your ovaries. If your place of employment finds out, does that make you a risk for insurance? Does that make you a risk for employment? I think I would just be more concerned with health issues rather than other issues. It is a difficult decision, but I have decided already that if I ever have it done, it will be a good thing to do. We're working on getting it approved by the insurance company now.

One of the reasons I am a little more aggressive about having the BRCA testing is because my mother was diagnosed with breast cancer last year, at age 79. My mom, thank God, is great. She now is 80 years old, and she was treated with a lumpectomy and radiation therapy. She has never had a recurrence. My mother is now on tamoxifen and has had zero side effects!

I think because I took the tamoxifen, I reduced my chances of something ever happening. I feel really good now that I took the tamoxifen. I feel that I won that part of the war. Statistically, it was the best thing to do. Would I do it again? Yes. Would I have a difficult time doing it again? Yes. Should I have done a prophylactic mastectomy? Fifty/fifty, I guess. If you get ten doctors in the room, five of them will say I should have done it and five of them will say not. I get very emotional when I think about it. So on one hand I feel victorious. On another level, you still feel scared. I think it's a fear that, once it's with you, it just doesn't go away.

I am married to a physician, and sometimes when I go to see doctors I am not intimidated by them at all. I can speak to them just as plainly as I am speaking to you. I know that people often don't want to take up too much of their doctors' time, or they don't want to keep asking the same questions over and over again. They want their doctors to think well of them. I could see how that might be a problem for some women when they have to make these choices, and

> *If I had to call the doctors, I called them. If I had to ask the same question 1,500 times, I asked the same question.*

they don't want to bother their doctors, necessarily. It just didn't concern me at all. If I had to call the doctors, I called them. If I had to ask the same question 1,500 times, I asked the same question.

The first life lesson that this has taught me was that you have to take charge of your own body. You can go to as many people as you want for opinions, but the ultimate decision has to be your own. To make a decision like this you have to feel confident that you have exhausted all intellectual avenues to discover what your options are. I went to the bookstore. I went to the library. I went on the Internet, anything that mentioned the word LCIS or tamoxifen, I guarantee you, if I could find it, I read it.

The doctor at Sloan-Kettering was the first one to tell me, "You take tamoxifen because it could save your life. All of the side effects, I can treat every single side effect. If you're having headaches, I can give you something for headaches. If you're having vaginal dryness, we can treat the vaginal dryness. If you're having hot flashes, we can treat the hot flashes. No matter what," he said, "I can treat those side effects." And as I look back on it, I think that was the turning point.

The overall effect that all this had on me, at first, quite frankly, was a very depressing one. It took the wind out my sails, and I couldn't just go on with life as if a change hadn't occurred. I didn't really know myself for a long time. You take a step back, and you realize how vulnerable you are. You feel very, very vulnerable. You feel the finality of life. You realize that you're just one little teensy-weensy person in this huge universe and how can you make a difference? I think it definitely had a very deep effect on me. It took me a while to redefine myself and to get to know myself again.

I've always been compassionate, but it's taken me to a new level of compassion for people in general. You know, if someone is in a bad mood or standoffish one day or is depressed one day, then there might very well be a good reason for it.

So, if I had to do it all over again, I would. Would it be difficult? Yes. And you just push yourself. I think ultimately it makes you a stronger person, and it makes you realize that you can do things that you never thought you'd be able to do, and that you could make decisions that you never thought you would have to make. It pushes you to a new level of maturity, and without a doubt it just makes you a more compassionate person.

Laura is a 62-year-old retired nurse. Her mother and sister had breast cancer, and a recent biopsy revealed that Laura had atypical ductal hyperplasia. She decided against treatment with tamoxifen.

I grew up in the Midwest in a small town. My aunt was a nurse. I knew that was what I wanted to do also. After high school, I attended nursing school in Boston. During those three years, my mother developed breast cancer and underwent a mastectomy. She recovered well and didn't need radiation or chemotherapy (which were not common forms of treatment then). I went on to work in nursing for over twenty years in pediatrics, neurosurgery, and also in oncology.

During much of that time, there was little we could do for children or adults with cancer, though toward the end of my career the treatments seemed to be improving. The surgery for breast cancer also was less radical and disfiguring, and it seemed that mammograms were helping to identify them at an earlier stage. My sister is a good example. She had a routine mammogram, and the doctor saw a few small specks of calcium that concerned her. My sister had a biopsy, which revealed a small area of breast cancer. So she had a lumpectomy and then radiation. She did not need chemotherapy, and the doctors feel that she is cured because the tumor did not spread to the lymph nodes or outside of the milk ducts.

I have had regular mammograms, and this year they found some abnormal calcium deposits. A surgeon performed a biopsy, and the calcium deposits were benign. But close by they found some atypical cells: atypical ductal hyperplasia. I read about this on the Internet, discussed it with my gynecologist and my surgeon. At their insistence I also went to see an oncologist. The oncologist was very nice and upbeat and told me clearly that I didn't have breast cancer in any form. He did tell me, however, that I am at a higher risk of developing breast cancer for several reasons, including my mother's and sister's history, and this breast biopsy. The doctor pulled out a calculator and put in information that allowed him to calculate my risk of breast cancer during the next few years and during my lifetime.

I realize that my risk is higher than most. I really don't deny it. My lifetime risk is significantly higher than most women's, though on the other hand my risk in the next five years is relatively low and is probably under 5 percent.

This risk does run through my mind, but I am a person who tries to deal with one day at a time and remain level headed.

This risk does run through my mind, but I am a person who tries to deal with one day at a time and remain level headed. The relatively low risk in the next five years is important to me.

The oncologist discussed with me that taking tamoxifen can reduce my risk of developing breast cancer. He reviewed information from a very large trial that showed that the risk of breast cancer can almost be cut in half by taking tamoxifen for five years. So I thought about it in detail, trying to weigh the risks and benefits.

Personally, I hate to take medications, any medications other than vitamins. I don't like antibiotics. I didn't take the birth control pill or any hormone replacement therapy, and although my cholesterol is slightly high, I am watching my diet carefully. I am concerned about what effects medications will have on me both in the short and the long term.

For now I've decided against taking tamoxifen as a preventative strategy. I have read about the problems that women have with hot flashes, which were a big issue for me years ago when I went through menopause. I am also concerned about the slightly increased risk of blood clots, because I have had two friends who had that problem who weren't on tamoxifen at all. I know that some women worry about the risk of endometrial cancer, but fortunately I have had a hysterectomy and so that would not be a worry for me.

I may reconsider this decision, and I do think about it from time to time. I see my breast surgeon and my gynecologist each once a year, and I have mammograms regularly. I also have a lot of confidence that if I do develop breast cancer, it will be diagnosed early and be cured, and that has given me some confidence to hold off on tamoxifen for now.

CHAPTER 20

Stories from Women

with Non-Invasive Breast Cancer

D uctal Carcinoma In Situ, known as DCIS, is the diagnosis of breast cancer located only in the breast ducts. It has not invaded through the duct walls, and it has not spread to other parts of the body. For women with DCIS, the critical aspect of treatment is making sure that the cancer does not recur locally in the breast. Fortunately, the risk of the cancer recurring outside of the breast is small.

Most women diagnosed with DCIS are advised to choose between lumpectomy with radiation therapy and mastectomy. A small minority of women with DCIS have lumpectomy without additional treatment. These women generally have very small areas of DCIS with a "low-grade" appearance under the microscope. Many women with DCIS also choose to take a medication such as tamoxifen, which may reduce the risk of local recurrence in the affected breast after radiation treatment and the risk of cancer developing in the other breast.

Joyce underwent lumpectomy followed by radiation therapy. She took tamoxifen and then was switched to a different hormonal therapy.

I thought only busty women got breast cancer. After all, my first cousin and aunt, both of whom survived breast cancer, wore D and DD, respectively. Boy, was I wrong.

I never had a regular menstrual cycle since I first began menstruating. During my senior year in college, I noticed I was growing hair in all the wrong places. I went on birth control for a couple years to regulate my hormones. My hair started falling out, and I discontinued the pills. Shortly thereafter, I started on hormone replacement therapy and continued for the next ten years. Later, I would learn that this ultimately caused my cancer.

I had just turned 35 in 1998 when, during a self-examination, I discovered a lump in my breast. Two weeks before I was to get married, a mammogram confirmed it. My family doctor recommended a highly reputable surgeon. The surgeon informed me that in almost all cases, lumps this size turn out to be benign and that I had nothing to worry about. Removal of the lump was scheduled after returning from my honeymoon.

Much to my chagrin, the lump in my breast turned out to be malignant. I met with my surgeon, a radiologist, and a highly recommended oncologist to discuss my options.

Given the size of the tumor and the fact that it was detected early (Stage I), lumpectomy followed by radiation was the agreed-upon treatment plan. After radiation, my oncologist recommended that I start taking tamoxifen. He told me that

> *After radiation, my oncologist recommended that I start taking tamoxifen. He told me that tamoxifen helps prevent the original breast cancer from returning and also helps prevent the development of new cancers in the other breast.*

tamoxifen helps prevent the original breast cancer from returning and also helps prevent the development of new cancers in the other breast.

Surprisingly, I got pregnant during my radiation treatments, so this precluded me from starting any medication until after my pregnancy. I began tamoxifen one month after my baby was born and discontinued it after twenty-two months when I started experiencing side effects that were unbearable. The drug had caused my uterine lining to thicken, causing excruciating pain, cramping, and bleeding. It was then that my oncologist prescribed Fareston, which I continued taking for an additional three years.

In hindsight, it's probably a good thing I was told the lump would most likely be benign. Otherwise, I would not have been able to relax and focus on the last minute details of planning my wedding, not to mention enjoying my honeymoon.

My husband, Duane, was diagnosed with colon cancer four months prior to my diagnosis. He, too, has been cancer-free for eight years. We both agreed that if our marriage could survive two cancer diagnoses the first year, we knew we could get through any turbulence in our marriage. I feel good about the decisions that were made regarding my treatment plan eight years ago and wouldn't do anything differently.

Nancy underwent mastectomy and reconstructive surgery. She then decided against treatment with tamoxifen.

In the fall of 1994, I was a 42-year-old wife and the mother of a high school freshman. I had graduated from college twenty years before with a B.S. in nursing. Always more of a tomboy, I enjoyed sports and outdoor activities. Being a nurse, I was kind of a health nut. I ate healthy, exercised, and was average weight. My aunt had had breast cancer in her sixties and was alive and well. I had no real risk factors for breast cancer, which is of course a fallacy, since most women have none.

Being aware of the importance of mammography, I had a baseline mammogram in my late thirties, another at 40, and then again at 42. I felt great, but something told me not to delay the mammogram. At that time, I was working in a family practice office, which was down the hall from the radiology department. The radiologist told me immediately that he had found microcalcifications in the left breast. He recommended a surgeon, who was also in the building, and briefly explained the needle localization biopsy procedure. At that point I wasn't in a panic, but I could have been. I was able to get in quickly to see the surgeon. My husband accompanied me on the first of many doctor visits. We made jokes about how weird it was with me exposed and my husband watching this other man do a breast exam.

It seemed like an eternity, waiting to have the biopsy, when in fact I was lucky with my connections to be getting in very quickly. With the needle placement, I had to have a radiologist do mammograms to locate

Survivors Tell Their Stories

the microcalcifications and actually place two extremely long needles in my breast so the surgeon would know the exact location.

Sitting and waiting was a bit frightful, as I was sure someone would bump into the needle. I was awake for the biopsy, which was probably a mistake. The smells are not the best. After looking at the tissue, my surgeon again tried to reassure me. He said there was a 97 percent chance that it would be benign. My husband was happy and thought I was nuts when I said I would wait for the biopsy results before I celebrated. Sometimes, we just have to listen to that inner voice, which was telling me that something was wrong.

Friday afternoon at work I finally got the call. Not the best way to find out you have cancer, but I appreciated knowing before the weekend. My head was going a million miles an hour as I tried to write down important information, what type of cancer, how large, etc. He gave me his home number and said to call him over the weekend if I had questions and that we would meet for an appointment Monday. Now in total panic, I called my husband to say I had cancer and that I was going home. I tried to call my pastor but didn't get through. So, in tears, I drove to our church and left a message for her to call. That night is a blur. I don't really remember telling my son or calling my parents or what my pastor said.

Saturday morning I was at the library, looking up anything to do with breast cancer. I took out several books and began reading diligently. Of course, my brain could only absorb miniscule bits of information. I read the same things over and over until I could process some of it. I was still in shock. I like things orderly, and I like to be in control. I was quickly spinning out of control. I also called National Cancer Information and requested information on ductal carcinoma in situ, which was the type of cancer I had. By Monday, I had a notebook with questions for my surgeon. My poor husband, who hates hospitals and doctors, came with me to all my numerous appointments.

Finding an oncologist was the first step. Two were recommended, and

> *I took out several books and began reading diligently. Of course, my brain could only absorb miniscule bits of information. I read the same things over and over until I could process some of it. I was still in shock.*

I chose one. Before meeting with him, still unsure of my decision, I spoke with a friend at church who had a neighbor who had just gone through breast cancer treatment. She raved about her oncologist and said he even came to her "end of chemo party." He was the doctor I had chosen.

I remember meeting with him in his office, notebook in hand and husband in tow. He basically explained that DCIS was the best kind of breast cancer to have, but that the type I had, comedo, was the worst kind of the best. Reading about it, I learned I would have a 30 percent chance of local recurrence if I chose a lumpectomy, which was what my surgeon was recommending.

Next I met with the radiologist, armed again with my notebook full of questions and husband again in tow. The doctor basically explained how radiation worked, but he didn't offer any extra information. Lawyers would have loved him on the stand. He did not answer direct questions. One of my concerns was how much damage the radiation would cause to my heart. He was not able to say 5 percent or 50 percent; he just concurred that there would be damage. Part of my decision process had to do with the fact that I was betting that heart disease would kill me before the breast cancer did.

I did not meet with a plastic surgeon before my surgery. I couldn't deal with the thought of reconstructive surgery at that time. I wanted the cancer out of my body right then. In the meantime, during my husband's and my anniversary dinner, my doctor called to say that the pathologist had discovered an area of microinvasion when reexamining the slides. Our lobster dinner sat on the table as I digested this latest information.

After much deliberation, I finally decided that I would be more comfortable having the mastectomy than the lumpectomy and radiation. It felt like a weight had truly been lifted once the decision was made.

After much deliberation, I finally decided that I would be more comfortable having the mastectomy than the lumpectomy and radiation. It felt like a weight had truly been lifted once the decision was made. I decided that if I had a recurrence and had to go back for more surgery, I would go nuts. I wanted to avoid radiating my left side. And, quite candidly, I wanted to be able to go home to Michigan for Christmas.

I had the mastectomy in November 1994. A year later I decided that

I would like to talk to a plastic surgeon about reconstruction. I realized that I was very self-conscious when wearing a bathing suit or anything that might reveal I was missing a breast. This time I was given only one option: a saline implant. I felt like I was being punished for being healthy. I didn't have enough fat to do the "tummy tuck" procedure. Now I had to decide if I really wanted to go through with several surgical procedures.

I did decide to have reconstruction, so now I have a "replacement." While it's not perfect, it has been a good fit for me. After the mastectomy, I also went for a second opinion to discuss the benefits of tamoxifin. While they felt I had a 95 percent chance of remaining healthy, tamoxifin could improve that by 1 or 2 percent. I wasn't willing to risk the side effects for such a small change and decided, with their blessing, not to take it.

Looking back, I know that my faith, my sense of humor, and the support from my family and friends got me through. I am thankful to have had breast cancer when I did, because it made me reevaluate my life. I have enjoyed taking more risks and doing things I never would have imagined, from taking a dory trip down the Colorado River through the Grand Canyon to riding in a gondola in Venice. Best of all, I enjoyed my son's high school and college graduations and have been able to see him grow into a wonderful man.

Would I make the same decisions today? Since I have had no further cancer and am much less concerned with the possibility of heart disease, I would most likely choose lumpectomy with radiation. I am also much less anxious about a diagnosis of cancer and wouldn't be as threatened by local recurrence as I was at the time of my diagnosis. Hindsight is always great.

Karen chose bilateral mastectomy and reconstructive surgery but decided against adjuvant therapy with tamoxifen.

I write this as I approach the one-year mark from when I was initially diagnosed with non-invasive breast cancer — DCIS. I was 44 years old and breast cancer was one of those things I never thought would happen to me. I maintained a healthy diet, exercised regularly, had three children (the first before I was thirty), breast fed all three, the first for one year, and had no family history. So I was shocked. The time was noteworthy, as I'd had my first mammogram on September 11, 2001, the day of the World Trade Center terrorist attack. In fact, I was leaving my appointment when I heard the news of the attack.

I am one of those people who has often found herself in the negative "1 percent" rather than in the lucky "99 percent." I see myself as a survivor. All of my boys were delivered by c-section, despite two valiant efforts for a vaginal birth. The second birth was the most challenging — it was then that my unluckiness in being one of the 1 percent was most vivid — the OB cut my bladder and then the urologist who was called in to repair the damage sewed my bladder to my uterus, requiring extensive repair surgery and a long recovery when my middle son was three months old and my older son was three and a half.

I know firsthand that bad things happen to good people.

I had experienced a variety of those types of situations in my life so I felt certain that the suspicious mammogram was going to be breast cancer. My view may also be shaped by the fact that both of my parents are Holocaust survivors, so I know firsthand that bad things happen to good people.

I understood research odds but my gut response spoke loudly. I was in a wonderful place in my life. I loved my job; I am tenured at a university and had just taken over as director for the family studies program, my passion. My children were at great ages: 15, 11, and 6, and I had just celebrated my twentieth anniversary with my husband. We shared family responsibility and had additional help at home. So when I received that call for a repeat mammogram, I knew only that I wanted to live and live cancer free.

Once the mammogram was confirmed as suspicious, I was in the radiologist's office at the breast center. This was truly a low point. What do I do next? Trying not to cry in front of all these strangers who suddenly looked at me differently (or so I felt), I didn't know what to do or who to call. One of the nurses or technicians suggested I call my GYN, which I did. They gave me a surgeon's name. I set up an appointment for five days later.

I received the biggest assistance from an oncologist who is also a friend. I was feeling so vulnerable that I didn't want to call him for a referral for a surgeon, but my husband insisted and was willing to make the call. He was able to help me get an appointment sooner with a surgeon he thought highly of. My friend/adviser was the biggest help in all the decisions yet to come.

I also received help in making decisions from a good friend who had been treated for breast cancer the year before. She was very knowledgeable and well read and wanted to give me so much information. She

She was very knowledgeable and well read and wanted to give me so much information. She also cared deeply for me and wanted to help. But it was TMI (Too Much Information)!

also cared deeply for me and wanted to help. But it was TMI (Too Much Information)! I was able to say this to her and ask for one book that she found informative.

One of the keys for me when making these decisions was to know myself—who I wanted to talk with, what I wanted help with, and when there was too much information. I am a very private person so each outreach was intimidating.

The breast surgeon was my next contact. I immediately liked her. She was to the point and had a surgeon's manner, but I sensed sincerity about her. I came to value sincerity above all as the next month unfolded.

She was to the point and had a surgeon's manner, but I sensed sincerity about her. I came to value sincerity above all as the next month unfolded.

There were times in my conversations with the surgeon when I felt things were moving too fast, and I didn't know if I was clearly communicating. But a few seconds or minutes later she would say something that let me know she had heard me. The core biopsy was scheduled for two weeks later. It was a long time to wait, not knowing if I had cancer and if I did, what type. During the biopsy I asked a lot of questions, and my husband wanted to come in and see the image and speak to the radiologist as well.

Perhaps the most difficult moment was calling the doctor's office to hear the results. I had read the book my friend suggested, so I had some background information to work with. The results were good/bad news: DCIS. The surgeon spoke with me about options and then scheduled an appointment five days later for my husband, David, and me to look at options. I had a lot of questions. I talked to my friend, and the night before the appointment I made an exhaustive, typed list of everything on my mind. David and I also talked about the role I wanted him to play. I was the talker, and then he added his questions.

By the time I arrived in the surgeon's office, I knew my decision would be focused on doing what I could to be fully living my life ASAP. I have always been a person who resisted medication or any intervention into my body.

This was no different; I wanted as little intervention from drugs or radiation as possible. I am very health-conscious and this was a guiding factor in all decisions. I was a small-chested woman wearing a 32A bra size all my life, and thus my identity about how I looked was more tied into being slender and physically fit than in being shapely. Another factor that came into the equation was that my husband's 47-year-old cousin died from breast cancer five months before my diagnosis. The story as we heard it was that they watched a suspicious lump and then it was too late. While my situation was very different, this information did have an impact.

One decision seemed to lead to another, and there were stumbling blocks. Some decisions were clear—a mastectomy versus lumpectomy and radiation. I envisioned a lumpectomy removing much of my breast, and I was opposed to radiation. I did not want to be in treatment that long, and I was afraid of the side effects. I did not want anything put into me but could handle removing something that was cancerous.

In discussions with my friend/adviser, the potential use of tamoxifen came up once again. This was overwhelming to me. The side effects scared me. That led me to consider a bilateral mastectomy. My question was, would aggressive surgery eliminate the need for prevention like tamoxifen?

Perhaps of most help after discussing this situation with my friend was talking with a woman who had had a similar diagnosis and had the bilateral mastectomy. She was a working mother with two children around the ages of my sons when she was diagnosed and treated. She told me about her decision-making process. I learned that she did not initially consider reconstruction, but a few years after the bilateral mastectomy she opted for the reconstructive surgery. This was critical information for me, as I was stumbling over the decision about reconstruction for the same "don't put anything in my body that doesn't belong" reason. Many people in my life were encouraging me to have the reconstruction, but I was resistant. Talking with someone who had similar ideas helped me a lot.

There were also those moments when something was said innocently that impacted my decision. For example, my boss at work talked about her administrative assistant who had a similar diagnosis. She'd had a mastectomy one year and then cancer was found in the second breast, so she had the second mastectomy a year later. The most influential part of our conversation was when I asked about reconstruction. She laughed and said she did not have the procedure. Sometimes she forgot to put the prosthesis in, and other days it slid so it stuck out over her shirt. The conversation was innocent on her part but eye opening for me. I went for a consult with a plastic surgeon shortly after.

Finding the right plastic surgeon was important to me, as I wanted to look like me, small chest and all. The first plastic surgeon and his office staff made me feel very uncomfortable. In fact, it was one of the few experiences after which I went home and cried. I called the breast surgeon's office, and the kind office manager made arrangements for me to see another plastic surgeon. He was very low key and what I needed. So I had two decisions made: bilateral mastectomy and reconstruction with implants at the time of the mastectomy. Other procedures for the reconstruction were not even considered. The thought of additional surgery—particularly abdominal or other muscular surgery—was more intimidating than the idea of putting something foreign in my body. I had been through abdominal surgery and never have forgotten my four recoveries. Plus it conflicted with my overriding goal to do this fast, with as little anesthetic as possible, and to get me back to living life as usual.

There was one final decision that I pushed for: the sentinel node biopsy. The breast surgeon was quite clear that it was totally unnecessary. I believed her but was still afraid. I felt that I was being so aggressive in other ways that I did not want to leave anything unexplored. It was very difficult to arrange the sentinel node biopsy, and it was a subject that was difficult to resolve while keeping the same surgery date.

I began to doubt myself and called the oncologist. I had to page her, which is something I rarely do. She was wonderful and helped me talk it through and feel OK about my desire to have the procedure. She and my friend/adviser also went that extra mile and helped navigate the arrangement of the procedure. It was such a gift to have that help when my courage and confidence seemed low.

The final decision was one to have genetic testing because of my Ashkenazi Jewish background. This was not a hard decision for me, as I worried about the link between breast and ovarian cancer. So after the surgery, I went for genetic testing and counseling and was found not to have that gene mutation.

My treatment is complete. I have had a bilateral mastectomy, and there was a tiny bit of the same type of cancer found in my second breast. I completed most of the reconstructive process, but when it came time for the nipple reconstruction and tattoo, I felt like I had had enough. Emotionally, I did not want one more procedure, no matter how benign a procedure it was. So I am reconstructed but nippleless and OK.

I look back on those many decisions made so quickly and am clear about what helped me make decisions, none of which I regret: my friend/adviser, the other oncologists, and the breast surgeon who listened and heard what I had to say. They problem solved with me. I was treated like a person with ideas and feelings, and the sincerity that was demonstrated and the time and patience so kindly given are things I will not ever forget, think of often, and will always be thankful for. My husband was also very helpful in my decision making. He kept his thoughts and opinions to himself and clearly would have supported any decision I would have made. But the gift to me was that he and I arrived at the same decision. His total support gave me that extra boost throughout the process.

At the time of my decision, I did not understand how anyone would not choose a mastectomy. To me, being free of the fear of cancer return was the prevalent issue. In retrospect I realize the enormous decision I made and frankly that is what I wrestle with. I did not know then that it would make such an impact on me, but the mastectomy and reconstruction have made an impact. I am different inside and continue to process the experiences I have had.

I got what I wanted, quick intervention that removed the fear of reoccurrence. I overlooked one thing, and that was that despite the relatively quick treatment for cancer, the internal process of dealing with my changed body and coming to terms with how having cancer (even non-invasive cancer) has influenced me,

> *I have no regrets and know that I would make the same decision again, but I understand how important this decision is, and I have profound understanding and respect for women who make different choices.*

continues to be something I think about. I have *no* regrets and know that I would make the same decision again, but I understand how important this decision is, and I have profound understanding and respect for women who make different choices.

Toby was 45 years old when she was diagnosed with a small non-invasive breast cancer. She underwent lumpectomy and received radiation but decided against tamoxifen. Unfortunately, Toby experienced a local recurrence of the cancer in her breast one year later and required a mastectomy. She still does not want to take tamoxifen. Two years after her mastectomy, she tested positive for the BRCA gene mutation.

I went for a regular physical with my internist, and he was horrified that I hadn't had a mammogram in five years so he wrote me a prescription. I put it off for a few months. My mother is 90 and has no history of breast cancer, and nobody in my immediate family ever had breast cancer. I felt confident, but I got a call a few days after the mammogram, from the internist, saying that something had shown up, and they wanted me to go see a surgeon to see whether I needed a biopsy. I talked with the surgeon, and we scheduled a stereotactic biopsy which is the least invasive. It's outpatient surgery with just a local anesthetic. I was not worried.

The surgeon called me around dinner time and said that in fact the biopsy came back positive and that he wanted me to come into his office the following week and we would discuss the options. So it was surreal. I got through the weekend somehow, and then I ended up having a lumpectomy on September 7, 2001. He took wide margins. It was a two-centimeter lump with large margins, and he again said, "Everything looked really good after the lumpectomy but you know, we'll have the final results in a few days. Come back to my office next week, and we'll talk about it." The day I was scheduled to go back, and I did go back, was September 11, 2001, and it was an incredible day. My husband, Carl, was in Manhattan on September 11, and all the phones were out so I was panicked all morning, not knowing what was happening to Carl, and the results of my lumpectomy were secondary. I heard from Carl at 1:30. I went to the doctor at 2:00.

When I got to the doctor's office I was the only patient there. No one else had shown up, and they brought a TV into the reception room, and the doctor and his receptionist were watching TV. This is so connected to my story. We were watching everything on TV, the doctor, the receptionist, and me, and I was telling them that my husband was there. And then finally, after about fifteen or twenty minutes the doctor said, "Well, we really should go back in my office and talk about the reason that you're here, which is for the results of the lumpectomy." That was a very strange juxtaposition of events for the beginning of my cancer. He said he took wide margins, and they were clean. He suggested I go see an oncologist and find out what I needed to do next.

The oncologist suggested that I take tamoxifen and that I have radiation. There was no need for chemotherapy because I had clean margins and it had not gone into the lymph nodes. He said that tamoxifen was a good preventive measure and radiation was a strongly encouraged follow-up to a lumpectomy. Honestly, I didn't want anything. I'm not opposed to medication but I like going with the least invasive treatment first. The thing with tamoxifen, and it's very vain, is my concern that it will chemically induce menopause, and I think I'm so close, probably within a couple years, of having it naturally. I just want to enjoy whatever comes naturally without inducing it. The other part of it is I think I am a total optimist. I don't panic, and I don't say, "Oh, my God, I'm probably going to get cancer again." It just seemed like taking tamoxifen and changing more about my body and my life was overkill. I kept thinking that the cancer itself was caught so early.

The radiation oncologist explained everything in a way that made me realize, it's only a few weeks out of my life. The side effects would probably to be minimal, if any, and so that seemed OK to me. Carl and I talked about it and were in sync the whole way. It's amazing; we are really different in a lot of ways but we came up with the same decision

Survivors Tell Their Stories

about radiation. The tamoxifen is one thing we did disagree on, but I didn't want to take the tamoxifen and he thought that was fine if it comes back and I catch it early. I absolutely go for mammograms now every six months, and I'll go to all the doctors every few months.

The radiation went great, and actually I ended making friends with all the people. I had no side effects from it. I didn't get tired. I didn't have the dried skin, the pink skin. My parents are survivors of the Holocaust and the thing that was absolutely the most upsetting to me was when you have radiation they mark you with permanent marker. Actually, I was very fortunate. The place I went uses a marker. Other places use tattoos so that when they line you up each morning for the radiation they pinpoint exactly where it is and they usually put in little blue dots, tattooed dots, and that I would not have done. My parents have the numbers on their arm, and I would not have done tattooing. Where I went was state of the art, and they just use permanent marker that goes away after six or seven weeks. It was just marker, but I hated seeing that. I hated getting undressed to take a shower and seeing these blue marks all over my body. I hated that, but that went away, so that was fine. So I was done. I had the radiation. I felt I appeased my oncologist.

I was fine, and that was January of 2002 when that was finished. I had a mammogram in August, and I was fine, 100 percent fine, so pretty much that was it. I didn't even think of myself at that point, at all, as ever having breast cancer. Just mentally it just wasn't my self-image. It just wasn't. So the first mammogram in August was fine, August 2002. Then I had the next one in February 2003 and, thinking also, you know, no big deal, and while I was still sitting there in the radiation center, they called me back to talk to the radiologist. He said, pointing to little spots on the image, "We think this is a little spot, we think this is a little spot, we think this is a little spot."

I went back to the surgeon, and he looked at it. He again, the optimist that he is, said this; he compared the August 2002 little spots with the original August 2001 spots and they were different. They looked very different, and he said, "Well, I think it probably is calcification because if this is what cancer looks like in you and this looks so different, then this isn't." So I said, "OK." We scheduled another stereotactic biopsy, and this is where I feel like, "I'm not being stupid." You know, "I'm being responsible, I'm checking it out." He biopsied each of the three tumors, and each of the three was cancerous. So when I got those results, in his office, a couple days after the biopsy, that's when it hit me, and that was probably the worst day. I was by myself. Carl is with me at home, but all of the medical stuff I have mostly done by myself. I never thought it was that bad that I needed somebody.

My father had throat cancer, which actually was not . . . well, it was cured. It was managed and then cured. We didn't know it was cured. We thought that's what he died of, but he died of melanoma. He had melanomas also. We were so focused on the throat cancer, for ten years, that the melanomas were not taken care of. They were excised, but we weren't focused on them as much as we needed to be. He had one on his arm that traveled into his lymph nodes. So he died of melanoma. I went with my parents to the doctors because they would get overwhelmed and because of the language difference. I learned with my father to keep a little notebook and write up the appointment and what the doctor said and what the follow-up was going to be, so I do that for me, too. So from the very beginning I've had just a little notebook that I carry to every doctor's appointment, and I write things down, and I don't tend to become emotional in a medical situation. I don't know how to explain because I am a really emotional person, but I really stay focused in that situation.

I just didn't feel that I needed that support in the doctor's office. I think if my husband went with me, it would feel like I would have to protect him, care about him, when we're in the doctor's office. So I would rather just deal with it by myself and tell him my version. So, yes, he's there for me but not in the actual doctors' offices. So when the doctor told me one year later that the cancer had recurred the second time, the only option was a mastectomy because you can't have radiation twice because too much radiation causes cancer. So, because I already had radiation I had no choice. The only options I had were whether I wanted reconstruction and how I wanted it, but having the mastectomy was not an option. So I left the office, and the first thing I did was drive over to see the rabbi, which is really weird because although my rabbi and I have a very nice relationship, I don't go to him for support. We've got more of a friendship relationship. I still don't understand why I did that, but I went to him. Luckily, he was in his office. We've know each other

Survivors Tell Their Stories

for many, many years, and I closed the door and I just, I told him, "I have to have a mastectomy," and I just burst out crying. That was really surprising to me that he was the one I went to, because I did call Carl from the car. You know, on the way over, I called Carl first. I talked to the rabbi. With the rabbi, it was a good place to just cry immediately, and maybe I did that because I didn't want to with a girlfriend. I don't know. I don't know but he was very nice.

I had to go teach. I went straight from there, came home and got my books, and taught for two and a half hours. Teaching for me has been a godsend. It's like acting. I just got so into what I was doing that I didn't think about the cancer. I was absolutely fine for two and a half hours, and as soon as I got into the car to drive home I started crying again. That evening Carl and I talked about it and again; we were so totally in agreement that I would have the reconstruction immediately. There really wasn't a lot of discussion about it. It was not should I have it now, should I have it in a few months, should I have it at all. It was, you know, absolutely have a mastectomy and reconstruction the same day, and the type of reconstruction was, I chose to have a TRAM flap. A TRAM flap is all natural, where the doctor makes an incision from hip to hip in the lower abdomen and uses the abdominal tissue and one of the two abdominal muscles, pulls it up through, the tissue and the muscle through the chest to fill out the skin that's left after the mastectomy. So the mastectomy surgeon takes out all of the breast tissue but leaves the skin, and the TRAM flap is refilling that skin with abdominal tissue and one muscle. It is all natural, and there is no chance of the body rejecting any foreign object or needing some future surgery to fix or replace anything, and you get a tummy tuck in the meantime, which I always think, oh God, be careful what you wish for. Because my whole life I've had definitely the Eastern European stomach, and my whole life I've, like, pinched it and thought, "Oh, if I could just cut this off." I thought, I'm not wishing for anything bad like that again, but you know, you get a tummy tuck. What he also explained that very first day was it's a much, much bigger surgery than having just implants, and it's a much longer recuperation, but once you get through it all, the long-term aspects of it are really positive in that it's all natural and your figure does get the benefit of the tummy tuck.

I just adore my plastic surgeon, and he's very cute. If you're going to spend a lot of time with a doctor you might as well like looking at him, and he's adorable and I just adore him. I really do. So then I never interviewed any other plastic surgeons because I had such absolute faith in my surgeon and my oncologist. If they both gave me the same recommendation, that was fine with me, and they were right. That's when the craziness began. I had about four weeks, maybe five weeks, between knowing that I needed a mastectomy and the actual surgery date. My friends all commented on how organized I was. I didn't break down. After that first initial going to the rabbi and crying, there were moments when Carl and I would sit together in the evening, and I would say, "Oh, my God, I'm going to have a mastectomy," or look at my breasts and think, "That's going to be gone in a month." I kept teaching. I did all the gardening outside because it was coming to be spring, and I knew that once I had the surgery, I wouldn't be able to do anything for months, so I did all my gardening. I went to a bath and bed shop and bought all the pillows I needed because when you have a TRAM flap you have to stay in a, kind of like a *W* position for weeks. You can't lie back. I went on the Internet, and I read everything I could find.

> *There were moments when Carl and I would sit together in the evening, and I would say, "Oh, my God, I'm going to have a mastectomy," or look at my breasts and think, "That's going to be gone in a month."*

I talked to an employee of the plastic surgeon's office, an older woman who was wonderful. She is there for helping you get through the day-to-day stuff. She knows I highlight my hair. She said, "Get your hair highlighted beforehand. First, it will make you feel good, second you're not going to be able to lean back to have it done." She said, "Go get your legs waxed," which I did, and I love it. She suggested that I get my hair permed. My hair is normally straight. She said, "You're not going to be able to lift your arm to blow dry for a couple of months, so do whatever you need to do to make your hair easy to take care of." So I had it highlighted and permed, so it was fun. She said, "You're going to have drains." "You're going to be swollen." "You're not going to be able to wear your clothes." "Go out and buy some things you'll like wearing." All of this to feel good. I love having her.

My oncologist takes care of me medically, and one day we talked about the medical implications and my prognosis for the future and all of that, and it was very emotionally heavy stuff. This was a month before the surgery. Then I went straight from his office to the plastic surgeon to talk about what I was going to do, and he's definitely not medically oriented in his conversation. It's more like, "OK, I can make you look however you want. Do you want to get bigger? Do you want to get perkier? Do you want to get rounder?" Insurance in Maryland pays for reconstruction on the healthy side to match. He said, "So let's see, do you want to go up to a C, or D, or this or that?"

That was the most confusing day to me because my oncologist had just told me, "I think you'll live to see your grandchildren." Then I go to the plastic surgeon, and he asks do you want to be a very perky DD when you get your grandchildren. It was too emotional. I can't go from, "Thank God, I'm going to live" to "How do I want to enhance my body?" because I never thought about plastic surgery ever, ever, ever. Well, then when I told my girlfriends about this, they all said, "Oh, yeah, get bigger, get perkier, I would if I were you." You know we're all at the age where everything is starting to droop. They thought I'd won the lottery, and they did that to make it more fun for me. So I went through a couple weeks of deciding how I wanted to improve. That's where Carl and I disagreed. Carl was always focused on the medical. He said, "I want you the way you are, and if you have to have reconstruction, just have the reconstruction to what you are and leave the healthy breast alone. Don't have surgery on something that doesn't need surgery." Well, we finally agreed that I would get "perky." I would stay the same size. I would not have an implant because to get bigger I would need an implant on the healthy side and it seemed kind of ridiculous if I chose to have the TRAM flap and this surgery to avoid an implant, why would I put one in when I don't even need one? I thought I'd get a little uplifted — that wouldn't hurt. So that's what we agreed on.

I was in the hospital. I was already hooked up to IVs. I am lying there ready to go in the operating room, and the plastic surgeon came once again to tell me what the side effects would be, like the consequences of these two surgeries, the TRAM flap and the lift or whatever it's called. I looked at him, and I started crying and said, "Can I still change my mind?" He's wonderful, and he said, "Yes." I said, "I don't want you to touch the healthy side. I just don't want you to do anything." The look on my husband's face was relief because he didn't want that, either. Carl burst into a big smile. The surgeon was there, too, because the surgeon does the mastectomy, then the plastic surgeon does the TRAM flap. The surgeon said, "You're making a good decision," and the plastic surgeon just laughed and said, "Well, I guess I get to go home earlier. It's less work for me." They were so wonderful. This was like ten minutes before wheeling me into surgery. I'm thrilled that that's what I decided. I think it just hit me then, I'm having this huge surgery here. I'm going to have scars, the whole thing of scarring. I am sure, in the recesses of my mind again, who my parents are was part of my decision. Because if you were scarred when you went through selection in concentration camps, if you were scarred or maimed in any way, you died. I am sure somewhere in my head I have internalized that scarring is not good. I just didn't do it, and they were wonderful.

I have done great, really great. I had physical therapy for two months, three times a week, for two months to just learn how to stand up straight and move again because things are in the wrong place, one of the muscles that helps us stand straight and stretch and do all that now is not there. I am regaining balance and am pretty much back to the way I was before the surgery.

We had a graduation party for both girls, because they both graduated, in August. I couldn't do it in June; I didn't have the strength. We had a big party here in August, and my cousins from out of town were staying with us. That was overwhelming. I cracked physically. I tried to go overboard to make a nice party, and it was so tiring. During the party we had about sixty-five people here. I went upstairs, and I just sat on the bed. "I can't do this, I don't want to go back down. I just want to lie down." I denied how much of a toll this has taken on my body — physically, not emotionally. The surgeon said it takes about a year after surgery to be back to normal, and my year is next week. It hasn't even been a year yet. So it was just a few months after surgery, and I'm acting like I can do everything — I'll wear my high heels, I'll have my sixty-five people over. It does take a toll. But I went back to work two weeks after the surgery. I could hardly stand up.

After surgery I was totally numb. I couldn't feel anything. Also, the skin over the TRAM flap developed blisters, and the doctor got worried about the blisters. I had what's called a skin-sparing mastectomy. Usually, with a mastectomy they cut almost like a football shape and take everything out. I wanted reconstruction, and all of my doctors were so concerned with how I would do physically afterward, which I really, really appreciated. So what they did for me was just take a little, the areola, and just a little bit bigger than that. A little bit around it and so it makes it more difficult for the surgeon to take all of the tissue out through this very small opening, but physically, aesthetically for the female, it's better. Afterward, you have to wait a certain amount of time, then they redo it; they make the nipple. They put a nipple on there and then tattoo the area to match the color of your natural one, and then there's no scar. I mean, you can't see it. You just can't see it, so ideally, with the TRAM flap, you can't tell if a woman has had reconstruction. You don't see any scars. The only scar would be that round circle, and that's tattooed.

With the skin blistering, we had to wait to finish the reconstructive surgery. I just had the nipple redone in January. Normally, it would be done about three months after the TRAM flap. They just want the patient to heal enough to undergo another procedure, but with me the skin wasn't there, and we didn't know what was going to happen. It's an incredible healing process to see what the body can do. All I did was take care of it with the ointments and the moisturizing that I needed to, and other than that there was no medical intervention at all. It just did it all by itself. It's a little discolored in parts; it's not evenly pink or white. But it's fine, and I keep thinking, I guess I am genetically a child of survivors.

I came home from the hospital Saturday night, and Carl and my younger daughter left Sunday afternoon to visit colleges. My older daughter Beth stayed with me for two days. She came home from college, and she was great. She did everything. Talk about cheer! I love being cheered on, and I'd go to the bathroom, and she'd say, "Mommy, you went to the bathroom, good job." We still joke about that. She was so adorable. She washed my hair in the sink, which was a huge ordeal. She put out the water for me. When Carl came back from the college visits, she had never done this in her whole life, but she yelled at him, absolutely yelled at her daddy for not taking care of me the way he needs to. She said, "You have to put out the orange juice for Mommy in the morning." "You have to . . . " I had flowers all over the place. "You have to water the flowers because Mommy loves flowers, and she can't water them. She can't walk around and water them, and you have to water them for Mommy." I told her I never had an advocate in my whole life, and she was my advocate.

> *I never had an advocate in my whole life, and she was my advocate.*

After my first lumpectomy and radiation, my oncologist wanted me to start tamoxifen to reduce the risk of a local recurrence and to reduce the risk of cancer in the other breast. After my mastectomy he again discussed it as a preventative for the healthy breast and he wanted me to take tamoxifen and I said no. It's cutting the risk and so he thinks it could prevent yet another cancer in the future. I tell him this every time, "When I start to go into menopause naturally, I promise I will take tamoxifen." He's always told me, "When you start, that's when the benefits start." So you can start at any time, although he suggests that I start it now. I'm 48. I don't think I have that many more years before menopause. I know I am in perimenopause now, so if I wait two or three years, is it going to be that awful? And he says no.

Beth was age 51 when diagnosed with a small-focus, low-grade DCIS. She chose lumpectomy and then decided against receiving radiation therapy. She presently is taking tamoxifen.

I went for my annual mammogram on October 30 and was sent on my way as usual. However, a few days later I received a message to return for a second, confirmatory, mammogram, which I did on November 7. My husband went with me. This time the doctor on duty showed me a string of little white dots on the X-ray and said I should have a biopsy.

After talking to my primary care physician, I made an appointment with a surgeon who'd been recommended a few years before to aspirate a cyst. I liked him then because he explained everything thoroughly and helped me make decisions, and when I went to him on November 15, I was not disappointed. He put the X-rays up and discussed them with me. He actually suggested that I not have surgery (though he said that surgeons "love to do surgery," he thought it wasn't necessary at the time).

Instead, he thought I could wait six months and have another confirmatory mammogram before doing anything. He really didn't believe it was cancer. He also said that he could do a rather complicated biopsy if it would ease my anxiety—complicated because the spot was very tiny and deep, that is, close to my rib cage. It could not be felt by me or by any of the doctors. And, he said I could wait until after the holidays to do anything.

I talked to my primary doctor, then I asked a few friends for the name of another surgeon for a second opinion. I called the office of one of the "best" breast cancer surgeons in the area (and a woman) and was put off by an obnoxious receptionist; I cancelled the appointment I was making. (I have since recommended this surgeon to others, and they had a more pleasant experience.) I then called another surgeon recommended by a friend and went to see him on November 22. When he examined me, it was obvious he hadn't looked at my chart. He palpated the correct breast first, then said, "Hmm, must not be that one," and moved to the other side. He ended by telling me about all of the state-of-the-art equipment he had and that I should schedule surgery with the nurse in attendance. He may specialize in breast cancer surgery and he may have been able to hide the scar better than my surgeon, but I had no confidence in him.

I told a few friends and neighbors about my situation and anxiety; they all said they would pray for me. I even ended up on a prayer list at the church of a friend's mother. I would describe myself as quietly religious. I grew up in a deeply religious family, but I don't attend church regularly. I believe in the power of prayer, and I prayed for guidance at each step.

I made an appointment to have the biopsy in early January with the surgeon I liked at the hospital five minutes from our house. Then I busied myself with Christmas, singing and making gifts. The biopsy was January 9. My husband went with me. They had to insert a wire in X-ray prior to surgery, to pinpoint the spot for the surgeon. All went well, though I had a violent headache the next day—apparently from dehydration. There was a thick layer of bandages that I quipped "made me look like a Picasso, with one breast up and one down." I'm in my fifties, and I hadn't had surgery since I had my tonsils out at age 7, so I didn't really know what to expect. However, one of my friends told me they had experienced a lot of bruising, so I wasn't too shocked when the bandages came off and I had what I thought was a huge scar and was really black-and-blue. I called the surgeon's office for suggestions to minimize the scar and bruising. My mental state was that all was fine.

That changed when the surgeon called me on the fourteenth at about 8 p.m. to tell me that he had the "best bad news" he could give me. "The lab results indicated an intraductal carcinoma; it is very small (8 millimeters), apparently has not spread, I think I got it all. It is a type of cancer that is not known to spread to the lymph nodes. The cure rates are excellent. No one dies of this type of cancer." He changed my appointment from the next week to the next afternoon so he could give me a better explanation, face to face. He recommended I take an antihistamine to help me get some sleep. His parting words were, "You are not going to die."

After I got off the phone, I went to the National Cancer Society web site and looked up intraductal carcinoma and printed the information to take with me when I went to see him. He looked at the printout and thought it was good. (Some Internet info can be pretty bad.) We used it as a starting point for our discussion of options. The cancer they found was in the margin of the biopsy. He said he thought that an oncologist would want additional margin to see if the cancer had spread. He also said that this type of cancer was treated with radiation, not chemotherapy, and my cancer was so small that I might not even need radiation.

Though I got a lot of support from my husband, sister, and friends, I was emotionally a mess; I cried at the drop of a hat. But at the same time I had a lot of confidence that I'd gotten correct advice from the surgeon. I called my primary doctor for a recommendation for an oncologist, and although the oncologist said he would manage my case, I needed a radiation oncologist. He also recommended a second surgery for extra margin, just as the surgeon had said. I scheduled the second surgery for February 6; the surgeon wheeled me down to surgery himself as I prattled about him being my knight in shining armor saving this damsel in distress. This time, when the bandages came off, I wasn't interested in the scar but in the sunken appearance of the breast; he said he'd taken "extra extra margin," and I was very distressed. (I'm not big, so a little tissue was a big percentage.) The tissue came back cancer free. The surgeon said the breast would reshape itself over the next year, and I should wait and see. His parting words might be construed as disconcerting, but in a way they were comforting: "You won't lose your hair with radiation, and I hope I don't see you again unless it is a social visit."

I was distressed about how radiation treatments would affect my job and my singing. I already was more tired after the second surgery than I'd been after the first, and the healing took longer. Even though I again was wearing my emotions on my sleeve, I discussed my anxiety with friends, and I started telling key people at the office that I might need to work at home or take more than the usual time off. I also confided in my chorus director, since I'm one of the assistants, and my absence could be a problem. And I set a short-term and a slightly longer-term goal: I asked the chorus director to allow me to sing in the Mothers Day concert no matter how many rehearsals I missed, and I planned to participate in a concert tour to Paris in June.

> *Even though I again was wearing my emotions on my sleeve, I discussed my anxiety with friends, and I started telling key people at the office that I might need to work at home or take more than the usual time off.*

I saw my first radiation oncologist on March 5. He said the small size of the cancer, the nonspreading type of cancer, and the large margin the surgeon took meant that whether I had radiation or not was up to me. Women with small breasts are good candidates for radiation without complications. He could not tell me what my chances of recurrence would be, just that it wasn't high, and though radiation would reduce the number, the delta might not make much difference. Also, if cancer did return, it could be the same type or a more invasive type. He wouldn't say whether I should or shouldn't have radiation. I asked him if I would be making a big mistake not to have radiation, and he said no.

I felt I wanted a second opinion, and from a woman, so I went to see the second radiation oncologist on March 11. She gave me statistics: 10 percent recurrence rate for Grade III cancer with clean margins (half of those are invasive, but four out of five invasive cancers are cured). My prognosis for recurrence was closer to 5 percent with low-end Grade II cancer, and that could be cut in half by radiation. Also, radiation has its own impact on cells. She said she thought I didn't need radiation. It was the best birthday present I've had in a long time.

Every doctor, from the surgeon to the oncologist, recommended that I take tamoxifen (or one of the newer preventive drugs) for five years, whether I had radiation or not. So, when I decided not to have radiation therapy, I decided to continue with my oncologist managing the preventive drug. Part of that decision was that I would have close monitoring for five years in case of a recurrence. It has been two years. I have a mammogram scheduled for next week. I'm still working, singing, praying, and cancer free.

church, teaching Sunday school, and being a wife, mother, daughter, sister, aunt, friend, and colleague.

Then I went for a routine mammogram, and the staff started scurrying around, and the doctor was saying, "Do you feel a lump? What did your doctor say?" And I'm thinking, "My doctor said nothing." So he rushed me to a sonogram, and I began to panic some. I'm thinking, "What are they doing? Do they see something? What is this?" And they were scurrying around and talking to each other.

My internist had me see a surgeon who tried to do an in-office biopsy with a needle. It caused excruciating pain. He said he couldn't get it. Several days later I had another biopsy procedure, and then I had to wait for the results. It was weeks because the doctors were out of town, and I was calling and saying, "When is he going to call me?" Finally, the surgeon called me about 10 p.m., and he says, "How you doing?" I'm thinking, "You know, buddy, you call me at 10 o'clock. This doesn't sound good to me!" My husband was out of town. The surgeon said, "I hate to tell you this when you're by yourself, but we found breast cancer cells." And then he said, "Do you have any questions?" I was thinking, "You just told me I had breast cancer. Let me see . . . OK, right now, I'm in shock." I said, "I don't know what questions to ask right now."

The first thing I remember thinking was, "How long do I have to live?" You never think of breast cancer for yourself, so you don't prepare. My heart was dropping out of my chest and going on the floor, and I was filled with negative thoughts and negative feelings. You know: "Oh my gosh, how am I going to tell my parents? They're too old for this. Why should they have to go through this?" In my family, we didn't talk much about disease. OK, diabetes, yeah. You better watch it, watch what you eat. They would say, "Sugar, don't eat all of that because you'll get diabetes." They could talk about other diseases but not breast cancer. And I think it's because you don't want to say the word *breast* because *breast* is so sexual. And you don't want to say *cancer*, because I remember growing up, somebody had cancer, and it was almost as if it was something contagious. So, growing up in Mississippi, they didn't like the word *cancer*. I also thought of my son, who had just started at the Naval Academy, and I thought "It's too hard for him to

Survivors Tell Their Stories

hear this. He is working too hard to hear this." It was just such a sinking, hurt feeling.

I reached my sister later, and she said exactly what I needed to hear. She said, "God has not given you just the spirit but a power of the blood and a sound mind." Somehow, that was like water thrown on my face. I was like, "Oh, you're right!" I was emotionally hysterical for half an hour to forty-five minutes before we connected, and when she said that, I said, "You know what? You're absolutely right." If I ever was a Christian, it was at that moment. It was as if I began to heal right then and there. All I knew was that it was a big journey ahead. I didn't really know how big the journey was.

My husband and I went to meet with the surgeon, and I asked him how many months I had left to live. This is what he said to me, and it was almost insulting: "Oh, you just have a garden variety kind of cancer." I'm thinking, "Cancer is cancer. What do you mean, a garden variety?" He said, "Well, I see this all the time." I'll never forget "garden variety." I said to him, "You just pick out of the garden and just go make your nice salad." He almost laughed. I'm thinking, "I'll be dead tomorrow, and he is telling me I have a garden variety." I'm thinking, "Cancer is C-A-N-C-E-R. These wild, crazy cells inside of me."

One thing I was thinking was, "Oh my God, they're going to cut both breasts off probably. What's my husband going to do? How is he going to handle it? Will he ever be able to touch me again?" We had just had our twenty-seventh anniversary. We were at the surgeon's office very quickly, and the doctor began this conversation about "You have to do this and you have to do that and these are some of the things that some women choose." He was saying, "Well, you know, you could have a lumpectomy, but there are some people who want a mastectomy."

I don't even know what his words were, I just remember my feelings about what he was saying: "You have to decide," and "You two need to talk together and make some decision, but we would like to get something done soon." He's saying, "You have to decide for yourself. Look at your options." And I'm thinking, "What options? What options do I have?" Well, I got Susan Love's book, and I talked with the surgeon and he said, "You have to make up your mind because we do need to

> *"How fast is quickly? What's going on?" I just felt bombarded.*

do something and we need to do something quickly." I was thinking, "How fast is quickly? What's going on?" I just felt bombarded. The whole idea of "get the cancer out" was frightening.

So I went home and said to my husband, "Willy, what are you thinking about?"

"I don't know."

"What do you think based upon what he thinks we ought to do?"

"I don't know, what do you think?"

That's what I got from him. He was saying, "I don't know."

I went to another surgeon and to a medical oncologist for a second

> *"I can't live with statistics. I really can't."*

and third opinion. I got more reading material, and I got on the Internet, and I looked at some statistics — and statistics never look good for cancer people. You know, you have a "10 percent chance of whatever." I was thinking, "I can't live with statistics. I really can't."

I met with a biologist on campus, and I showed her my biopsy report. We talked and talked. I had a friend who had gone through this and died. And then I talked to my assistant pastor at church and about five or six other people at church. You know, a lot of people had gone through this, and I had made a conscious decision to let their stories be their stories. In other words, they weren't going to move me any kind of way, because people had all kinds of horror stories and told me, "I wouldn't take this, if I were you." But no one's me. I'm who I am. I also had books, and I was reading, reading, reading. By the time chemotherapy came around, I couldn't read anything, so I am so glad I read beforehand.

The night of the diagnosis, I knew nothing, so I felt real good about the lumpectomy, like, "Oh, I'm just doing this to save my breast," because the surgeon was saying things like, "Well, some people want to save their breast." A lot of what he was saying to me was implying, "I know you're going to feel real bad about this, and I know that you're going to feel vain about your breast." And I'm thinking, "Why are you saying this to me? Just give me the medical facts."

I chose to have a lumpectomy. I did a lot of reading about that, too,

Survivors Tell Their Stories

and I thought, "Why have a mastectomy when they could remove the cancer with a lumpectomy?" In fact, if I had needed a mastectomy, that was no problem, either. I did have one situation where a person told me, "I just told them to cut it off, even though they suggested I could have a lumpectomy, because I didn't want to be radiated." But then it occurred to me that every woman must make her own choice. Lumpectomy seemed like a reasonable thing to me.

The radiation experience was frightening. All that equipment over you, and the staff runs out of the room and leaves you in there. They can't even be near the place. Then I needed chemotherapy. When I went for my first appointment with my oncologist, my plan was to have as normal a life as I could. I had no idea about the doctor visits, and everyone's in there lined up, and it is so crowded and everyone's sick. I began to think everyone has cancer because the offices were so packed you barely had room to sit!

So, I decided I was going to settle down into this. Whatever comes is what I'm going to accept. But I needed time to get there. I didn't want to feel rushed. Because people just were rushing me. This thing about cancer, they rush you. But my oncologist was different. He spent so much time with me, I felt guilty. I was thinking, "Do you have any other appointments? How do you have this much time to give to me?" He was so nice, so wonderful, and I felt so affirmed by him. He talked to me, and he was drawing charts and breasts and this and that, and I'm thinking, "Thank you for giving me something." I was glad to have some facts and figures. The doctor walked me through the chemotherapy process that he recommended, and I started treatment soon afterwards.

A few weeks later my hair started to fall out. One morning my mom asked me if it was falling out yet, and I said, "No, I haven't lost it yet." But by that evening, I was pulling it out. It was the day that it was to come out. It was not attached to my scalp anymore. I was like, "Look, Willy!" I mean, it was almost fun. We had decided that we were going to do this ritual and just shave my hair. Chemotherapy was interesting. Fridays I just felt sick as a dog. On Tuesdays and Thursdays, I felt OK enough to go teach. There was only one time that I was lecturing and I thought, "I can't say another word." You know, I just felt tired, and I just finished the class.

I surrounded myself with positive things. I was reading about cancer, but I was also reading holistic kinds of things, about being at peace and spiritual kinds of things. I also made some lifestyle and career changes. I got off of every board I was on. It was too stressful. And I said, "Now, guess what? This is my life, people." Before this, I was giving too much and the school was taking too much, so I took my life a notch down. I thought, "They say they can't do without me. But if I died of breast cancer, they would do."

I did not take tamoxifen because they didn't find me estrogen positive, though they wanted me to be estrogen positive. It was like, "Oh, phooey, you're not estrogen positive, we can't put you on tamoxifen."

How is life different as a result of this experience? I am very different person. I think I live what I believe a lot more than I did before. I was leading this hurry-scurry, scattered life. People took too much out of me. I gave too much. You know how they have this book out, *Women Who Love Too Much?* How about *People Who Give Too Much?* I was giving too much. People acted as if they needed me, and they were taking from me in ways that I wasn't receiving. Because if people feel as if they are receiving from you, you always stay on the giving end.

I'm thankful for being able to settle in with this. I'm more at peace. I'm a better wife at home. I think, "Just let him be." You know, he's a lot freer. He just bought a sports car.

Now I say, "Yesss! Do it!"

Before, I would have thought, "Who does he think he is?" But now I say, "Yesss! Do it!" I want my life to be enhanced now. I am not going to be a contributor to any negative life. I'm just not going to do it. I'm going to just enjoy what I have each day. Despite it being cancer, I still received a gift. There is nothing that can be done that can conquer me. Nothing. Even death. You see what I'm saying. So, it's like each step of the way, there's nothing that could win. I win through this.

Anne, a choreographer, was 75 years old when she chose to undergo mastectomy without reconstructive surgery. Several of her lymph nodes were positive for cancer. Anne decided to take tamoxifen. Her oncologist encouraged her to consider chemotherapy, as well, which she declined. She also

underwent a breast reduction on her other breast one year after her mastectomy. She contributed the following story ten years later, at age 85.

It was more than a year since I'd had my last mammogram. I was very busy taking care of my husband, who had recently gone through brain surgery, and I had just completed months of rehearsals for a musical. I had a performance scheduled, and while performing, I noticed my body just didn't feel right and I could not move well. Frustrated and disgusted, I went back to the dressing room and changed into low-heeled dance shoes. Nothing helped. I couldn't believe that I couldn't trust my balance. I gathered at that time that it was stress, but it just made me more aware to get moving, to take care of myself, and to get that mammogram taken.

The doctor looked at the new mammogram and mentioned that he saw something, but he said I could wait until the next time to see if there was any change. I decided, after about a week, that I was not about to wait for another year and I took the X-rays to my surgeon. As soon as I saw them on the screen, I said, "Oh—that's cancer." But the doctor said that no one could tell that for sure until a biopsy is taken. But I was sure. I added that I wanted the entire breast removed. Somehow it didn't seem to disturb me much. I felt: if it is cancer, fix it, and I'll get back to all my activities. When people ask me did I ever think, "Why me?" I always reply, "Why not me?" I'm not any different from anyone else. To me, you accept it, and since you have no alternative, you just adjust.

The biopsy showed multiple lesions, and out of twelve or so lymph nodes examined, two showed cancer.

> *When people ask me did I ever think, "Why me?" I always reply, "Why not me?" I'm not any different from anyone else. To me, you accept it, and since you have no alternative, you just adjust.*

The doctor came to me with a sad expression. I wasn't surprised at the diagnosis, but I could see how much it bothered him. I tried to cheer him up. I assured him that we would just get going and do what had to be done. I had classes to teach and many shows to put on all over the area, in nursing homes, senior centers, and so on.

The surgeon recommended a mastectomy because there were several different areas of cancer in my breast. After the surgery, I had prolonged problems with fluid accumulating under the skin. While I was recovering, visits from friends who had breast surgeries and the American Cancer Society helped, but my outlook was pretty well established already. The situations that were occurring brought out my sense of humor once again. As an example, when my daughter had to make a sudden stop in the car, I said "Wow! I am swishing all over!" The fluid went forward, backward. It almost felt like a little swimming pool inside my chest. I was going for the draining two to three times a week. I drained for a full eight weeks. The doctor said that was the maximum, and I had the maximum.

At that time, a friend of mine also had a diagnosis of cancer. She said that because of my unbelievable attitude, she was going to go to the same surgeon and oncologist I had, and follow everything I did so that she would come out of this feeling just fine, just like me. That was quite a compliment.

It's odd, how people think you did something special. That's me: I look at things, address them, face them, and act upon them. Not too many second thoughts on anything, once my decision is made.

I went for a fitting for a prosthesis and bra. Yech! It felt like I was trying on a hundred pound sack!

I look at things, address them, face them, and act upon them. Not too many second thoughts on anything, once my decision is made.

Anyway, I got fitted and was proud that I looked pretty normal. No regrets of any sort, just always busy checking if I was keeping the prosthesis pretty even with the remaining breast.

After one year, still feeling a bit lopsided at times, I decided to have surgery to reduce the size of my other breast. But I decided against having surgery to rebuild or reconstruct the side of my mastectomy because by this point I was comfortable with the prosthesis. I went from a size fifteen prosthesis to a size two, an A cup. That felt so much better.

The surgeon and oncologist suggested I have the chemo and radiation from March until June. My son asked me to please get a third opinion. The third opinion suggested that I did not warrant chemo or radiation. He said that since only two lymph nodes were affected, it could do more damage to my heart. I already had undergone two angioplasties a few years before, and angina was still something I had to deal with. I decided to take his advice, and to me, take my so-called chances as to whether the decision would work in my favor, in the long run, or even the short run.

My oncologist put me on tamoxifen, which I took for about five years. It is now ten years since my surgery, and I am doing just fine. I still teach dance, perform, and continue as a choreographer, as I have done for the past fifty years.

Never forget that a sense of humor can be seen (if you look) in the most unexpected happenings in one's life.

I have to add that the doctor's close supervision of your progress as the years go on can make a big difference. Also, it is important for the patient to recognize and follow up on any doubts they have. Never forget that humor can be seen (if you look) in the most unexpected happenings in one's life.

Eva was 48 at the time of her first diagnosis and has been treated with lumpectomy and radiation, chemotherapy, and hormonal therapy. She developed cancer in her other breast just over one year later and made similar treatment decisions along with her doctors.

Sometimes I feel that my life is a movie. I stand outside the scene that's unfolding. I am watching it as I participate in it. Looking back at my past, I often think, "Did I really do this?" or "Did this really happen to me?" Sometimes I am proud of what I did, and sometimes I resent what was dealt to me. Usually, as a director of my story, I take control, believing that having handled many difficult situations before, I can handle this one too, and it all will end happily.

This was my first thought on an ordinary April morning when, taking a shower and soaping my body, I felt a pea-sized bump on the side of my breast. "It's a bump, not a lump," said my brain, immediately moving into a fighting mode. "What's going on? I recently had a mammogram that showed no irregularities. I'll call my internist, and we'll take care of this annoyance."

I made an appointment to see my family doctor. With no particular alarm, he sent me to a surgeon for a biopsy. This minor procedure was performed within a day or two. I felt in control of the situation, not delaying anything. Still, there was a nagging thought about why this was hap-

> *I thought I did all the right things: living a healthy lifestyle, eating lots of broccoli, nursing our sons, and exercising. I didn't have breast cancer in my family.*

pening to me. I thought I did all the right things: living a healthy lifestyle, eating lots of broccoli, nursing our sons, and exercising. I didn't have breast cancer in my family.

The surgeon said to come see him a few hours after the biopsy. I was glad it was on the same day. I wanted to hear the news as soon as possible. My husband came along, and we both listened anxiously to the doctor's friendly, assured voice. The results were positive for cancer, he said. It is cancer. In my mind, just for an instant, it felt like the blade of the guillotine fell, and it was all over. But the next instant I came back to reality, having taken a deep breath. My husband held my hand in great concern as we were given several options.

> *In my mind, just for an instant, it felt like the blade of the guillotine fell, and it was all over. But the next instant I came back to reality, having taken a deep breath.*

Since this was a small tumor in the lower quadrant of the breast which had not spread anywhere, I had the choice of lumpectomy or mastectomy. He explained that some people even have a double mastectomy because this type of cancer (lobular breast cancer) can recur in the other breast, mirror image. He could perform either of the surgeries. He suggested that I get some other opinions. He explained that after the surgery, there should be radiation and/or chemotherapy. He mentioned the name of an oncologist who would be part of the special team that would take care of me, along with him and my family doctor. Later I found out that these three men were not just colleagues but personal friends as well.

That night, my husband took me to a quiet restaurant for a special dinner. As we were discussing this difficult situation, I cried softly, out of fear. The thought that covered me like an unwanted blanket was that I did not want to die as my mother had. I was born in 1941, in Budapest, Hungary, and my family suffered a great deal during World War II, not just as Hungarians but as Jews. As I was growing up, many stories were told to me in hushed voices about the death camps, the ovens into which babies were hurled, and the suffering of my Aunt Clara, who survived the concentration camp of Bergen Belsen, and my Uncle Imre who, be-

Survivors Tell Their Stories

ing near death from starvation, was shot and killed in a Hungarian labor camp.

In March 1957, when I was sixteen, my mother was not feeling well, and soon she was in a hospital having a hysterectomy. I hardly knew what that was, but I still remember the large, barren room with many beds. My father was told the awful news, right away, that my mother had ovarian cancer, which was discovered at the time of surgery. She had about seven months to live. My mother was 46 years old but looked much younger, with short brown hair, bright dark brown eyes, and a slender figure. She always wore elegant but simple clothes. My father adored her, I idolized her, and she was loved and respected by her parents and siblings. The tragic news hit everyone very hard, but only my father knew that she did not have long to live. I knew about cancer, the awful word *krebs* in German, and I watched helplessly as she endured her radiation treatments. She was hopeful to the end as she suffered in silence, taking morphine shots for pain and waiting for a miracle to get well. But nothing helped. I went to school occasionally, spending a lot of time with my mother, but neither of us was realistic enough to know about saying good-bye. None of us expected her to die, so young, so soon, before realizing her lifelong dream of living in America.

Now, even as I was facing breast cancer, I knew I did not have a death sentence. There were treatments, and I was going to do everything possible to get through this. First of all, as a librarian and curious person, I researched the treatment options. I perfectly fit the profile of a person

There were treatments, and I was going to do everything possible to get through this.

who could and should have a lumpectomy. This sounded ideal to me. The surgery was scheduled within days. At some point, I asked my surgeon why he suggested mastectomy as one of the options when lumpectomy was sufficient. "Why?" he said, "Because I am a surgeon, and surgeons like to cut." I understood that, but I was glad that I chose the treatment that was right for me.

Fortunately, the lymph nodes were not affected; the cancer had not spread. Because of my general good health, there were no complications, and I recovered swiftly. When I saw the oncologist, we had an instant rapport. This was very important because I was to be in his hands from now on. I had complete faith and trust in him. He explained the treatments to come, the medications, the radiation, the chemotherapy. I decided to continue my job at the library with the support of my coworkers. I made one phone call to a librarian who had throat cancer and asked her about the chemotherapy. I will always remember that phone call. This woman was not an upbeat person, perhaps because her situation was hopeless (which I did not know). She described hair falling out in the shower, on the pillow, in clumps, on the brush. It was very frightening. Hair was always an important thing in my life, so the idea of becoming bald felt weird. One thing was sure: I did not want to share my baldness with the world by wearing scarves or turbans. I found out before my chemotherapy began that there was a shop that specialized in wigs for cancer patients.

I was ready for radiation and chemotherapy. I found radiation unstressful. True, it was a daily routine, and I had to drive to a hospital for treatment, but then I drove straight to work. The young man who administered the minute-long laser beam was a very friendly person, and we clicked right away, so each day we told each other jokes and funny stories. This really was wonderful because before the treatment I usually had to wait, and the corridor was full of sad people with bald heads or on stretchers, and the room where the radiation took place looked like a space ship from a science fiction movie. The room's darkness was both peaceful and intimidating, but my technician and I always had a cheerful time. I always left with a smile and drove to work with my favorite entertainment in the car—books on tape.

Then came chemotherapy. I remember the tingly feeling I felt as the medicine flowed through my body, uncomfortable at first but then painless.

The people I came across in the fight to conquer the spread of cancerous cells were very kind and caring people, which made my journey bearable. I was also fortunate to have a colleague at work who had been through breast cancer treatments and was very understanding and pragmatic. With her daily support, as well as the support of my family and doctors, I felt very strong. I believed, and still do, that I am a "survivor," a strong individual, determined to conquer—with help—this chapter of

Survivors Tell Their Stories

my story, and move on. And so, months went by, mostly uneventfully, and fortunately I did not feel tired or nauseated.

When the treatments were over, everyone was elated at my success. Thank God, it was over. My hair gradually grew back, and it was in lovely soft curls! I was happy. This was in the summer. Little did I know that in the first month of the new year, I would get another surprise. As I was getting dressed, I pulled my sweater down, and I touched my breast—the other one—and felt a pea-sized lump. Oh, no, I thought. Just as Dr. Webster had predicted, here was the mirror image growth. Shocked as I was, I now knew what to expect. I knew the ropes, I knew the medical staff, and I knew the treatment.

So, back to the doctors. The biopsy this time showed that the cancer had spread into the lymph nodes and all the treatments had to be stronger. Still, I was not frightened because of the oncologist's supportive care. Unfortunately, this time the radiology technician and I had no rapport. It was strictly business, short and serious.

Radiation was not noticeably different this time around but the chemotherapy was. It was a more aggressive course because the cancer cells were more likely to be spreading at a faster pace. For starters, my hair fell out after the first treatment. But I was ready with my wigs. One day, after all the treatments were over and I was in the waiting room for a checkup, I saw a middle-aged lady whose right arm and hand were huge. I asked the nurse what was wrong with her. She explained that she had lymphedema, which can happen after the lymph nodes are removed. This picture stayed with me. A few days later I noticed an infection around my thumb nail and my hand was getting puffy. I rushed to the doctor's office. There, for the first time, I cried. He was very surprised because all through the two sets of treatments I did not cry once. Now I fell apart. I had the image of that woman in my mind and told him about my fear. He assured me that nothing like that woman's situation was likely to happen to me. That was my biggest trauma!

More than ten years have gone by since I had breast cancer. At the time of my cancers, my two sons were in their early twenties. I told both about my illness but not in an alarming way. I remember that I did not want them to feel frightened as I did when my mother was sick. I recently asked them about those days and what they remember, ten years later.

Rob said he was aware of my having cancer but because of my positive attitude he was not worried. Andy was going to college at that time and lived at home, closer to the situation. He also remembers a sense of optimism and casualness from me. He remembers that on a special occasion he commented on how good I looked, and when I mentioned the wig to him he said he did not realize I was wearing it. Andy remembers a feeling of concern during my illness but not fear or apprehension about the future.

I am now a grandmother and have retired from being a full-time librarian. I try to enjoy life every day. Occasionally, I read about people's experiences with cancer, such as Lance Armstrong's biography, *It's Not About the Bike.* I understand the way he handled his illness, and I think he is a wonderful role model. I enjoy sharing my experiences with anyone who asks me, bringing, I hope, an optimistic outlook to an initially frightening experience.

In the end, I learned to see what's important in life. I am spending time with my family and friends and doing the things I enjoy or always wanted to do but did not have the time or opportunity to do before. I take care of myself physically, by doing some kind of exercise almost every day; intellectually, by taking classes at a local college; and emotionally, by playing with my grandchildren and seeing my girlfriends often. And often, I count my blessings.

Katie, at age 41, underwent mastectomy, reconstructive surgery, and chemotherapy.

I was a 41-year-old single woman with a highly stressful career. I was taking a leave of absence from my work to get some much-needed rest and to allow myself to process my grief at the loss of my parents. My father had died two years earlier, and my mother had died that January, both after lengthy illnesses. I had provided much of their care.

During my time of rest, I made two decisions. The first was not to make any big decisions about anything in the immediate future. The second seemed like a small decision: to get a physical examination. Within three weeks, following a routine mammogram, I was sitting in a surgeon's office making life-altering decisions.

The day of the mammogram, the radiologist told me the films were suspicious and that I should contact my physician. That afternoon, I saw my gynecologist, who examined me again without feeling any abnormal growths. He called a surgeon in the same medical office center, made arrangements for me to be seen immediately, and sent all the reports with me. The surgeon examined me and told me we needed to set up a biopsy.

What I remember most is the numbness and the loneliness. I did not allow myself to think of the possibilities before the biopsy and decided not to share any information with my extended family until I knew something definite. The one person I told was my friend, June, who is like a sister to me and who had been such a sustaining help during my parents' illnesses and deaths.

I did not allow myself to think of the possibilities before the biopsy.

June took me to the hospital for the biopsy, and I remember how afraid we both were, but we didn't talk about it. The needle-placement biopsy procedure was very painful, primarily because the tumor was so deep. Unfortunately, I was not given any sedative to help me relax. The biopsy was done using local injections. My body did not respond optimally to the medications to numb the area, so I felt much of the surgical procedure.

The next week, June took me to the surgeon's office, and I told her to just wait while I went in to get the report. In a very professional and concerned manner, the doctor told me I had breast cancer and that I must make some decisions. His nurse was in the room with us and at that point she told me she would get my friend for me. The surgeon again repeated some of the report and then gave me the name of an oncologist, a radiation oncologist, and a plastic surgeon. I was told to meet with all three and then return to him to discuss my decision about a lumpectomy or mastectomy.

My reactions over the next weeks fluctuated between disbelief, dread, and inward agony. I remember thinking I just wanted to leave, to escape. I wanted to get on a boat to Bora Bora and isolate myself until I felt strong enough emotionally and physically to deal with this. I remember praying to God that I was

I wanted to get on a boat to Bora Bora and isolate myself until I felt strong enough emotionally and physically to deal with this.

very willing to face this but not now. I felt so fragile, like I might shatter into a million pieces and never come back together again.

I made my appointments with the recommended physicians. Each was extremely kind, open, encouraging, and informative. The meeting with the radiation oncologist was the determining one in my choice of surgery. He showed me the mammograms and educated me about the tumor and what we could see on the films. He explained what we were seeing and said that either surgery was possible. As I viewed the films, I saw other white areas that looked very similar to the tumor area and asked about them. He responded that these were why I really needed to decide between the two surgeries. The areas I saw could possibly be precancerous, he explained, and I might need to have other biopsies in a couple of years and repeat the same process. I remember telling him that with that information, then I did not have a choice to make. I could not repeat the emotional torment I was in, nor risk the spread of the disease.

I did not want to read anything about breast cancer or seek out additional information. Part of this, I am sure, was a form of emotional protection and denial. The one person I spoke with who was a breast cancer survivor was not helpful to me. She minimized her own experience and told me that the chemotherapy was really nothing. Additionally, she seemed to imply that if I followed her suggestions about dealing with cancer that I could breeze through the process. This only angered me, and I knew she had no idea what this experience was like for me. I decided at that time not to seek out support groups or talk with anyone except medical professionals. I checked the credentials of the doctors who had been recommended to me and felt confident in their training and expertise. I was treated as an individual by each doctor. They answered all of my questions, they took time with me, and I felt that what happened to me mattered to them.

I did not want to read anything about breast cancer or seek out additional information. Part of this, I am sure, was a form of emotional protection and denial.

Their recommended course of treatment was mastectomy. Reconstructive surgery was favorably indicated, and I was encouraged by the possibility of having a TRAM flap procedure—using my own tissue as replacement for the breast. I would be able to have the reconstruction as part of the mastectomy procedure. For me, this made the surgery much more acceptable, and I wanted to do the surgery immediately.

Following the surgery, my oncologist discussed with me his recommendation for aggressive chemotherapy. I dreaded the chemotherapy much more than I had the surgery, but I was willing to go through the treatment to try to insure as best I could that I would not have to repeat this process.

I would be able to have the reconstruction as part of the mastectomy procedure. For me, this made the surgery much more acceptable, and I wanted to do the surgery immediately.

My six months of chemotherapy were extremely difficult, emotionally and physically. I'm sure that part of this was due to my postsurgery exhaustion and the continued grief I was experiencing, which now included grief over my own health, femininity, and sexuality. We were forced to change protocols several times during the treatment, and this was unsettling and disappointing. With the treatments, I felt and looked like I had cancer. The reality of cancer finally hit. I could not deny it any longer.

With the treatments, I also had to learn to give myself injections to maintain my blood count. Because I was experiencing nausea with the chemotherapy, my oncologist told me about a psychologist who was successful in training patients in self-hypnosis to prevent the nausea. This not only proved extremely beneficial in the treatments but also gave me a professional whom I felt could assist me in working through the emotional trauma.

One of the most difficult parts of the experience for me was going through this alone. While my friend June was so helpful by being with me on the first night after each treatment, she lived ninety minutes away and had her career and her own family to care for. A few other people from my church were helpful when they could be, but for the most part, I was alone. The man in my life at the time lived many miles away and was not able to be present with me except on rare occasions. The loneliness and sense of just barely holding together were predominant. I basically held on emotionally one hour at a time, for months.

Ironically, one of the most helpful experiences was when I received a call from the oncologist's office following my regular blood work. The nurse told me that my counts were dangerously low, that I was to go to the hospital immediately, and that the doctor would be in to see me that afternoon. I checked in at the hospital and was placed in isolation, where I received several IV fluids. Rather than being frightened or depressed, I was actually relieved. For the first time since my treatments began, I felt like I could relax and feel cared for. I didn't have to worry about trying to care for myself. The five days in the hospital were a much-needed respite.

After my treatments were completed and I was declared "cured," I set about to discover what my "new normal" was about. My strong belief is that no one can walk this journey and go back to "normal." We find a new normal, based on our changes and experiences. For me, this was a tremendously refreshing and enlightening venture. As I journeyed, I changed physically, emotionally, and spiritually. Physically, my appearance changed, I plunged into immediate menopause, and I had many scars and new discomforts to accept and incorporate into my new life. Emotionally, I had to abandon the dream of giving birth to a child, and I had multiple layers of grief to dig through. Spiritually, I realized that for me, the disciplines of faith that I had taught for years were of less help

> *My strong belief is that no one can walk this journey and go back to "normal." We find a new normal, based on our changes and experiences. For me, this was a tremendously refreshing and enlightening venture.*

for me than was a simple but profound experience and recognition of being in the presence of God constantly. My faith tradition teaches that God supplies strength for all our needs. My experience verified this belief, but God's strength came only at the precise moment of my need and in the precise amount needed. I was not transported out of the trauma, or even away to Bora Bora, but I experienced God's presence with me in all of the hellishness of the journey.

As I was approaching the end of treatments, my one constant prayer was that since I was having to go through this, somehow I needed to discover ways to use the experience for good. And I can report today that the growth journey continues with exciting ventures. Sunrises and sunsets are especially wonderful! Shortly after my recovery, I resigned from my position and began a new academic journey of earning another master's degree and a Ph.D. in the field of integrative counseling psychology, which combines behavioral science and spirituality.

Today, I am married to a wonderful man I met three years ago, and I am enjoying my new venture of learning to be a life partner and a stepmom. And I recently was awarded my Ph.D., having done my research in optimism and spirituality as aids to adjustment for women with breast cancer. The journey continues. I know that there will be other times of trauma, grief, and difficulty. But I believe that because I've experienced breast cancer and have learned the life lessons offered, I am better equipped for the rest of the journey.

Davi, at age 56, had a very small invasive breast cancer. She chose lumpectomy and chemotherapy. The tumor was very small, and therefore the decision regarding chemotherapy was a complicated one.

It was the Saturday before my son's graduation from high school. He was graduating on Sunday, and I had my mother-in-law from California visiting us. I always did a breast checkup, usually once a month, in the shower. Sometimes I'd miss a month but not often. I was in bed and I rolled over and somehow I felt, I don't know quite how, but I felt it, a tiny, tiny little bump, and so I did a breast check lying down, which I had never done before. For some reason I thought—and I understand now that this is incorrect—that you only did them in the shower, standing up. It was definitely little, kind of felt like a pea that moved around—

It was definitely little, kind of felt like a pea that moved around—a very, very tiny pea.

a very, very tiny pea but having never felt that before, it definitely alarmed me. At that point I didn't tell anybody, I just called my doctor and they paged him. He said to be in his office Monday morning at 8:30. So it was a hard weekend to get through because I was supposed to be happy because my son was graduating from high school. I didn't tell anybody because I didn't want to alarm anyone. I was a little bit nervous.

I was waiting on my doctor's doorstep Monday morning. My doctor palpated my breasts and said yes, indeed, he could feel something very, very tiny. He said I had two choices. He was sure it was what they call an adenoma and that these were very common in women my age and that they were benign. He said, "You can go home and come back in three months, or I can do a biopsy (aspiration) right now." I was actually shocked that my doctor would tell me I could wait three months. Imagine how many women go home and don't come back until it's too late! It's unconscionable to offer that as a choice.

Well, I come from a family of doctors. My father was a doctor, so I have no fear of anything medical, and I said, "I'm not going home and waiting three months. I want a biopsy right now."

An aspiration is not pleasant because it's painful, and he did it without anesthetic. He sent off to his lab what he got, and he said he'd call me and let me know. I went home, and I waited about a week. Of course, I was nervous but not so nervous anymore because he had told me that it was probably benign. Then a week later he called me to say that the results had come back inconclusive, and he was sending me to another doctor who does nothing but these aspirations. She stuck a long needle into my breast without anesthesia and pulled out fluid, and it was very painful. But, you know, you grab onto something, you grit your teeth, and you know it's going to be over fast.

> *I said, "I'm not going home and waiting three months. I want a biopsy right now."*

I remember her telling me before I left her office that something did not look normal. About a day later I heard from her, and she told me that I needed to see a surgeon immediately, that he should do a biopsy, and I should not take no for an answer. So that had me concerned. She said she was not going to say that these were cancerous but they appeared to be abnormal. Maybe her word was precancerous, so I still wasn't all that concerned, but I was beginning now to get a little worried. I made an appointment with a wonderful surgeon, and I got in to see him immediately. I guess when you have something like this they make time for you, and I was seen within a day or two. He looked me over and immediately scheduled me for surgery, but he said, "I don't think this is anything to worry about. I think this is an adenoma." Once again, he was not terribly concerned. So I went home feeling pretty good.

The biopsy was easy because they give you something. But I wasn't asleep. My husband went with me. It was an in-and-out procedure, and the surgeon is a very funny guy so, you know, a lot of laughing and talking in the operating room. I felt very comfortable. I didn't feel anything because with the local anesthesia the biopsy itself was not terribly painful. I was up and walking around that same day. It was just tender.

He called me as soon as they got the pathology back. It must have been within a day, and instead of saying, "Come and see me," he said to me, "I am so sorry. I am so sorry." He said, "I am so sorry to have to tell you this, but you have cancer. You have breast cancer." I almost dropped the phone.

We determined at that point that we would do a wider excision to get everything out that might not have been gotten out with the biopsy, so I went back in for a lumpectomy. He did the lumpectomy and what I had was a 0.6 centimeter nodule containing infiltrating carcinoma with ductal and lobular features. The single sentinel lymph node was negative for any evidence of tumor. During the wider excision, breast tissue measuring 7 by 4.5 by 2.5 centimeters was removed and showed no evidence of residual infiltrating carcinoma, but there was extensive residual atypical ductal and lobular process.

The healing took much longer with this wider excision. It was very tender. I could not jump up and take a walk right away. It hurt a lot. I probably just expected it would be the same thing, and I should have realized it wouldn't be because they took out a lot more breast tissue.

Now the problem was we really didn't know what to do with me. I could have gone either way in regard to the chemotherapy. We had hoped that I could take tamoxifen, but the tumor was not estrogen sensitive so that wasn't an option. Chemotherapy would reduce the risk of the cancer coming back later in life but the tumor was very, very small, and so the risk of recurrence was very low. My oncologist is a firm believer, at least I think I understand him, and this is how I am, in being aggressive and in doing the one thing that's going to give you the best shot at coming out of this. He wanted me

Now the problem was we really didn't know what to do with me. I could have gone either way in regard to the chemotherapy.

to be comfortable in my decision so he sent me, along with my husband, to another oncologist, who said it was a no-brainer, that even though I had a tiny cancer, he explained, it was like a dandelion. A seed could have just blown around and be somewhere in my body just waiting to hatch. So he strongly advised chemotherapy.

The worst part of it was the chemo, and that was followed by radiation. Chemo was once every three weeks, but I began to become very debilitated. I lost a lot of weight. I weigh probably about 108 on a good day, and I dropped to ninety-two pounds on my worst day. I had no appetite whatsoever. I was so nauseous, and I tried every medicine in the book. The only thing he found that worked a little bit was what we called "fake marijuana." It's a green tablet. It's based on marijuana, and it gave me a modicum of appetite but really next to nothing. I would take a bite here and a bite there.

I had great support. The school district where I work, all the interpreters, they brought food over once a week. Everybody made their own thing, so I would try a little of this and a little of that. I might not eat it all. But my husband was there to finish it all off, and this meant I didn't have to worry about cooking.

I knew that my hair was going to fall out, and I had gone to my hairdresser to cut my hair short. I had long hair (like I do now), and he cut it real short. That probably was the saving grace. I would recommend every person who's going to have chemo do that or even go get your head shaved because when it starts to come out, it is frightening. It comes out all over. You wake up, and it's in your bed. It's all over your clothes. I saved it all. I put it in a bag. I still have it. I did not get a wig. I went and looked at wigs and decided it wasn't me. I knew in a strong wind I'd be fussing with it. I didn't want that so I made scarves for myself. I got those bandanas, and I jeweled them. I used to paint, and now I turned to making scarves. To this day my youngest son says, "Mom, you looked so glamorous in the scarves, why don't you wear them now?" But now I have my hair back in abundance.

After the chemotherapy, there was a one-month break, and then I started radiation. During the radiation I was a little tired but not compared to the chemo. I'm normally a hyper person — I have tons of energy — and I was a little tired with radiation, but it wasn't bad. I didn't feel any pain, and I understand that some women can, the breast is tender. In comparison to the chemo, it was a piece of cake, so I wasn't complaining.

Looking back on the experience, my sons were away at college and weren't around to see everything, and I'm thankful for that. They've always seen me as take charge and lots of energy and go, go, go, and by the time they did see me, I more or less had my health back. Jed, my oldest, had to come home from college and kind of babysit me when my husband was out of town on business, but that was early on, before I was well into the chemo and had lost a lot of weight. So I think once my kids knew the cancer was out, that I was doing everything possible, and that I had an excellent, excellent prognosis, they didn't dwell on it. They see me today; they see that I look fine, act fine. As my husband likes to say, "She's as bitchy as ever"—meaning, "She's got her health back."

When you're considering choices, the choices need to be proactive. You can't put your head in the sand and just think this is going to go away, because it's not.

With chemotherapy, there is a light at the end of the tunnel. You know it's not forever. You pretty well know how many weeks and months it's going to be, and you get all your hair back, you get your strength back, and you put your weight back on. To me it was just a bad dream. I am so

You can't put your head in the sand and just think this is going to go away, because it's not.

glad I did chemotherapy, and even while I was doing it, it never entered my mind to stop. I knew I would just bite the bullet and, as the Nike ad says, "Just do it."

Debbie was 37 years old when she was found to have a very large tumor occupying a large portion of her breast and multiple large, firm lymph nodes were felt in her armpit that were believed to contain metastatic cancer. Debbie was treated with preoperative chemotherapy and had an excellent response to treatment and then underwent a mastectomy. That was thirteen years ago.

At the age of 37 I was diagnosed with breast cancer. I can't say I was surprised because I had long suspected something was not right. My husband felt a lump in my left breast when I was 33, and cancer ran in my family, but no one had been diagnosed with breast cancer. At the time I was frightened and went to my HMO right away. The doctor told me I had fibrocystic breasts and not to worry. When I requested a mammogram he told me that my breasts were too firm at my age and nothing would show up on a mammogram. Upon hearing what I wanted to hear and blindly accepting the premise that he was a well-trained doctor who would not put my life in jeopardy, I accepted his diagnosis and went on with my life.

Over time my breast became more and more painful, and the lump grew. Still I accepted the diagnosis. I was tired much of the time and again went to my HMO to see if I was anemic. The doctor told me that anyone with my schedule would be exhausted. I had a 4 year old, worked full time, went to graduate school part-time, and was doing a field placement twenty hours each week. Again, the diagnosis made sense to me, so I accepted that I was going to be tired and stopped complaining. Over the next three years, my breast became increasingly painful. The lump continued growing. My breast began to dimple and my nipple inverted. The pain kept me awake at night, and I began sleeping with a heating pad because it seemed to help. I was in so much chronic pain at that point that I had to get some relief. I changed my insurance plan and made a commitment to myself to see a private OB/GYN as soon as I graduated in the fall.

I followed through with my commitment and in mid-August saw a private OB/GYN and went for my mammogram. As I undraped my breast for the mammogram, I knew immediately by the look on the technician's face that I had cancer. Although she didn't say anything, she couldn't hide her shock. A few weeks later the doctor confirmed my suspicion, and things began to move very quickly. From the doctor's office, we called a surgeon, who agreed to see me the same day, in between surgeries at the hospital. He seemed to understand how anxious I was to get some answers, and he scheduled a biopsy for the next week.

As part of my job I had worked closely with a consultant psychologist for eleven years. His wife was a social worker specializing in grief therapy. I talked with her, and she cautioned me to see an oncologist before I agreed to any surgery. She assured me that advances were being made every day in cancer treatment. I talked to her about so many things that I regretted and wished I could go back in time and change. I cried for my son more than for myself. I wished I had not spent four years of

Survivors Tell Their Stories

my only child's young life in graduate school. I was angry with myself for spending so much precious time at work instead of with my son. I was angry that I waited to have a second child because now my son would be an only child, and I didn't ever want him to be lonely.

Most of all I was terrified that I would not live to raise my 6-year-old son to adulthood. He was so young to have to go through this trauma. Worry about him was excruciating. I felt so guilty. Ann consoled me and most importantly instilled in me confidence that, through modern advances in cancer treatment, I could be kept alive until my son graduated from high school. This thought kept me going. She referred me to an oncologist she had worked with and respected.

> *Most of all I was terrified that I would not live to raise my 6-year-old son to adulthood. He was so young to have to go through this trauma.*

The oncologist and his staff also seemed to understand how stressed and anxious I was after my diagnosis, and they scheduled an appointment immediately. I brought my mother and husband to the appointment. The oncologist was very calm and confirmed that the mammogram appeared to show calcification indicating a cancerous tumor. He reassured me by explaining what would be learned by the biopsy and told me that he knew and respected the surgeon. He patiently took time to answer all of our questions. I felt much more confident after talking to him.

I requested only local anesthetic for my biopsy because I get nauseous after general anesthetic. After some pleading on my part, the surgeon agreed. During the procedure, he joked and talked and kept the mood lighthearted. We laughed and listened to music, and the procedure was over quickly. He explained to me that the tumor was approximately the size of a racquetball and appeared to be cancer. The sample was sent to the lab, and the results went to the oncologist.

At my next appointment with the oncologist, he explained how treatment was dictated by the type of cells found in the biopsy. I remember mine had estrogen receptors, and that was a good thing. My mother took copious notes of everything the oncologist said. Because of the size of the tumor, he suggested chemotherapy before surgery, which at the time was a new approach. Part of his rationale was to shrink the tumor before surgery and then perform a less disabling mastectomy. Soon afterward I started chemotherapy.

The oncologist warned me that he was going to treat the cancer very aggressively. I was all for that.

I was very open with my diagnosis and treatment with all my coworkers. My colleague's wife, the social worker, explained that how I handled my condition would determine how others responded to me. She was absolutely right. My friends and coworkers waited to see how I talked about my situation before they decided how to treat me. I had tremendous support from family, friends, and coworkers during my treatment.

> *I was very open with my diagnosis and treatment with all my coworkers. How I handled my condition would determine how others responded to me.*

I was fortunate to have doctors during my cancer treatment who believed in having fun in the midst of tragedy. Each doctor was open, warm, outgoing, lighthearted, supportive, and optimistic. They were never glum, cold, or self-absorbed. Whenever I had to be hospitalized, they supported me by visiting almost every day. I never felt alone or scared and was confident that they cared about what happened to me.

Despite my optimism, I was amazed to watch the tumor shrink from the effects of the chemotherapy. Over the months of treatment, the tumor grew smaller and smaller. My breast seemed to deflate. I didn't have to imagine the effectiveness of the chemo because the results were so clearly obvious. I had read that sometimes doctors weren't sure whether the chemo was effective until after the treatment was completed. In my case, the treatment was clearly effective. I could see it working. Seeing proof that the cancer was being destroyed allowed me to maintain my positive attitude. I worried less and wasn't as frustrated by the side effects of the chemo.

> *Seeing proof that the cancer was being destroyed allowed me to maintain my positive attitude.*

In January the tumor was barely palpable by the oncologist. I stopped chemo to build up my immune system for surgery. I had a mastectomy in February. All my lymph nodes were removed. While some of the lymph nodes looked irritated and might have been cancerous at one time, none of them tested positive for cancer. I never imagined such good news.

One month after surgery, I restarted chemo and then radiation, which ended soon after.

Today I am free from cancer. It's been thirteen years since my diagnosis. I am truly blessed. I'm grateful to so many people who supported me during my cancer treatment. Most of all, I credit the oncologist for keeping me alive to watch my son graduate from high school and begin college this year.

Barbara was age 50 when diagnosed with breast cancer. Barbara underwent mastectomy and breast reconstruction. She then received chemotherapy.

The first thing I felt was numb. I was in the radiology office for a routine mammogram, but they found something suspicious. Even after taking two additional pictures, I still didn't understand the implications when they asked me to wait around while they fit me in for a sonogram. Then the technician told me that there was a large solid mass in my left breast that was suspicious and that I should call my gynecologist immediately. I was alone, and I had to drive home and get on with my day, since I was having a party in my house that evening.

That was very hard for me. I remember crying all the way home and wishing there was someone—anyone—I could talk to, and yet I really didn't want to talk to anyone because that would make it somehow more real. I guess I was hoping or trying to believe that it was really nothing—just a cyst, or something benign. I really hadn't felt the lump myself up until the time they showed me where it was, so maybe they were wrong.

I remember crying all the way home and wishing there was someone—anyone—I could talk to, and yet I really didn't want to talk to anyone because that would make it somehow more real.

When I got home, I spoke to the gynecologist, who was a new doctor for me. I remember feeling that she was very cold, that there was no emotion or sorrow in her voice when she matter of factly gave me the names of several surgeons I could call to schedule a biopsy. I felt doubly hurt by her unfeeling attitude and decided then and there to go back to my old gynecologist. That was the best thing I could have done because his reaction and caring attitude helped me deal with the ups and downs of the next few weeks. I picked a surgeon and spoke to a reconstructive surgeon, who spent at least half an hour with me explaining my options should I be diagnosed with breast cancer. My afternoon improved greatly, and I was even able to tell my husband, Jan, without crying. We were able to take comfort in the knowledge that whatever happened, we could go through this together.

The next couple of weeks were very hard—the uncertainty, the worrying, and the wondering what the outcome of the biopsy would be and where we would go from there. This all happened around the holidays, so we were somewhat distracted by the festivities with family and friends. We even went on a short trip to Williamsburg, Virginia, and were able to enjoy the time away.

After the biopsy, I thought maybe I was in the clear, since it was done on a Friday and afterward, the surgeon came in and gave me the feeling that it might be benign. However, that evening, just after Jan went out to do some work at the office, I received a call from the surgeon saying the biopsy looked bad but that he wouldn't have confirmed results from the lab until the following Monday. Again, I was alone to hear the news, and my emotions ranged from anger to sadness to fear. How I got through that weekend I'll never know. It seemed to be the longest two days of my life. Again, Jan was there for me, helping me to see the good in all this—that if I did have breast cancer, the fact that it was found early would be the silver lining in a very dark cloud.

On Monday evening, I got the bad news. It was cancer, and I needed to make some decisions. I made an appointment with both the surgeon and the oncologist I had picked. The surgeon presented me with the options, and I chose to go with a mastectomy with immediate reconstruction. I was happy that I had already picked out the reconstructive surgeon because it was one less decision I had to make at a very stressful time. The oncologist also spent a great deal of time with me and my husband, explaining the treatment I would likely have once the mastectomy was done and we knew the extent of the lymph node involvement.

I spent the next few weeks on the Internet, exploring different web sites to learn as much as I could. I learned about the treatment options, the things I might experience as I went through the treatments, and also my reconstruction options. During this time, I again met with the reconstructive surgeon, who explained the reconstruction process and presented me with choices. I chose to do a TRAM flap reconstruction because I liked the idea that my own body tissues would be used to re-

> *I chose to do a TRAM flap reconstruction, because I liked the idea that my own body tissues would be used to replace what I had lost with the mastectomy procedure.*

place what I had lost with the mastectomy procedure.

The weekend before the surgery was very hard. Part of me wanted to go in the hospital and get this disease out of me, and part of me was scared to death. I had never had such an invasive procedure before, and I wasn't sure how I would react to losing my breast. But, by Monday morning, the day of the surgery, I was surprised at how calm I was. All I wanted to do was get this thing done with so I could move on to recovery.

After several hours of surgery, I woke up to find myself bandaged. I was pretty out of it that day, but, surprisingly, the next day I woke up to find that I really wasn't in much pain. I had a morphine drip that I could control. I really didn't need much pain medication, and the next few days went by pretty quickly. Coming home, I almost cried when I saw that Jan had set up the family room as a bedroom so I would be as comfortable as possible. He also stayed home with me for the next two weeks, looking after me and tending to the drains that needed emptying and measuring. I learned that there was no lymph node involvement and was anxious to get on to the next step of chemotherapy. I didn't give much thought to the lost breast at this time because I was focused on completing chemotherapy and the next surgery to create a nipple for my new "breast." I knew that the surgery would have to wait until after the course of chemotherapy treatment was completed, and I was in a hurry to start, so that all of this would be over as soon as possible.

I had four courses of chemotherapy, Adriamycin and Cytoxan, over a three-month period. I would take the chemotherapy on a Friday afternoon and feel fine until Sunday, when I would get somewhat nauseous. I never threw up, but I felt extremely tired for the next few days, and I lived on anti-nausea medication. Even losing my hair was not so bad. Before I had the surgery, I went to Amy's Salon, where I bought a wig that looked a lot like my hair and hairstyle. At work, no one even noticed that I was wearing a wig. They all thought it was my hair, and that made me feel really good. While I missed having hair, it was easier in the mornings to put on the wig and go, since it was already styled. It did get hot, however, and in the evenings, at home, I always took it off as soon as I could. My daughter had a harder time seeing me without hair than I did. I guess she saw it as a sign of my illness and was constantly reminded that I had cancer. She was only 17 when the breast cancer was diagnosed, and she took it very hard. I do think, however, that it brought us closer because I always talked to her about how I was feeling and how I was getting well in spite of the way I looked.

> *My daughter had a harder time seeing me without hair than I did. I guess she saw it as a sign of my illness and was constantly reminded that I had cancer.*

After the last chemotherapy treatment, I developed a fever, and my white cell count went down so low that I had to be hospitalized for a few days. I found that to be very difficult, since I wanted to get on to the reconstruction of the nipple, and I thought that this would delay it. It was also depressing and a little scary since everyone who came into my single room had to wear a mask. Also, the IV was hard to insert, since the chemotherapy had really messed up my veins. I cried when the nurse had to insert the IV into my forearm because that was the only good vein she could use. I couldn't wait to get out of the hospital and get on with the rest of the treatment.

Finally, it was time for the second surgery to reconstruct the nipple. The surgery went quickly, and I was home that evening. Now I was done, other than the office procedure of having the areola tattooed so that it looked real. I should have been so happy, and at first I was happy. But then, a few days later, I fell apart. I didn't understand at the time, but I became depressed and Jan got concerned. He insisted that I speak to a psychiatrist when I said I didn't want to live any more. The psychiatrist put me on Serzone even though I told him I couldn't take that kind of medication. This medication took away my appetite and made me feel even worse. So Jan took me to my

> *Now I was done, other than the office procedure of having the areola tattooed so that it looked real. I should have been so happy, and at first I was happy. But then, a few days later, I fell apart.*

general practitioner who prescribed Paxil and Neurontin. After a few days of this regimen, I began to feel more like myself.

After talking to a therapist, I came to realize that what I was feeling was common. I had spent the last several months in a fight for my life and had the support of the general surgeon, the reconstructive surgeon, and the oncologist to help me. But now, all of this was behind me, and I was alone again with my fears that the cancer might return. My support system was gone, at least in my mind, and I was feeling very alone. I joined two support groups. Jan came with me to one support group and helped me get through the uncertainty and fear that I was feeling. Between these groups, Jan's support and love, along with that of the rest of my family, plus the therapy, I was able to stop the medication after seven months and get on with my life.

> *I had spent the last several months in a fight for my life and had the support of the general surgeon, the reconstructive surgeon, and the oncologist to help me. But now, all of this was behind me, and I was alone again with my fears that the cancer might return.*

These days, I continue to see my oncologist periodically. I have a clean bill of health, and I am almost five years out from the time I was diagnosed and had my mastectomy. I am feeling great and looking forward to lots more years of health and happiness. My newest family member, my granddaughter, is helping me to realize how precious life is and how little time we have. It is so important to make every moment count and recognize all the good things that come our way. Now I see breast cancer as a glitch on the radar screen, and I have put it in perspective. I have so much to be thankful for and to look forward to and great friends and family who helped me get to this point.

Lillian was 65 years old when diagnosed with breast cancer. She was treated with lumpectomy and radiation therapy. Lillian also received adjuvant chemotherapy.

I had my first experience with a breast aspiration in 1964 at age 30, six months after the birth of our son, David. Little did I dream it would be the first of many needles and three biopsies between then and March

2000. Getting so many needles put in me made me think that if I had something to drink I would spout like a fountain.

Over the years, one of my gynecologists believed in routinely giving his patients thermograms, but I don't think this was done by too many other doctors. My thermograms usually showed areas of heat, which was indicative of something to watch. In looking back, the interesting part of having the thermograms was that the doctor said he would not be surprised if I had a problem some day with the left breast, not on the right side where I had had two biopsies and many aspirations. He turned out to be right on the money.

My cancer was found during a routine GYN checkup and confirmed with a biopsy. I elected to have a lumpectomy, and the sentinel node and two others tested positive. I was told that my cancer responded to treatment well and that if there is a good cancer to have, this was it. And make no mistake about it, being told you have cancer is a life-changing experience, not just for you but for your whole family. The fact that my sister had died just nine months before of cancer that began as lymphoma in the breast made it more so. A barrage of tests was ordered, followed by consultations with the surgeon, two oncologists, and a radiologist. My husband Bill and son David accompanied me to all the appointments, and we made a cassette recording of all of them. Family support was invaluable then and remains so to this day.

And make no mistake about it, being told you have cancer is a life-changing experience, not just for you but for your whole family.

It was recommended that I get a mediport, and this was a wise move because I was hospitalized after each of my first three chemo sessions for three to five days and had two blood transfusions and two platelet transfusions. I shudder to think of all the extra needles I would have been subjected to during these stays and my eight treatments if I hadn't had that mediport. My treatments were administered on the "sandwich" schedule—four chemo treatments followed by thirty-five radiation treatments and four more chemo treatments. The only negative point of this approach was that I lost my hair twice and was subjected to the hot wigs for a longer period of time. Through it all, maintaining a sense of humor was good for my outlook and managed to give me some form of "exercise" through smiling.

Another time-consuming part of all this was the number of office visits for blood checks and injections. Time-consuming things help you forget about the unpleasant things that come your way, and you gladly take the tamoxifen every day for five years. One memory that remains is the weird feeling you get when you see the chemo entering your system for the first treatment. And there is still that period of nervousness during checkups, and especially during mammograms.

> *Time-consuming things help you forget about the unpleasant things that come your way.*

I cannot say enough about the compassion of all the doctors and staff. They were always available when needed, even at 3:00 a.m., and we became friends. My outlook on life has been altered and my faith in God strengthened during this period. I feel I was helped by all the prayers said on my behalf, not only from my church but the churches of my husband, son, siblings, and friends and relatives. Maybe it is a growing older change, but I find material things have less and less value. I thank God for each day given me and for the care of wonderful doctors I see regularly and for the miracles of modern medicine. My prayer is that all cancer patients could receive the care I did and that this epidemic of breast cancer will soon be eliminated from the face of this earth.

Becky was diagnosed with breast cancer at age 38. She chose mastectomy with immediate TRAM flap reconstruction. Becky also received adjuvant chemotherapy.

I was 38 years old when I discovered a lump in my left breast. I was performing a self-exam in anticipation of my annual checkup with my gynecologist. The lump was large, about the size of a walnut in its shell, and felt as hard as a rock.

My gynecologist confirmed the lump, and I scheduled a mammogram and ultrasound for the following week. While I was somewhat concerned, I was not alarmed based on my relatively young age and lack of family history of breast cancer.

After those tests were complete, I went about my errands for the day. By the time I got home from the grocery store, I found a message on my answering machine from my gynecologist saying that I needed to see a surgeon that same afternoon. Unfortunately, the mammogram indicated microcalcifications, and the ultrasound showed a solid mass. Now I was alarmed, and I made hasty arrangements for my neighbor to keep an eye on my children (then aged 5, 8, and 11), and my husband agreed to pick up my test results and meet me at the surgeon's office. It seemed that we had boarded an accelerating roller coaster and hadn't had time to fasten our seat belts.

> *It seemed that we had boarded an accelerating roller coaster and hadn't had time to fasten our seat belts.*

A biopsy was set for the next Monday. Because of the size of the lump, I was not given a choice as to the type of biopsy. An excisional biopsy to remove the lump and some surrounding tissue was called for. Lab results confirmed invasive ductal carcinoma with a four-centimeter tumor (about an inch and a half).

Here again, I did not really have a choice as to treatment. The biopsy indicated unclean margins, so additional tissue had to be removed. The biopsy had left a significant cavity in my breast. The best surgical option for me was a mastectomy. This was followed by chemotherapy consisting of four rounds of fairly heavy-duty drugs: Cytoxan and Adriamycin. I suppose I had the option of doing nothing, of letting nature run

> *The biopsy had left a significant cavity in my breast. The best surgical option was a mastectomy.*

its course and praying for a miraculous healing. But with many years of life ahead of me and three young children to care for, this was never a considered option.

Where I did have realistic options to consider was in the follow-up care. Prior to the mastectomy, I visited with a plastic and reconstructive surgeon who provided me much needed light at the end of the dark tunnel. He explained that in my case, reconstruction could consist of an implant or a TRAM flap. The implant option was that after the removal of all the breast tissue and some lymph nodes, a starter implant would be inserted prior to closing the incision. This would be gradually inflated over time, giving the skin a chance to heal and stretch. Eventually, the initial implant would be replaced with a permanent one which would have a more lifelike look and feel. The TRAM flap option would consist of sculpting a new breast from the tissue taken from my abdomen. The muscle, fat, and supporting vessels from my abdomen would be rerouted under the skin of my chest and used to fill in the space previously occupied by breast tissue. The benefits of the TRAM flap are that the breast is reconstructed during the same surgery as the mastectomy (so I wouldn't have to go home breastless), and you have more realistic-looking results, no artificial materials remaining in the body, and a free tummy tuck. The cons of the TRAM flap are longer surgery, slower recovery, and some weakening of the abdominal muscles.

After discussions with family, friends, and other breast cancer patients, I decided to go with the TRAM flap. My recovery took about four to six weeks, but I am very pleased with the results. I had two follow-up procedures to improve the appearance of the reconstruction, both of which were outpatient surgeries with very easy recoveries.

After finishing chemotherapy (and yes, I did lose my hair and wore a wig for about nine months), I decided to take tamoxifen. My tumor was estrogen receptive, so tamoxifen would decrease the likelihood of recurrence for me. Again, this was not a difficult decision to make to stay healthy.

After ten years, I consider that I made the appropriate choices for my diagnosis and place in life. Others will be faced with similar choices and will no doubt follow different paths, but I do not second-guess any of the decisions I made to restore my health and wholeness.

Beth is a 53-year-old minister. She chose lumpectomy, received chemotherapy, and then received radiation therapy.

On a beautiful day in April, I left my office to drive to the gynecologist, wondering if keeping my appointment would be a waste of her time and mine. Six months earlier, I had gone through both a routine physical and a mammogram and had been assured that everything was fine! But my doctor prescribed a low-dose birth control pill to ease some other problems. "While on these hormones, I'll need to see you every six months," she told me. Six months! I had hoped to follow a more liberal regimen—

Women with Invasive Breast Cancer 297

a physical yearly and a mammogram every two years—at least until I turned fifty. I had little fear of breast cancer. After all, my mother never had it, and I had given birth to and nursed three babies. I thought I was one of those candidates whose low risk didn't warrant much concern.

I am a parish pastor. Earlier that day I had welcomed the parents of our church's preschool for a program and was formally dressed in my clerical collar. The doctor's assistant looked at me and asked, "So what do I call you? Father?" I laughed and told her "Beth" would be fine. She asked if I was married, and my chart answered her question. "Oh, I see you have children. So you can have sex, huh?" In as serious a voice as I could muster, I deadpanned, "Oh yes, I can have sex. I just can't enjoy it!" We both laughed.

Later, as the doctor began to examine my breasts, the assistant began to relay that conversation. The doctor didn't laugh. Her hands stayed in place, sensing a problem. "I wonder what this is about?" she asked. "Is it a lump? I didn't feel anything in my self-exam!" I responded with sudden seriousness and alarm. The doctor placed my fingers on the lower half of the left breast. "It's something," she said, as I felt for the first time the "marble" growing inside me. "It may only be a cyst, but I want to schedule a mammogram right away."

That appointment was scheduled for two days later. I tried to assure myself that there were many options—and malignancy was only one of them. But my brain swam with memories of the woman who had been my childhood next-door neighbor and "second mother." She was diagnosed with breast cancer in the early 1960s and had died months before my graduation from college. I had made a small contribution in her memory to cancer research. Would it be coming back to help me now?

Waiting and dealing with the unknown was probably the hardest part of my early cancer journey. Much as I tried to calm myself, my mind still wandered toward the worst possibilities. My husband and I held on to each other and tried to take it "one day at a time." We determined that, until we knew more, we would share nothing with our children, our parents, our congregation, or our friends. We prayed together and put ourselves in God's safekeeping.

My husband and I held onto each other and tried to take it "one day at a time."

Survivors Tell Their Stories

A scripture passage proclaims, "In all things, see good!" I began to contemplate: What if my gynecologist hadn't put me on hormones and ordered me back in six months? The cancer had been growing inside me for years. How much more time could have passed before I discovered it?

Though I was nervous, I also felt surrounded by God's care as I met with the surgeon. Both he and his assistant extended compassion as they asked for information and tried to answer my questions. The surgeon didn't want to say too much before the biopsy was completed, but I sensed he knew already that we were dealing with a malignancy. He noted a swelling in my armpit. "It could be from an infection somewhere in your body," he said, but I knew the more ominous possibility . . . a spread of the cancer to my lymph nodes.

Several days later my husband and I sat in the surgeon's office and heard the report. The cells removed during the biopsy proved to be malignant. I thought of our children . . . three sons—a college junior, a high school senior, and an eighth grader—and a daughter about to finish fifth grade. For the first time, tears flooded my eyes. "I still have an 11-year-old at home," I said. The confidence and immediate assurance in the surgeon's voice is something I will long remember: "This is curable!" His assistant put her arm on my shoulder. My husband squeezed my hand. I had never expected the words *cancer* and *curable* to be in the same sentence. But in that moment I found the calm to face whatever lay ahead.

> *I had never expected the words* cancer *and* curable *to be in the same sentence. But in that moment I found the calm to face whatever lay ahead.*

Because the lump was in the lower outside quadrant of my breast, I was a good candidate for a lumpectomy. The surgery was scheduled for the following week. We decided to share the news with our congregation on Sunday morning, but since that was Mother's Day, we delayed phoning my out-of-state mother and my in-laws until Monday morning. Knowing the news would be hard for her to receive, I also sent my mom a letter, putting in writing what the surgeon had said: "This is curable!" We sat with our three children at home and explained as best we could what would happen to mommy. Our oldest son heard the same news when he finished his college finals and came home later in the week. I found it helpful to be as open and reassuring as I could be. This also opened the way to a lot of love and care that surrounded me and my family in the following weeks.

Surgery removed the cancer that had invaded my breast and one sentinel lymph node. My husband and I then visited an oncologist. After examining me, he spent two hours with us—answering questions, explaining his recommendation for the chemotherapy that would attack any errant cancer cells in my system, assuring us that my prognosis was promising, and agreeing that the second opinion we desired was a prudent measure. We made appointments for further tests, including a CAT scan, bone scan, and echocardiogram. Some of these fell on our twenty-fifth wedding anniversary—certainly not the way we anticipated celebrating and yet each providing a special gift: assurance that I was healthy and ready to take on the chemo!

In order to keep family and friends informed, we opted to send a group e-mail after surgeries and treatments. I also found that sitting at a keyboard and sharing updates was a good way to journal my thoughts, feelings, and experiences. These e-mails remain a diary for a time that three years later seems almost surreal. They remind me of the wonderful care I received . . . the humor along with the drugs that infused me with healing . . . the lows and the surprisingly frequent highs during those months. I have since returned to a normally healthy and active life. I have counseled various women and a man who have been diagnosed with breast cancer. Reading these e-mails helps me remember and share some of their fears and struggles.

I am in the business of equipping others to trust in a higher power. I believe God works through people—medical professionals, research scientists, family and friends—to bring healing. My heart is truly filled with thanksgiving for all that was done for me, and for the life that continues to invite my participation.

Luba, 48 years old, chose mastectomy and decided against having reconstructive surgery. She received chemotherapy and hormonal therapy.
Four and a half years ago when I was 44, I went for another routine mammogram after not having one for one and a half years. Here's the

brief synopsis of what happened. A suspicious looking density was found behind my left nipple and my primary care physician suggested that I follow up with an ultrasound on both breasts. Multiple cysts were found on both sides and since I had cysts aspirated before, I wasn't too concerned. However, the density behind the nipple concerned me a lot, so I had a true needle biopsy done by a surgeon with shaky hands. The lab results of that biopsy were negative, and I was told to just relax but my gut said to pursue this further. I always listen to my gut! Thankfully, my primary care physician errs on the side of being conservative and agreed with me to not just relax and gave me a referral for a biopsy.

This time the surgeon that I had tried to get initially was back from his golf vacation and did a biopsy on my left side in March 1998. He would only take my call for results of the biopsy after I got home from work, and I knew that was a bad sign. Sure enough, the diagnosis was infiltrating lobular carcinoma. I remember details now because I am a stickler about getting copies of pathology reports and operative reports for my records and keeping track of what goes on with me medically. What followed was a nerve-racking week of going for tests to see if the cancer had appeared anywhere else in my body (bone scan, blood work, CT Scan, chest X-ray, and liver ultrasound). I had preliminary meetings with an oncologist, recommended by a friend who had a wonderful experience, and a surgeon who specialized in breast surgery. As each test result came in, I breathed another sigh of relief because they were all negative.

Only when I knew those results and had met with the doctors and had a plan in mind was I able to tell my teenaged daughter what was going on with me. She was so tied up with her life and activities that I wanted to be able to give her the information without all the unknowns. My husband was involved in the process with me from the

> *Having access to all the information as it became available made me feel just a tad more in control of this disease and helped me make decisions.*

beginning and went through all the anxiety and tension with me. Having access to all the information as it became available made me feel just a tad more in control of this disease and helped me make decisions. At no point did I feel that anyone was pushing me in a direction that I was not in agreement with. It seemed to me that given the nature of the type of breast cancer I had, my decision for a mastectomy was a natural one for me.

What convinced me was knowing that the cells had roamed outside the actual tumor and that the tumor was not well defined and that the disease was not contained to the area just behind the nipple but that vagrant cells were marching (I had visions of them in single file) to the other parts of my breast. I talked things over with my husband, who said it was essentially my body, and we joked that I still had another breast left, anyway. I went to see the surgeon, who gave me additional information about research findings that no longer said that there was any advantage to having a mastectomy rather than a lumpectomy. Was I aware of that?

My response was that I wanted to get rid of as much of the breast tissue as possible for my peace of mind, so that I would not have to constantly worry about whether some cells were left to do their damage.

So, basically, it was getting information, being treated respectfully regarding my opinion, talking to friends who have had cancer experiences, and firmly believing that I would get through this, that helped with the decision to go ahead with the mastectomy. Yes, I was "young," but I was in a stable relationship,

> *I wanted to get rid of as much of the breast tissue as possible for my peace of mind, so that I would not have to constantly worry about whether some cells were left to do their damage.*

and my husband really understood what was involved here, so the whole physical image issue was not a major one.

My daughter was also supportive and while she was upset, she handled things in a mature, understanding way. She later told me that because I was so sure that I would get through this successfully, she was not very worried. It wasn't until a year later, when all three of us participated in the Race for the Cure in D.C., that she told me it hit home how serious my illness was and that she could have lost me to it. That shook her up more than when I was actually going through treatment.

In meeting with the oncologist, who spent an inordinate amount of time with my husband and myself and who explained and illustrated my cancer type, we talked about treatment options postsurgery. Radiation was not indicated in my case, and I was relieved by that, since I have a fear of radiation, having been exposed to more than my fair share of X-rays since I grew up in a time when being X-rayed was considered a fairly harmless way of checking teeth, diagnosing TB, and even fitting shoes. The fact that I would not require radiation again strengthened my conviction that mastectomy was the way to go for me. The issue, and it wasn't a major one, was whether to have reconstructive surgery.

Since I am a fairly small-breasted woman and didn't have lots of extra abdominal fat to get rid of, and I didn't savor the thought of more hours in surgery building up breast tissue, I said no to the reconstruction option. I could foresee more complications of more surgery and felt that doing it would only be for vanity reasons, and it wasn't that important to me.

Since I am a fairly small-breasted woman and didn't have lots of extra abdominal fat to get rid of, and I didn't savor the thought of more hours in surgery building up breast tissue, I said no to the reconstruction option. I could foresee more complications of more surgery and felt that doing it would only be for vanity reasons, and it wasn't that important to me. The surgeon explained the prosthetic options to me, and I was confident about taking that approach.

When I came home after the surgery, I was visited by a kind soul from the American Cancer Society who brought me a packet of information about postmastectomy exercises and a complimentary bra. She asked me for my age and my bra size over the phone and showed up at the door the next day bearing a size 44B bra, having confused my age with my bra size. Since I'm a 34B person, we shared quite a laugh! After surgery, I recuperated for one and a half weeks and then returned to work, knowing that chemo treatments were to begin in about three weeks. Since my lymph nodes were all negative and the cancer was stage I, the chemo was an insurance policy to assure that any stray cells were oblit-

I was visited by a kind soul from the American Cancer Society who brought me a packet of information about postmastectomy exercises and a complimentary bra. She asked me for my age and my bra size over the phone and showed up at the door the next day bearing a size 44B bra, having confused my age with my bra size. Since I'm a 34B person, we shared quite a laugh!

erated. I was more than willing for that to happen and began the series of four chemo cycles in mid-April. Since we had plans to go on our annual beach trip in July, my plan was to be done with the treatments by then. The oncologist encouraged a positive goal such as a vacation to make the treatments go better.

There wasn't much discussion about which type of chemicals to use, since this was rather standard procedure at this point. Yes, the hair fell out, the wig was purchased and gave me a look that I've always wanted, and I worked throughout the treatment time, scheduling them on Thursdays so I could work on Friday. When I felt tired and nauseous, it would be on Saturday, then I could rest on Sunday and go back to work on Monday. The fatigue was not overwhelming, but it wasn't until about a year or more after chemo that I felt my energy level returning to normal. I'll never forget going on a gentle boardwalk ride at the beach on a windy day, holding onto my wig with one hand and onto the restraining bar with the other, hoping my bandana would not fly off, followed by my wig. Having continued working throughout the chemo treatments and having a vacation goal really helped me get through this time. I was also happy with my wig and wore it daily to work.

The next decision-making phase came after the chemo was finished and I was about to start tamoxifen. Unfortunately, I had a complication from the chemo IV; a blot clot formed in the arm vein that was used to draw blood one day. Since I was told about the side effects of tamoxifen and one of them was increased chance of blood clots, I was not a good candidate for it until that blood clot cleared up. I began to take Coumadin in August of that year to try to break up the clot. This process was worse than the whole breast cancer process because I had to constantly go for blood tests and keep a heating pad on my arm, knowing all the time that my estrogen levels were not being kept down, which could conceivably feed any stray cancer cells. The oncologist decided in October that we needed to address the estrogen issue and discussed with me the possibility of giving me shots of Lupron, a hormone suppressant. Since I was not yet menopausal and knew my cancer had estrogen-positive receptors and would eventually respond to tamoxifen, I agreed to the Lupron shots until the blood clot cleared up and I could begin tamoxifen.

By January, ultrasounds on my arm showed that the clot was almost gone; I stopped the Lupron shots and began on the tamoxifen. I continue on tamoxifen to this day, and in March I will have reached my five-year mark since my mastectomy.

Given my proclivity to form blood clots, I also take a low-dose aspirin daily to keep my blood from getting too sticky. I also get regular mammograms on my right breast, meet regularly with my doctors, and try to eat well. Cancer is a pervasive presence in my family: my father died of bladder cancer at age 63 and my mother died of colon cancer at 73, and several other members have had it. So my thinking was that in my case, it was an issue of when, not what. Now that I've had the diagnosis, the when is answered, and I continue to be vigilant about my health and keep my attitude positive and optimistic.

My advice to anyone embarking on this journey of breast cancer is to inform yourself of exactly what your condition is, talk to others who have walked the walk before you, have real life goals ahead of you, try to maintain as much of your normal schedule as possible, and surround yourself with competent medical people. Make your decision based on all of the information you can get and consult with your closest family and friends. Ultimately, however, the decision must be one that you are comfortable with, since it is your life and your body.

Ruth was 60 years old when she was diagnosed with breast cancer. She chose to undergo a mastectomy and was treated with chemotherapy and then tamoxifen. Ruth also decided to have a prophylactic mastectomy.

I know it's odd to start with a hernia when discussing breast cancer, but I popped a big one on a day in May while lifting a case of flyers at the post office loading dock. That was the start of the year that never should have happened. During the time when I was consulting with doctors on what to do about the hernia, I noticed a texture change on my left breast during breast self-exams—not a lump, but a difference. Surgery for the hernia was impossible since I had three parties for one hundred people scheduled in July, including my mother's ninetieth birthday at my home, and recovery time would have made those commitments impossible. So I watched the texture, which stayed pretty much the same, and I kept on going. I operate a busy pet store and fitting everything in was already a problem with a seven-day-a-week job, but by September things were settling down and I started stocking for the holidays.

In late September I woke up to a lump where the texture change had been, the same place where many years before I had had mastitis (an infection in the breast). My doctor was away, but I made an early afternoon appointment with another doctor.

In her office, I told her I needed some antibiotics for mastitis and then watched her face as she examined me. On impulse, I said, "It's malignant, isn't it?" Caught off guard, she answered "Oh, yes," and then she realized what had happened. I had already determined what it was. She was really upset by answering as she did, and I had to assure her that I would cry that night after I got home from work.

The next stop was the surgeon, who looked at the situation that was not an infection but clearly a lump. Before I realized what he was doing, he did a needle biopsy and confirmed it was malignant. By now I wanted to go ahead with a mastectomy. I also wanted the hernia fixed. The surgeon would not do both at the same time but agreed to a sequential hernia operation two days after the mastectomy. So in October, after a month of great anxiety about wanting the cancer out, I had a mastectomy, and two days later an abdominal hernia repair on the hysterectomy incision with the addition of mesh. The hernia was much worse than the mastectomy.

Now came the consultation with an oncologist, even though I was node negative. I had a short list including a reference from my last customer on Sunday, who had told me about an oncologist when I told him I was having a mastectomy on the following day. Why, you say, did I choose based on a customer's advice? The customer turned out to be the chief of breast cancer at the National Institutes of Health. Was that luck?

The only time I needed a friend along was during the first oncologist visit. The oncologist explained why chemo was recommended based on the aggressive nature of the tumor, and I decided to do it but not until the first of the year. The most interesting part of the appointment was when the oncologist explained that while Adriamycin would be used at a dose intended to not cause heart damage, it could not be repeated, because "your heart remembers."

Chemo was awful, although I missed only one day of work (remem-

Survivors Tell Their Stories

ber, the store is open seven days a week). "Chemo brain" [some degree of cognitive blurriness after treatment] is real. I'm nine years out from my treatment, and I think my mind function gradually improved in measurable ways for the first four years after CAF (Cytoxan, Adriamycin, 5-Flurouracil). I have lymphedema in one arm, and this is a huge obnoxious problem brought on by breaking the affected arm four years out and then breaking the windshield with my hand in a car accident eight years out.

> *I decided to do a prophylactic mastectomy when removing the chemo port. Breast cancer is the best cancer to get. Breasts are not essential body parts, and* WE LIVE.

I decided to do a prophylactic mastectomy when removing the chemo port. Breast cancer is the best cancer to get. Breasts are not essential body parts, and WE LIVE.

Laurie is a registered nurse and was 41 years old when diagnosed with breast cancer. She chose to undergo mastectomy and six months later had a prophylactic mastectomy of her other breast and reconstructive surgery.

I am 46 years old. I am a wife, married twenty-one years, and mother of three sons, 12, 17, and 19 years old. I have been a registered nurse for nineteen years, and currently work part-time in an emergency room. I am enrolled in school part-time, taking classes in American Sign Language. I volunteer part-time at a nonprofit organization, spending time at a community center for the deaf. I paint in watercolors when I can squeeze it in and paint commissioned work now and then. I work out at a health club two to three times a week. Now for my story.

Thursday, December 16, 1999. This is a day that will forever be engraved in my mind. This day started out like all others: I woke up and jumped into the shower. I had never done monthly breast exams on a particular day of the month, but about once a month I checked my breasts while showering.

I had never had cystic breasts, and my breasts were small. As I passed my soapy right hand over my left breast, I felt a small lump above my left nipple. I was surprised and immediately thought cancer. After getting out of the shower, I called my family doctor for a prescription to have a mammogram. I had been given a prescription in the spring after

I had never had cystic breasts, and my breasts were small. As I passed my soapy right hand over my left breast, I felt a small lump above my left nipple. I was surprised and immediately thought cancer.

a pap smear but never followed through. At that time I had also had a manual exam of my breasts by a nurse practitioner, which had not found anything. That evening when I was in bed, I told my husband about my lump and mammogram scheduled for the morning. He didn't say much. On Friday, I had a mammogram. After the mammogram the radiologist recommended a sonogram, which I had. He then came to speak with me. He said I should call a surgeon that day to schedule a biopsy. Again, I thought cancer. I went home and started calling surgeons. If one had told that they could perform a biopsy that afternoon I would have gone. I felt an urgency to get it out of me. After calling four or five surgeons, I finally found one that could see me the next week. I had never heard of this surgeon but didn't care.

My appointment was for Monday, so I had all weekend to think about what I already thought was cancer. Monday morning I went to see the surgeon. He felt my lump and looked at the films from my mammogram. I told him I thought it was cancer because I could see the "finger like projections" on the films, which I had read about. He said he was not convinced it was cancer. The soonest he could do a biopsy was Thursday, the 23rd, two days before Christmas. He planned to remove the entire tumor, and he said if it had clear margins he might not need to do any further surgery, whether or not it was malignant. As I left his office, his secretary again told me the doctor did not think for sure it was cancer. This did not lessen my fear.

On Thursday, I went to an outpatient center in a hospital for my biopsy. The thought of the surgery didn't bother me at all. I couldn't wait to get the tumor out. After the biopsy, I woke with an elastic bandage around my chest, which I was supposed to leave on until Saturday. My surgeon told me he would be away the next week, and I could call or go see his partner for the biopsy results on Tuesday. On Friday, I remember going to my brother's annual holiday party. I was not in the mood. I was sore, had my elastic bandage on and could think of nothing but the results of my biopsy. Christmas came and went fast. I tried to hide my fear and

Survivors Tell Their Stories

never told my children anything at that time. Tuesday morning came not too soon. I went to my bedroom and called the surgeon. I told him I wanted the results over the phone. He calmly said the tumor was malignant, about one and a half centimeters.

He told me to contact a radiologist to discuss radiation therapy and a plastic surgeon to discuss reconstructive surgery. I told him I already knew that I didn't want radiation. He told me to contact one anyway, that I should at least talk to him. I went into the living room to tell my husband. I said, "I have cancer" and started crying.

I went back to see my surgeon with my husband the following week to get the details of my cancer. He said the margins of the tumor were not free of cancer cells and he would need to remove more tissue. He said I could have a lumpectomy or mas-

I told him I already knew that I didn't want radiation.

tectomy and that I would need to have chemotherapy. If I had a lumpectomy, I would also need radiation therapy. He told me my tumor was invasive, and that was bad; my tumor was poorly differentiated, and that was bad; and the tumor was estrogen negative, and that was bad. The word *bad* went through my head over and over again. I left crying. I was to call him back and let him know if I wanted to have a mastectomy or lumpectomy.

My visit to the radiologist went as I thought it would. He informed me of all of the positive and negative aspects of radiation therapy, but mostly positive. He told me if I had a lumpectomy with radiation and the cancer came back, I would still have a breast to remove. (Just what I wanted to hear.) He said the procedure is not uncomfortable and is for five days a week for only eight weeks. He described side effects like feeling tired and being red and tender at the site of radiation and surrounding area. I didn't care what he said; I had my mind made up before I went. I would not have radiation. In my past experience as a nurse, I had seen some bad results after radiation. This may be the exception, but I was not going to take that chance. In addition to this, I was not willing to go through eight weeks of radiation after having surgery and chemotherapy over three months.

My visit to the plastic surgeon went quickly. I started crying when I told him why I was there. He was positive and sympathetic. He took a quick look at my breasts and abdomen. He told me that I didn't have enough abdominal fat to have the muscle and fat from my abdomen transferred to my chest for reconstruction, but I could have implants if I chose to have a mastectomy. He showed me a book of photos with reconstructive breast surgery that he had done. I liked him even though we had a very short visit.

I called my surgeon and told him I wanted to have a mastectomy. I knew this from the start. I wanted the least possible chance of the tumor returning in my breast tissue. The surgery was scheduled for mid-January, the soonest possible date. I broke the news to my sons that I had breast cancer. I knew they would worry, but, of course, I had to tell them. I told them I would need surgery followed by chemotherapy and that I would lose all of my hair. I think everyone was in shock. We didn't have any long conversations, just some questions and answers.

> *I called my surgeon and told him I wanted to have a mastectomy. I knew this from the start. I wanted the least possible chance of the tumor returning in my breast tissue.*

I was not overly nervous the morning of the surgery—in fact, I couldn't wait to get it over with. I drove to the hospital myself so that my husband could get my sons off to school. He arrived at the hospital before I went into the operating room. One thing that sticks in my mind is that a recent cancer patient, who also was a nurse, came to speak with me. She was angry about having cancer and told me what a horrible experience she had with chemotherapy and losing her hair. She was not comforting at all. I only stayed in the hospital overnight. I could have stayed longer but was anxious to go home. My recovery at home was quick. My mother came to help, and my sister-in-law stopped by to cook dinner.

I was scheduled for chemo beginning in early February. I had four courses, one every three weeks. I didn't return to work because I was too upset about the whole experience of having breast cancer and knowing I was going to lose my hair with upcoming chemo. I'm self-conscious about my looks and hated the thought of facing anyone I knew when I was bald. I didn't even want old friends to see me. I vividly remember my first chemo. I went to my oncologist's office with my husband. An IV was started. I watched the red fluid, Adriamycin, drip by drip into my vein. I also received IV Cytoxan. All went well, and I thought, "This isn't bad." That evening my husband and I went to buy a new car. I began to feel lightheaded during our transaction and needed to sit down. I don't know if it was a mental or physical response to the day and my first chemo. I still couldn't believe it was happening to me. The following day I had the terrible taste in my mouth that came after all four doses of chemo. To me this was the worst part of the chemo. I could taste the chemical in my mouth and also felt like I was breathing it. It was the reason I dreaded the following three doses. I also felt like I had the flu for one or two days after each chemo. I took my anti-nausea medication and never vomited, but I never had much of an appetite for about a week after each chemo dose.

I remember losing my hair. I found out I have a nice little round head. I wore a wig when I went out and a hat with a headband when in the house. I never let anyone see me when I was bald, not even my family. I hated looking like I was sick and thought I had the typical cancer patient look. I became pale, thin, and hairless.

> *I wore a wig when I went out and a hat with a headband when in the house. I never let anyone see me when I was bald, not even my family.*

It was during my chemo that I decided I wanted a mastectomy on my remaining right breast. I wanted to decrease my chances of getting cancer again, at least in my breast. I was not high risk for getting breast cancer in the first place. I was average weight, watched my diet, exercised regularly, had no close relatives with breast cancer, had a baby before thirty years old, and breastfed three babies. I thought that if I could get breast cancer once, with no risk factors, I could certainly get it again. The thought of surgery again didn't bother me at all. When I told my oncologist that I wanted to have a mastectomy on my remaining breast, he told me he would support whatever decision I made but to wait at least six months before deciding. I told him I would not change my mind.

After my last chemo dose, at the end of April, I began thinking about my hair growing back. I couldn't wait to feel somewhat "normal" again. It didn't really start coming in until August. My family went to vacation for a week at the beach in August, and I wore a hat the whole time. I still had not started working again. I received disability pay, but benefits were running out and I knew I would soon need to return to work. The week after I finished my chemo, my neighbor knocked on my door. She told me she had an aggressive breast cancer with a ten-centimeter mass. I felt so bad for her, knowing she was headed for a much longer battle than I had.

I didn't want to return to the same job I had left when my cancer was discovered nine months earlier. I was not quite sure what I wanted to do. I just knew that I wanted to be happy with my job and my life. It was at this time that I decided to pursue something I had thought about for many years. I signed up for an evening class in American Sign Language. I don't know why, but it was something that had appealed to me for years. Whenever I saw deaf people using sign language, I felt I wanted to learn how to sign. I also took a part-time nursing job. I love my sign language class and have pursued it with hopes of one day becoming a sign language interpreter in the medical field.

By October I hadn't changed my mind and couldn't wait any longer to have my second mastectomy. I was sorry I didn't have it at the same time as my first one. My oncologist supported my decision although he said I was not at high risk for breast cancer again. (I thought, I never was in the first place, and I still got it!) I went to the same surgeon and told him about my decision. He was not supportive. In fact, he tried to discourage me, but my mind was made up. If he didn't want to perform the surgery, I would find another surgeon. He told me I could take tamoxifen, but I still felt this was not to my benefit. He agreed to do the surgery. Again, I was not scared. I was home the day after the surgery, and all went well. I had the expected discomfort. I had implants placed in both breasts at the time. I had previously had an expander placed in my left breast. The biopsy on my breast tissue showed abnormal cells, which would probably have developed into breast cancer.

> *I went to the same surgeon and told him about my decision. He was not supportive. In fact, he tried to discourage me, but my mind was made up. If he didn't want to perform the surgery, I would find another surgeon.*

Looking back on my breast cancer experience, I am happy with the decisions I made. I think my biggest fear was for my children. I didn't want them to watch their mother die. I know it was hard for them to see me look so sick. I thought about them growing up without me if I were to die. I still think about the cancer returning but don't dwell on it. I still try to take care of myself. I don't know if I would have ever pursued learning sign language if not for going through that experience, so I can see how something good has come out of it. I try to make the most of every day and do what makes me happy, but sometimes, like everyone, I get caught up in life's chaos.

Kimberly was 38 years old when diagnosed with a breast cancer that was large and considered locally advanced. She chose to undergo bilateral mastectomy with reconstructive surgery. She received chemotherapy and radiation therapy but decided not to undergo a bone marrow/stem cell transplantation.

I had come home from a tennis match and noticed something strange when I looked at my right breast. I noticed that the right nipple was bleached out to the color of my skin, and I thought it was very unusual, so I got close to the mirror, lifted my whole breast up and realized that I felt a large mass. My mom had had breast cancer and I had been monitored at an earlier than usual age, and I found it unusual because I had had a mammogram approximately two to three months before and everything was fine.

So the next morning I called my primary care physician and went in immediately, and he said that I needed to go immediately and see a surgeon. About an hour later, I went to the surgeon's office. He decided to do a needle biopsy at that moment, and when he did nothing aspirated. He said that I needed to have a biopsy done, so I went to an outpatient center the same day. Well, I was concerned. I was very concerned. I just said, "OK, let's take whatever the next step is." So we went to the outpatient center. He did the biopsy and before he finished sewing me up the phone rang in the operating room. He left my side and answered it and then came back and told me that it was malignant, before I was even off the table. He told me to get dressed and to meet him in his office in one hour.

It made me think back to when my mom had breast cancer many years before. When she was diagnosed, I was 21 years of age. She went into surgery, and the surgeon came out and made me make the decision for my mother whether to take both breasts. At age 21 I didn't have the understanding that I do today. And the doctor said that because I was her only next of kin, I had to make that decision, so I made it. My mother's cancer was caught at a very early stage and she did not have to go through any treatment, so she went through reconstruction approximately six to eight weeks later and that was the end of her ordeal. My route, of course, was a lot different. When I went to the surgeon's office, that same day, with my mother, I sat across from him, and the surgeon told me that I had stage IV inflammatory breast cancer and that I was a goner and that I was to get my papers together because I wasn't going to be here long.

I thanked him very much and said goodbye, and at that point that's when I decided to take matters into my own hands and to research as to what to do. That led me to an oncologist, with whom I decided that the best treatment was to go through chemotherapy so that they could try to shrink it because it was such a large tumor. They both felt that the way the surgeon handled the situation was very unprofessional. I wanted to move on, because I'm not the kind of person who's going to dwell on what another person has done. I don't believe it should have been handled that way, but we were beyond it. Now we needed to take care of what needed to be taken care of. So I went through five and a half months of chemotherapy. It was explained to me that it was necessary to shrink the tumor before I could even have surgery. It was a very aggressive tumor, and that was the reasoning behind the treatment plan. I didn't question that.

I had three daughters, and I was a single mom. I could count on my mother for any kind of medical support, but she also works full-time and lives a busy life. I had been married for fifteen years and had just separated from my husband one month before I found out I had cancer. My biggest concern was about my children. I was afraid of losing them because of my medical condition. I wasn't as concerned about the cancer as I was the welfare of my children. I needed to do whatever was necessary so that I would be there for them. And my strength came from my children, knowing that I needed

And my strength came from my children, knowing that I needed to take care of them and doing whatever was necessary — so if I needed to do whatever the most aggressive treatment was, then I was going to do it.

Survivors Tell Their Stories

to take care of them and doing whatever was necessary—so if I needed to do whatever the most aggressive treatment was, then I was going to do it. This was not about me—this was about my children.

For support I talked to the pastor of my church. I did talk to another woman who was a breast cancer survivor about what she had been through, and that was a lot of support in itself. I talked to people at a research hospital, and I had a friend at the National Institutes of Health (NIH) who was able to give me a lot of information. I'm the kind of person who wants to understand what the drug does. Yet I will have faith in my doctor; you know, that's why I'm seeing the doctor.

When I started the chemotherapy I was told that eighteen days after starting chemo I would lose all my hair. So I bought two wigs. One wig looked exactly like my hair, and I wore it before I lost my hair and you could not tell.

Every time I went through a treatment, it was a three-day process. I would feel bad for three days, but for some reason, at the end of that third day, suddenly it was like, *boom,* I was back, and I was like I had never gone through anything. People were wonderful. I used to be a leader in USTA tennis and played with women from all over. Those women got together and coordinated everything to be sure that there were groceries in my home. I could never return the kindness that was shown to me. The support came from women in the tennis community and my church. It was overwhelming.

I finished the chemo, and it was time to have the mastectomy. I was in the hospital for three days. They did a double mastectomy. They said that because the tumor was so large there wasn't any question as to whether the left breast was at risk to develop cancer, so they did a prophylactic mastectomy. Knowing what my mother had been through, I

I looked at it and said, "I'm alive. Thank you. I'm here." Not, "Oh, my gosh, look at me."

knew what to expect after surgery. I know how she felt emotionally after she had the surgery. I was taken aback, too, when I saw myself the first time I was unwrapped. I knew that it was very bad, and I knew that this was the way that it was going to be, so I was prepared. I can't tell you that it wasn't shocking to look at. It was. But for me, I looked at it and said, "I'm alive. Thank you. I'm here." Not, "Oh, my gosh, look at me."

I had the six and a half weeks of radiation, Monday through Friday. The radiation, that was very different. That was something that I had never experienced because my mother had never gone through that either. She hadn't gone through chemo or radiation. I had no choice whatsoever. When I was going through it, you could see the burn marks on my back, it was so strong, and one of the nurses said it looked like third-degree burns. She used to treat it each day with some sort of a salve and wrap me in dressings.

I would focus on other things when receiving radiation. It was as if I had a photograph album of my life and of my children. I would lie on the table, and my eyes would be closed and in my mind I would see picture after picture, but these weren't pictures in any albums. They were pictures of things that I remember about my children that were happy things, and they might be from a long time ago to current things, but I just found that I focused on my children and the happy things.

After radiation I was asked if I wanted to have a stem cell transplant. I said no because they felt that they had gotten everything they could get, the cancer, and I felt there wasn't any reason to do it.

The reconstruction started about thirteen months after the double mastectomies with silicone implants. The reason I did it was not for cosmetic reasons. It was because that prosthesis was heavy, and I was too young of a woman to wear that for the next fifty years. I had complications all the way through. From one surgery to the next, there was always a problem. The implant eventually had to be removed. Four months later I had TRAM flap surgery because they could not do an implant on the right side. They said that the radiation had a lot to do with why the implant didn't work, so when they went in, it was actually a good thing. When I went in, they removed a lot of scar tissue. They did a TRAM flap procedure where they cut me from hip to hip, and they took the stomach muscle and channeled it up and reattached it through my right chest wall. My right side is the TRAM, and my left side is an implant. The TRAM is very soft, because it's your own skin. The left side was done with saline at the time, and it was hard as a rock. The way I wear my clothes it's not as noticeable, and it's not important to me right now.

I also started taking tamoxifen. The benefits of tamoxifen outweigh the risks. As I said to my children, I was going to do whatever I felt was the best, and that was why I made the decision to go on the tamoxifen.

My mother had cancer, and I had cancer, and my children have such a big concern about whether they're going to have cancer. I have mixed emotions about whether I should find out if I carry the gene. I don't feel clearly about it, and if I don't feel clearly, I don't feel it's something I should do. I do not want my children to worry all through their lives, "Oh, my gosh, I have this gene, this is going to happen." They need to live their lives, and then if that should come about, then we deal with it.

I'll share something that happened to me that I hope other women will understand. Being a single mom for a number of years, I really never thought that I would remarry. I didn't look for it. But then I met a very nice man who is now my husband of three years. When our relationship grew, and I fell in love and knew that he loved me and cared about my children, the time came in our relationship, over a year after we had been together, when it became physical. The first time for him to see me without my clothes on was such a very emotional and scary thing to me. My husband is a blessing. When he saw me for the first time and saw those scars, I remember him looking at me, touching the scars and saying how thankful he was that those scars

We look at each other and say, "Today is a gift."

were there because if it weren't for those scars he never would have known me. At that point, how much more I loved this man whom I already loved. He put my fear and embarrassment at ease. I finally realized that I had been strong for myself, but this was a time where all my emotions, strength, and everything were set aside, and what I was feeling was coming from way deep down. From that point on he was my biggest supporter, besides the girls, and he shared everything else with me as far as the reconstruction and so forth. To this day we look at each other and say, "Today is a gift."

I'm happy that my children look at me as a strong woman. This experience has also shown them that they are strong. They also have faith. My children grow stronger from what

I burst with joy at being able to tell people that having breast cancer doesn't mean the end of your life. Life can be everything you want it to be.

they've seen me go through. I burst with joy at being able to tell people that having breast cancer doesn't mean the end of your life. Life can be everything you want it to be. I'm walking proof that my life is better than I thought it could ever be — not that I don't have ups and downs, not that I don't have good days and bad days, but overall, you can live life to the fullest.

Regina was 49 years old when she was diagnosed with breast cancer. Her mother had bilateral breast cancer, and both Regina and her mother are positive for a subtle change in the BRCA gene which may have predisposed them to this disease. Regina was treated with lumpectomy and radiation, and then she received adjuvant chemotherapy.

I'm 53 years old. I work for the federal government, and I have for thirty-two years. I'm at the National Institutes of Health. I have one child who is 19 years old. I teach aerobics part-time; I like doing needlework and talking to my mom.

I found it myself. I found two lumps. I was having this itching, burning sensation. One day I was scratching (it was an internal itch) when I found two lumps, called my doctor, went in to see her, and she found them. I had the mammogram, which showed I had two distinct lumps. My doctor was on vacation when they were found with the mammogram. The radiologist wanted to do a sonogram, but I had to wait a week because my doctor was on vacation and radiology needed a referral from her. The sonogram just confirmed what the mammogram showed.

The radiologist wanted to do a sonogram, but I had to wait a week because my doctor was on vacation and radiology needed a referral from her.

I don't remember fear. I just reacted and knew I had to do something. And I didn't tell anyone initially, and then I told my son. He had seen his grandmother go through it, and I said, "Brandon, I found a lump, and I'm going to have to go into the hospital — it's just outpatient — to see what's going on." He was a sophomore in high school. He didn't react, but I think that is a boy thing. I didn't tell my mom at first. It's like being pregnant — you don't want to tell anyone in your first trimester because of the possibility of losing the baby — so that was my way of dealing with it. I wanted to find out exactly what was going on before I shared it with someone.

In my heart, I knew, I think because of being exposed to it when I was young, with my grandmothers. I had a sense of knowing me, my body, what was going on, and what could be happening. Years ago, the doctor would say, "You're at risk. It doesn't mean that you are going to get it, but you're at risk." When my grandmothers were diagnosed—my father's mother and my mother's mother—I felt more at risk. So when I found those lumps, I didn't want to alert anyone until I knew all the facts.

I had an appointment to go for a follow-up the day my results came in, and the doctor's office didn't have a chance to call me beforehand. I had a two o'clock appointment. The doctor's assistant came in with the doctor, and he's talking to me as if I knew something was wrong. I went in for my follow-up appointment, and the doctor is talking to me about the pathology report, and I'm looking at him, like, "Oh, OK." I'm very slow in reacting, and I wouldn't cry. I didn't get upset, and I remember everything so well. We went into his office, and he did the diagrams. He went into the whole scenario; he was very thorough. Even though I hadn't been warned or prepared before the appointment, the manner in which he handled the whole situation was excellent. There was a calm about him. You know, I deal with doctors all the time in my work at the NIH, and I guess because he is a seasoned doctor, he's dealing with this all the time. He's a surgeon, so he's dealing with all kinds of operations, not just breast cancer or lumpectomies or mastectomy.

When I went about the biopsy, he talked about everything. "If this is what we find, you have choices." So all of those were presented, and I think I had in my mind a lumpectomy. The surgeon explained that there's no true difference in treatment outcome between lumpectomy and mastectomy, and I remember him saying that because of my age and my physical health, he felt a lumpectomy would be best. I remember thinking that the mastectomy is pretty big surgery, and I'm an active person, I don't think I could just sit around at home recovering.

The surgeon did the lymph node biopsy—a sentinel node procedure. He injects you with isotopic dye, and the dye goes through, and wherever it stops there is a possibility of an abnormality, which is removed and sent to pathology to do their thing. I liked the idea of the procedure because it was, "We will not be removing everything, we will be removing only what this procedure indicates might be abnormal." I knew that something might be done, that there was a possibility, but he couldn't tell until he looked at the lumps. He explained to me that if what was found was cancerous, then he would have to go in to complete that part.

I went into the hospital, had the lumpectomy and the lymph node dissection, and the nurses came right in. I was comfortable in the hospital until an hour or so before leaving, but I had a bad experience with a nurse who was attending me at that time. They gave me a shot of Demerol right after surgery, and then I got another shot that morning, and I started having pain. I have a pretty high tolerance for pain, but I was not happy with the nurse who was attending to me. Eventually, the nursing assistant came in, and I asked to get my nurse. She came back in a half an hour and said that the nurse wasn't around and she would go find her. The nurse came in and said I couldn't have a shot, that I had had my limit. She said, "I'll be right back," and then she was gone forever. My mom showed up to take me home, and I was still waiting for some help.

I came home, and I was soaked with blood because the drain was not working well. My son was there, and I told my mom to go home because I could see she was already upset. I was thinking that I could handle the drain because they had me work with the drain tube at the hospital, and I could do it with my left hand. I ended up calling a very close friend, though, and she came with gauze and gloves and changed all the dressings and taped it really well. I went in a day early to get the drain out.

I suspected it was in the lymph nodes because the surgeon described the cancer that I had as a fast, aggressive form. I had invasive carcinoma, and he explained that it develops in the mammary duct, and it literally just "bursts out," and that, in terms of timing, I was fortunate in reacting right away. I thought, "Well, maybe that burning, itching sensation I was feeling before I felt the lump was this cancer growing within the duct, and when it came out, more could have been there, but by reacting when I did, it prevented more problems."

My oncologist talked about the whole process of chemotherapy, what goes on, and he asked me if I would be interested in participating in a clinical trial. I said yes. He explained the drugs that were used and how my treatments might differ by being part of the clinical trial.

I got all this paperwork, some seven or eight pages about the clinical trial. I read through it, and I decided, yeah. You were part of team A, B, or C, and you didn't know what group you were part of. I thought that my participating might help someone else—somebody younger, somebody older, everybody reacts differently. I looked at it this way: no matter whether you were part of the trials or just receiving a regular treatment, based on your diagnosis, you would be getting the best treatment, no matter what. I look at the trials as a way of helping other people, because they say one out of eight or one out of nine women are diagnosed with breast cancer.

> *I got all this paperwork, some seven or eight pages about the clinical trial. I read through it, and I decided, yeah. You were part of team A, B, or C, and you didn't know what group you were part of. I thought that my participating might help someone else—somebody younger, somebody older.*

I had several tests before starting the treatment. I had the echogram, and I had the CAT scans. I started my treatment, and I didn't feel uncomfortable. Because I saw my mom go through the treatment, I knew I was going to be hooked up to an IV. I knew there was a possibility of not feeling well because I had seen how a person reacted to it. But the physical part of the first treatment was a breeze. One day during treatment, my nurse asked if I would mind sharing the room with a new patient who was very anxious abut her treatment, and I said, "No problem." Mom was with me. The new patient's friend was with her, and her anxieties were just extreme—she got sick when they hooked her up to the IV anti-nausea medication. We became friends. We exchanged phone numbers, and she still calls me now and then. The treatment area is a big room with two large recliners, and a sofa, so two people easily share the room. The staff is very sensitive to the personalities, to the manner in which people come in and how they are relating. They have a psychiatric nurse who is available two times a week. I only went to one support group during my treatment, and I found it very depressing. It had ladies who had been diagnosed years ago and had finished treatment.

I knew I was going to lose the hair, and what bothered me was loss of my eyelashes. I went to a department store to find a foundation to cover up the change in my complexion, and I got a wig before I lost my hair. It came down far enough that it hid my eyebrows. I didn't have my head shaved. I had already started wearing the wig before. I think it was the nurse in the oncologist's office who said to me that I might want to start wearing my wig before treatment, to get used to wearing it and to have people get used to seeing the change. I told people that I had a "bad hair experience." Having the treatments on Friday, I was sick on Saturday and Sunday. Monday I would get up because my son was going to school, and I still tried to do the same routine—getting him up, ready for school. He was driving, so I didn't have to drive him to school. I actually invited him to go with me one time for a treatment. He went all the way to the doctor's office. He drove, and then we were in the waiting room waiting for me to go back, and he said, "Mom, can I go get something to eat?" I said, "Sure." I think it was a lot for him to just even go to the doctor's office, but I wanted him to see inside the office and see the people.

Bonnie grew up in Taiwan and moved to the United States as a young adult. She was 41 years old when diagnosed with breast cancer thirteen years ago. She chose to undergo a mastectomy without reconstructive surgery, though now she is considering having a breast implant.

I was working as a nurse in our local hospital's orthopedic unit. One of my patient's daughters told me that her mom had a big lump in her breast and called me to check it. It was very hard and suspicious and I notified the doctor. I really had not performed a breast self-exam often, so later that night I started to check my own breasts and then I found a small lump. I saw my doctor, was referred to a surgeon, and after a biopsy this proved to be a breast cancer. So that patient is my angel because she reminded me to do the breast exam, which I probably would have delayed otherwise.

That patient is my angel because she reminded me to do the breast exam, which I probably would have delayed otherwise.

When I learned that I had breast cancer after the biopsy, I made a de-

Survivors Tell Their Stories

cision that I wanted a mastectomy. If I had chosen to have a lumpectomy, then I would have needed to do the radiation, but after mastectomy the whole tumor would be removed. It was also an easy decision for me to not undergo reconstructive surgery. At that time the most common procedure was to place a saline or silicon implant. I didn't like either idea because I worried that a saline implant could break and silicone had a bad reputation then. I had been a teacher in Taiwan, but I came to the United States and studied to be a nurse. I cared for many women who had had a mastectomy, and so it was a more comfortable decision for me to make.

Psychologically to only have one breast, it has not been that much of a problem for me. Now, thirteen years later, I am reconsidering having a breast implant. I have been swimming regularly since I was 46 years old, and now I'm 54. It's an inconvenience to put a prosthesis in my bathing suit, and then the swimming is not easy. I have been thinking that if I have a breast implant, I may also want to have my remaining breast reduced in size to match the shape and size of the implant. Although it has been many years since my mastectomy, my health insurance will still pay 90 percent of the bill for the surgery. I think that after reconstructive surgery, I would be able to swim like other people.

My husband doesn't say much about my having additional reconstructive surgery. He is not a person who talks, and for a while after my surgery I was very lonely and frustrated, but now I'm getting better because I'm swimming, doing yoga exercises, and I'm pondering God's words. If I have reconstructive surgery, I may have a different image, and it may be better for our relationship. But truly if I have the reconstruction, it will be for me and not really for my husband.

Kathleen was age 45 when diagnosed with breast cancer. She was treated with lumpectomy and radiation as well as chemotherapy.

I was diagnosed with breast cancer when I was 45, a mother with five children ranging in age from 25 to 16. Not that a diagnosis of cancer can ever come at a good time, but this one couldn't have come at a worse time. Our family had a series of tragedies that year, and my illness was the "crowning blow." My husband's sister was dying at age 50 from colon cancer, two of our sons had lost good friends on Pan AM 103, and two close friends had died of cancer. With a name like Kathleen O'Connor, I guess you could call it "Murphy's Law."

My tumor was found during a mammogram, and I saw the surgeon the same week. After he determined that it was not a cyst, a lumpectomy was scheduled for the following week. The surgeon insisted that the surgery would be "a breeze." Quite to the contrary, it was emotionally draining and pretty uncomfortable. It reinforced the adage that there is no such thing as small surgery. Right after the surgery, the surgeon informed my husband and me that the tumor was definitely malignant and that we should make an appointment with him to talk about my options. We were stunned at the diagnosis, and it was especially difficult for my husband. I wasn't prepared for the physical sensation of raw fear. As a hospice caregiver for many years, I thought I would be better prepared for a cancer diagnosis — I wasn't! I guess one is never prepared. For several days after my surgery, I really was scared that I, like my mother, would die young. I prayed, and through grace, I got a grip on myself.

I don't think there had been many studies on mastectomy versus lumpectomy at this time. The surgeon said either of those options was appropriate for me. The "plus" of going with the mastectomy was that it would require no radiation treatments. He said that many women felt that removal of the breast gave them the greatest peace of mind that all the cancer was gone and "couldn't come back." He thought that I would also be a good candidate for a lumpectomy and recommended that I make an appointment with a radiation oncologist.

Even though he had removed the tumor during the initial surgery, the surgeon wanted to go back in and make wider margins and take out some lymph nodes to determine if the cancer had spread. The tumor was bigger than he had first thought, and that was worrisome; everything got blown up in my mind. The surgeon was noncommittal about which surgery I should have. He kept saying it was totally my decision. I barely listened to what he said after he mentioned the increased tumor size. Thankfully, my husband did listen to him and felt positive and encouraged me to think about the lumpectomy. I made an appointment with a radiologist oncologist to determine if she felt I was a candidate for radiation and a lumpectomy. I also made an appointment with the plastic surgeon to get information on reconstruction if I decided to have a mastectomy.

My appointment with the radiologist was like something out of *The Three Stooges*. I arrived at the appointment with a written report from the surgeon's office. The radiologist needed the actual X-rays to determine my appropriateness for radiation. I was such an emotional, stressed-out mess that this seemed like the end of the world to me. But

> *She needed the actual X-rays to determine my appropriateness for radiation. I was such an emotional, stressed-out mess that this seemed like the end of the world to me.*

God love her, I got my X-rays and went to her house that evening, and she looked at them under her kitchen counter lights and said I'd do great with radiation.

In the meantime, every well-intentioned breast cancer survivor called me to tell her story. Several had had mastectomies and encouraged me to just "get it off." It was too much information for me, and I went back and forth about mastectomy versus lumpectomy. My husband's roommate from college was a general surgeon, and I went and saw him about what he thought I should do. Unlike my surgeon, he strongly recommended that I go with the lumpectomy. Of course, he was talking to me as a good friend, not as a patient. He said he had removed too many healthy breasts where the pathology showed after the mastectomy that there was no other cancer in the breast but the lump he had removed at diagnosis. I wanted to keep my breast, but I wanted a guarantee that all would be well. He looked right at me and said "Kathy, you could leave here and be killed going home on the beltway. There are no guarantees in life." Boy, did I need to hear and think about that! I know that there are no guarantees in life, having lost family and friends unexpectedly. But in my panic and fear, I forgot that I needed to make a decision based on knowledge and then trust in my doctors' and my own ability to meet this challenge.

I decided to go with a lumpectomy and radiation. My husband wholeheartedly agreed with my decision. I chose the lumpectomy/radiation treatment for several reasons. My surgeon had told me that there were clean margins around my tumor. He felt that he had gotten it all. I trusted his judgment, and I wanted to keep my breast. Having nursed my children and always been pleased with my breasts as a woman, I did not want to lose one unless it was absolutely necessary. I had had such a positive experience with the radiation oncologist, who was so knowledge-able but also so warm and compassionate. Letting me come to her home to look at my X-rays went well

I trusted his judgment, and I wanted to keep my breast.

beyond the call of duty. The meeting with the plastic surgeon only reinforced my decision.

One of the best things my surgeon did was put me in touch with one of his patients who had had a lumpectomy several years before, a nurse at my surgeon's hospital. She was supportive, and it was calming to talk to her — much better than talking to a myriad of friends who gave too much advice. I talked to her several times during this decision-making period, and she was an angel in helping me make decisions and being positive.

My next stop was to go to an oncologist. I did not know if I would need chemotherapy after my surgery. I made an appointment with an oncologist and carried with me all the records from the surgeon and hospital.

The oncologist had not gotten back all of my pathology, but he wanted me to have chemotherapy. He told me to think of it as my insurance policy and encouraged me to stop my fatalism and take control of what I could control. He recommended Bernie Siegel's book *Love, Medicine, and Miracles*. It was a great book for me to read at that time. I decided that this was a challenge that I had been given, and I needed to meet this challenge as best I could. I wanted to know that if I did have a recurrence, I had done everything in my power at the time of diagnosis. If the cancer returned, I wouldn't have any "what ifs?" I decided to go with chemotherapy. The oncologist explained the protocol. My pathology showed that I had a very aggressive type of breast cancer and had to have chemotherapy anyway, but I had already made the decision.

I was blessed in my care with a great medical team: the surgeon, the radiation oncologist, the oncologist, and warm, empathetic nurses. I also have a loving husband, family, and friends. I controlled what I could control — my attitude and the choice of physicians. But ultimately, I needed to trust in my physicians, their knowledge and experience. And

I must add, trust in God, that regardless of the outcome, I would handle it with as much courage and grace as I could muster.

Seventeen years later, I am a "professional grandmother." Sixteen children call me "Nonna." I am thankful for the care and treatment of my physicians. I am thankful every day.

CHAPTER 22

Stories from Women with
Advanced Breast Cancer

Today, breast cancer is generally detected early, but sometimes it is not.
Sometimes the first diagnosis is metastatic breast cancer. Other women
develop recurrent cancer after primary therapy.

Although advanced breast cancer remains a serious disease that often requires
prolonged treatment, great strides have been made in its medical management.
Women with advanced breast cancer face treatment choices that are guided by the
following factors:

1. Where is the cancer located? Is it in the bone or in the internal
   organs?
2. How much time has passed between initial therapy and diagnosis
   of the recurrence?
3. What is the pace of the illness? Is it symptomatic and progressing rapidly, or is it asymptomatic and changing slowly?
4. How effective was previous treatment, and what were the side
   effects?

5. What is the woman's age, and what other medical conditions does she have?
6. What treatment options are available?

There is no simple equation for designing a treatment plan. With her doctors, each woman must weigh the risks and benefits of different options and consider the quality of life she will have with each choice. Women facing the same diagnosis often make different decisions and may make decisions that differ from their doctors' advice.

Yvonne was 47 years old when her breast cancer was first diagnosed. She received chemotherapy and initially did well. But about three years later, she developed headaches caused by brain metastases. She was treated with radiation and has done well for over three years since then.

One evening I went home and as usual cleared the day's mail. Out popped a card from my HMO that read: "When you are 40 you need to have an annual mammogram." The instruction was clear. I took it along with me to the doctor and got the authorization to have a mammogram scheduled.

Bear in mind, I have always been a healthy person. That is why this was my first mammogram. The process was simple, but the look on the technician's face was one of deep concern. I picked up on it and asked, "What's wrong?"

"The doctor is coming in to see you," she responded. I said out loud, "Lord, please do not let this be what I am thinking, but if it is, give me the strength to deal with whatever comes my way." He heard, and he answered.

That is where my journey into the world of breast cancer began. My family physician is small in stature but has the biggest heart. He gave

My family physician is small in stature but has the biggest heart. He gave me great comfort. He looked for the best surgeon he could find and made the appointment himself.

me great comfort. He looked for the best surgeon he could find and made the appointment himself. My surgeon was the greatest. He was reassuring and kind. I will always remember the words he spoke to me on my first visit: "If this area is what they are concerned about, I wouldn't worry too much, but let's do a biopsy and see." The next week was unbearable. I had shared the information with only a few people.

Well, here comes the big day. Results of the biopsy. I had gone to the doctor's office alone. The doctor said, "This has bowled me over." I felt sick. I knew what was going to be said next. The tears just came rolling down like an overflowing dam. I wept.

I asked, "Why now? Why now?" Repeatedly. The doctor responded, "I don't know what else is going on, but one thing I do know is that this is major stuff." Amid the tears, I called my daughter to come and take me home. All I wanted to do was to go to bed and sleep forever.

She is my only child, and she had never seen me sick. I knew she would be scared and worried, so I tried to regain some level of composure and tried to reassure her that I would be fine and that I would get better. My concern shifted from myself to her. How would she manage without me? There was no easy answer.

As a woman of faith, I put my faith into action. I called on God for help, for guidance, and for a great team of health professionals who would be kind, gentle, and considerate. He heard, and he answered, and he sent me the best team of oncologists you could ever ask for.

I paid a visit to my family doctor, who said, "Yvonne, I have the very best oncologists for you. They are very, very good."

I had several consultations prior to my surgery. I was extremely fortunate to have both my oncologists and my surgeon located in the same building and on the same floor—everything works together for good.

Before surgery I had put together my small group of supporters. Team leader was Trudy, my daughter, and there were three other close friends who would accompany me on doctors' visits and have input in every aspect of my treatment. They became my ears, my brain, and my memory.

On a wider scale, my small prayer group became my family. Karen, my trusted friend (you always need to have one of those) was my encourager, my prayer partner, and the one who saw to it that my faith was intact and my spirit lifted high. She took care of and organized help for all my needs. With the assistance of Pamela, my personal RN, I was able to deal with medical emergencies as she took charge of my personal care.

It was time for chemotherapy. The horror stories came from every angle. Thank God, I did not have any of those horrible experiences — none of the dreaded nausea. My friend Max was a tower of strength. He transported me to chemotherapy treatments and because he had personal experience with chemotherapy and its effect on the body, having had several family members who had died from the disease, his support was invaluable.

No one can prepare you for the hair loss. It was the worst part of the sickness. Every time I ran my hands across my head and felt those clumps of hair filling them, all I could do was cry, most times uncontrollably. I felt like I was losing control of myself. It was devastating. It was worse than losing my breast. I was not ready for the baldness, so I had a wig styled to match my usual hairstyle, complete with the gray strands.

Whether it was the tamoxifen or the chemotherapy, I do not know, but I went spiraling into menopause. That was rough. I was not ready! I was looking forward to having a smooth transition just like my mother and older sister had, no fuss, no discomfort, no hot flashes, none of that stuff! Sorry, that was not going to be!

With the encouragement of my oncologists, and based on their recommendation of a very good surgeon, I decided to have reconstruction and chose to have a TRAM flap. I was pleased with the results. The timing of breast reconstruction and the method and type of reconstruction you choose are personal matters. Do your research, consult with your doctor, and in the end go with your gut feeling; you can't go wrong.

> *The timing of breast reconstruction and the method and type of reconstruction you choose are personal matters. Do your research, consult with your doctor, and in the end go with your gut feeling; you can't go wrong.*

How has breast cancer changed my life? In too many ways! The most significant change has been in my attitude towards life. I now live each day as if were the very last one. I can never be sure. I can no longer trust my body. It is fragile. It can fail at any time.

I now pay attention to my body. A pain in my head might not just be a pain. It could be a brain tumor or something else; it happened once, it can happen again. Every day of my life is a day of celebration, another day that I have survived breast cancer. When those cancer cells metastasize wherever and whenever they choose, my oncologists and I deal with them and see them as bumps along the road. I now live a life of humility, completely surrendered to the Almighty.

It took three years for my body to settle down, and the cancer to give me a break. I refuse to let cancer win the fight. I can proudly state that I am now in my eleventh year of survivorship although I cannot say that I am cancer free or that I am in remission. In 2005 I started to feel severe pain in my right leg (always my right side—I wish I knew why). Radiation was ordered for the lower area of my femur, but in spite of these treatments, six months later the pain was escalating and my gait was abnormal. As a result, another round of radiation was ordered for the upper level of the right femur: still no easing of the pain. As a matter of fact, the pain got worse.

Now I was off to see the orthopedist: cortisone shots, X-rays, MRIs, bone scans, and nothing showed up. To get on with daily living, I had to resort to using a cane; my quality of life had now been reduced to a bare minimum. The situation seemed dire. My trusted oncologist said, "This is cancer. We have to find someone who can find the appropriate treatment."

So off to the orthopedist oncologist I go. A comparison of a new bone scan with the images done six months prior revealed a hairline fracture in the femur. Surgery was ordered to place pins in the femur to stabilize the bone. Once again I had to call upon my faith to sustain me and give me the strength to face yet another period of pain and difficulty while the healing process took its course.

I move forward on my journey in the hope that a cure will be found for breast cancer while I can still celebrate and revel in the moment.

During the early years of my illness, I read or heard that the survival rate for single women was significantly lower than that for married women. As one who has been single all my life, somewhere from deep within I resolved that I would not add to that statistic. I was going to be strong, I was going to eat well, I did as much exercise as I could, and above all, I kept a positive attitude and glorified the creator, every day, for all his goodness and his grace. It is by no means easy. It takes a measure of strength far beyond your own—a supernatural strength is what keeps you going.

My advice to the newly diagnosed is this: first and foremost, you must be proactive. Find a well-known oncologist, one who is an expert in the field and committed to doing everything in his or her power to help patients. You must be comfortable with your oncologist and all other health providers to whom you will trust your care. Ask questions, seek answers, use all the facilities and sources of information available to you. As far as it is possible, deal with the situation in a positive manner. Knowledge is power, and *faith* gives strength. Be thankful for each new day, and love your friends and family and show them that you care. Every day that you see the sunshine or feel the gentle breeze is one more day that you have survived breast cancer.

> *My advice to the newly diagnosed is this: first and foremost, you must be proactive.*

Ann was 48 years old when she was diagnosed with metastatic breast cancer in 1993. She was treated with chemotherapy and then underwent a stem cell transplant. The cancer went into remission but recurred three years later. Ann received several years of chemotherapy and now is doing well on a hormonal therapy.

I found the lump while I was in the shower. It was in April. I was not yet 50. There was no breast cancer history in my family, so I didn't worry about it. I told my husband that I found this lump, and we let it go for a few days. Finally, he said, "I don't know why you're not dealing with that." So I went to my gynecologist, and he felt it, looked at it. It was fairly large, and you could really see it.

I went from the gynecologist to have a mammogram, and it happened that the person who gave me the mammogram was a former student of mine. How embarrassing! She was mature, far more mature than I was. She really was in charge of this process, and she said, "You need to have a sonogram, and I don't want you to wait." She had already done a tough mammogram, and I said, "You're really hurting me." She said, "This is for your family. I need to do this." She knew what she was doing.

She sent me down the hall for the sonogram, and the doctor who read that sonogram was young. He came in with an envelope that was sealed and said, "This is the report." And he was jumping. I mean, he couldn't stand still. He was jumping all around, and he said, "This is the report. I want you to take this to your gynecologist right away, and it's sealed." And I thought, "Of course, I'm going to open this." I got to the car, opened it and read it, and was devastated. I went back to the gynecologist.

My gynecologist said, "I want you to go to a surgeon and talk to him," which I did. My husband was with me. The surgeon said, "Let me aspirate it." And then his demeanor completely changed. He said, "This isn't good. We need to take it out as soon as possible."

So in May he did a lumpectomy. It was an in-and-out surgery. He only took out the lump, and he must not have liked something he saw because when he met with us afterwards, he said, "I want you to have tests. I want you to have chemotherapy. I am going to give you the names of three doctors to see. This tumor is fairly large, but even if it weren't, I would still want you to have chemotherapy. You need to do this. I would tell my wife to do this."

I began a battery of tests. When I went for the bone scan they found what they called a "hot spot" in my spine, and then they set me up for a different kind of X-ray, and then we waited for my surgeon to call. He called, and he said, "You have cancer in your spine."

I completely fell apart.

We met with the first oncologist for two hours, and it was just dreadful. He said, "You have a stage IV breast cancer. You will not survive this. We have no way that's proven to cure you, and these are your choices: you can have chemotherapy and just do the regular round, and that may extend your life for a while. You can have a bone marrow transplant, autologous, and it will be dreadful. They take you down to your death, and then try to build you up, and you may not make it, and I don't know if you want to live what's left of your life that way." I guess doing nothing was the third choice.

My husband was there, and he has been phenomenal through the whole thing. This always makes me cry. I really think it's much harder for the caregiver than it is for the person dealing with it because you know how you feel. They don't know how you feel, and their imagination is much worse for them. And they don't have a lot of control. He really needed to control the situation, and he couldn't.

We went to see another oncologist, and his attitude was completely different. Completely different. "Yes, we have bad data results, and, yes, you have a chronic disease, but we can treat it. We treat diabetes. It's a chronic disease, and this is what I think you should do." There it was: a plan! Something to hold on to, a goal and the message that I could do

> *We went to see another oncologist, and his attitude was completely different. Completely different.*

this. He wanted me to do chemotherapy to get the disease under control and, in the meantime, to meet with a doctor to prepare for a bone marrow transplant.

If you give me a road, I can go down the road. Just don't throw up stop signs. My oncologist was so confident that this was the path and that he could keep extending my life, and that's all I wanted.

> *My oncologist was so confident that this was the path and that he could keep extending my life, and that's all I wanted.*

I met with my school principal, and she said, "You need to decide if you want to retire or not." And I had never even thought about it. I had twenty-seven years in the school system, and I thought I'd go to at least to thirty. I wanted to be a principal, and that was the track I was on. That's what I expected to do. Anyway, she said, "You will get a medical disability retirement, and you need to decide what you want to do."

Initially, I kept working during the chemotherapy, but it was exhausting. I remember doing an interview one day. We were hunting for a new resource teacher in Special Ed. I was conducting the interviews with a panel after school, and I didn't think I would ever make it through.

Then one day my husband came home and said, "I want you to retire." I was surprised, but he was right. His point was that my position was entirely too stressful for my health. Not having had the experience of being a principal of a school will always bother me a bit. But it's a fair trade for the good health and life I enjoy.

Finally, it was time to go for the autologous bone marrow transplant. I was there for three weeks and slept through most of it. But, as you get better, it's harder to sleep. You feel itchy inside. It's hard to relax. Just the smell of food makes you throw up. But the nurses were incredible. There was one who would come every night and rub my back until I could relax enough to try to fall asleep. I came home for Thanksgiving.

I couldn't make anything for Thanksgiving dinner. I started to run a fever, and after Thanksgiving I went back into the hospital briefly.

Finally, I could spend the night in my own bed. It felt so good. I did have to keep going into the hospital regularly. At first my husband took me every day, and then once a week. Gradually, you are weaned away, and finally you're at the point where you can go to radiation, and I was OK through that. All of this took the better part of a year. The doctors told me I wouldn't be better from the transplant for a year, and they were right. When I hit the year mark, I suddenly felt better.

All that was done, and I was good for almost three years. Then, right before Christmas this time, my oncologist called and said my blood markers had suddenly shot up. The cancer was back.

I started again on chemotherapy. I had a bad reaction to it. It was Christmas Eve, and we always had our Christmas on Christmas Eve. My mom was there, and I was so red and swollen. It wasn't from the chemo. It was from the other stuff, the steroids they give you before the chemo. I hadn't told her about the recurrence yet, and friends were over. She said, "Ann, why is your face so red?" and I looked at my hands. "Don't ask me this." Later, I told her. We just dealt with it. We took it in stride, and it was OK.

We started everything. I was doing Taxol every three weeks, went through the whole hair thing again, and then finally started Herceptin. They said I should get in a trial for Herceptin because the tumor was HER-2-Neu positive, which meant I was expressing the kind of protein that makes the cancer aggressive. Herceptin, this new monoclonal antibody, can attach itself to that protein. So I was the first person in my county to take it.

I started with it, and they were real freaky about how I was going to react to it. Some people had bad reactions. I didn't. Then I switched to Taxol every week because the new theory was that if you keep your level up, it doesn't affect your body as much. So you take smaller doses, but you take it every week, so you don't have this up and then down and then up. I went for treatment every Wednesday for three or four years, so the people on staff are all really good friends now. And it became just part of my life. I didn't mind it. I liked seeing all the women. We talked of books and movies and recipes and life and what we're doing, and it was just that group of people I met with every week.

I stopped the Taxol a year and a half ago. I saw a new doctor who hated taking me off of Taxol, but I was starting to have side effects. I fell over a number of times, and that was from neuropathy in my feet. Twice I was carrying my granddaughter and fell. I just rolled over. It was amazing. Well, they gave me medicine for that, and I got a little bit better. I still did drop things. I didn't even know I was doing it. And I forget things. I missed two lunch dates with the same people.

I went off of the Taxol, and I took myself off Herceptin because it was affecting my heart. When you have a chronic disease, the longer you live with it, the more power you feel, the more you are able to read your own body and mind and know what you need to do.

There are other medicines I could use, and so if I have a problem with the cancer coming back (and it can), I'll have options. So now it has been a year, a year and a half without chemo and a year without the Herceptin. Now I take a pill every night, a hormonal therapy called Arimidex.

At the beginning of this journey, I read a lot. I got Susan Love's book. I did talk to some other people. I got the PBS stuff. I looked at the NIH website that would give me professional reviews and things. I did that. I went to a nutritionist for a while. I went to a support group for a while. They came and picked me up. I wasn't supposed to be driving yet. I went twice, and I just hated it. I hated it. All they talked about was cancer! I wasn't in the mood for what I perceived as a pessimistic attitude.

I have two other friends whom I met at the doctor's office, and we meet regularly for lunch. We kept up with each other's health, but that is never the main topic of conversation. We have that bond, but we enjoy each other on other levels.

I have the wonderful distinction of being a stage IV who has survived for over ten years! From

That's my main advice to other breast cancer patients: recognize and appreciate the wonderful aspects of each day. Enjoy your life. Enjoy today.

many standpoints, this has been a very good experience. I don't feel bad or angry about it. I don't feel robbed of anything. In fact, my life has been enriched because of it. I am a different person because of it, and that's a positive thing. I appreciate life. I truly understand that every day is beautiful. I try very hard not to say, "I can't wait until tomorrow." That would mean that I wasn't enjoying today. I work at not wishing my life away. That's my main advice to other breast cancer patients: recognize and appreciate the wonderful aspects of each day. Enjoy your life. Enjoy today.

Madeleine was 43 years old when she was diagnosed with metastatic breast cancer in 1993. She was treated with chemotherapy and then underwent high-dose chemotherapy with bone marrow transplantation. She also had a stem cell transplant. She was on tamoxifen for nine years. She is now on Aromasin.

I was diagnosed with stage IV cancer in May of 1993. It was discovered because I had swelling under the arm and had gone to the gynecologist thinking maybe she might find something. She did not find anything. In February, I had just gone to get my mammograms, and the results were fine, as usual. I had also been going for yearly breast exams, and when the gynecologist examined me she found nothing. She gave me a prescription, thinking this would help the swelling.

I was into physical health, and I thought the swelling was because I had been cutting the grass and maybe I had overdone it. I was taking Advil but two weeks later it still wasn't going down. I always felt there was something underneath my arm—nothing visible, but just something. My gynecologist had said, "In two weeks, if it doesn't get better, call back." I called her back and nothing helped, so she sent me to see a surgeon.

I made an appointment with him and he did find a lump, a very small, small lump. On the mammogram he wasn't sure if he even saw anything, but it didn't matter at this point. So after that we set up an appointment for me to go get a biopsy, and we did that and that came out very positive, of course. You know when the doctor calls you, it's not good news. It was about 3:30 in the afternoon. Dr. Fox calls me, and he says that I should make an appointment to see him. I was by myself, and I said, "OK, what happened?" and he would not tell me. I said, "Look, right now I am imagining the worst anyway, so you might as well tell me if you found anything." And he said, "Yes, you have breast cancer." It was not his choice to tell me on the phone. I made him tell me because I knew I had breast cancer as soon as he called me.

I called my husband, and I said, "You've got to come home." He said, "What's wrong, what's wrong?" I said, "Come home now, just come home now." Then he came home. I told him. He hugged me. Then, of course, I had to tell my kids.

Each one of them handled it in a different way. My oldest son hugged me, and then he got real quiet and went downstairs to clean up his room. That has always been an issue with me, and I knew that was how he was handling it. Then, my daughter got home, and I told her, and being a girl she was more emotional. She started crying and yelling, "No! Not you, Mommy, not you, Mom, not you." And I said, "Yes, yes, me." Then we had a cry. Then I told my middle son, who doesn't accept anything easily and who tries to avoid anything that is painful to him. He just said, "Mom, you're going to be all right. You're going to be all right. Don't worry about it. You're going to be just fine." I said, "OK." That was the end of that.

I called my sister right away. She was crying, very upset. We're very close. I have four brothers and one sister and we are all very close. After those three days, I did not hear from anybody. They were trying to call, but I didn't want to talk to anybody. It was not the time for me to talk to anybody. All my life I've always been the strong one in my family. I had to be the strong one, you know what I mean? We lost our mother when she was very young, in her thirties, you know, like 36, and my dad at 58, so I've always been the strong one. I always helped others, whether it was a customer, a friend, somebody in the family, I was always the one who was there for them. All of a sudden they were crying for me, and I did not want that.

I was always the one who was there for them. All of a sudden they were crying for me, and I did not want that.

I was worried about them worrying about me, and I was worried about my kids and my husband because nobody was really discussing it. We were just kind of feeling it, just trying to go on day by day. I really wanted life to be normal around me. My daughter would say, "Mom, if you want me to stay home tonight I will stay home." I said, "No, don't stay home, because if you stay home that means you think I'm gonna die." Or if you're going to keep visiting me then you think I'm going to die. Just let life be as normal as possible so that I can live a normal life as well as do all my other things that I knew I had to do. So that was my main thing, just living a normal life and having everybody around me living a normal life.

I didn't want people who didn't visit me before to come over and visit with me. I had asked my sister to tell everyone the news, but I did not want anybody to call me. "Don't call me. I don't want to hear from anybody. Just let me try to deal with this right now." I really thought that I could beat this without telling anybody. That was before it was that bad, before I knew it was stage IV. I thought, "OK, I'll go for treatments and not tell anybody and then just go on."

I had surgery again, and I had a whole lot of positive lymph nodes. I then had gone through a number of tests arranged by the surgeon, and I remember my next appointment with him. We sat in the office, and he was telling me that this was stage IV, and it had gone from the breast and the lymph nodes to the liver. I knew when he said that it had gone to the liver that that was going to be it for me, you know. He started telling me what he suggested that I should do, and then I didn't have to think about it. I knew I had no choice. I had to go through the bone marrow transplant and the stem cell transplant.

As far as the choice between lumpectomy and mastectomy, he suggested to get just a lumpectomy done. Since the cancer had gone out of the breast it didn't really matter. I chose that. As far as choosing the bone marrow transplant, I knew my chances of dying were very great. When I had seen the transplant doctor she said, "30 percent make it and 70 percent don't." This was ten years ago. So I said, "OK, I'll take the 30 percent. I'll do that." I chose to take the most aggressive, the most painful, the longest treatment that I could get, regardless how much pain, regardless how much time I would be off, regardless of what I had to go through. I had to go through the worst in order to get back from this.

I am not a reader, but I started reading. The more I read and the more I asked, the more scared I became. So then I decided that I'm different from you. I'm different from them. I'm different from everybody; I'm going to make my own decision. I'm going to do it my way with the information that my doctor had given me. And I stopped reading at this point. I took one day at a time, one treatment at a time. You have one pain at a time. One day in the hospital. Everything was always one day at a time. I didn't want to worry about tomorrow.

> *I took one day at a time, one treatment at a time. You have one pain at a time. One day in the hospital. Everything was always one day at a time. I didn't want to worry about tomorrow.*

My doctor recommended that I receive chemotherapy before the bone marrow transplant, and he wasn't sure at this point whether or not the chemo would get rid of all of the cancer. We decided to just try it. I started my treatment, and I had to get a course of chemo. I was very sick with the chemo. From the first drop, I started throwing up. Even when they were giving me the anti-nausea medicine, I was throwing up because of that.

I went through a series of that, and after I was done, I was actually in remission, even in the liver. So that was very encouraging with me. I think it was like four months, and I was fine. Of course, at that point I probably could have stopped doing anything. Then I said, "No, if I stop now it may come back, so I'm going to keep on going." I went ahead and scheduled an appointment for a bone marrow transplant. I knew this was my full-time job now. I also had a stem cell transplant after the bone marrow transplant.

I was in the hospital three and a half weeks, and I went through the procedure to remove and store my bone marrow. After they did the bone marrow removal, I was really in pain, and I was really crying. I was like half asleep and dozed off, and I remember the transplant doctor came in, and I was crying and crying. I said to the transplant doctor, "I always wanted to live until I was 100 but now I am willing to settle for 99," and she started crying. She had tears in her eyes, not really bawling, but she had tears in her eyes, and then I realized that she was really a very warm person but she had to be tough on the outside. She had to be tough for us.

I then had the high-intensity chemo. After that I was weak for months. I think even picking up a pencil would have been too much for me. I was that weak. Plus I wasn't eating because I was throwing up twenty-four hours a day. Even a green pea would have been too much for me to eat. I just couldn't handle eating anything. It was like torture when someone put food in front of me, even just a teaspoon for me to try to eat, and that went on for a while.

One morning at the hospital, I became paralyzed for about fifteen minutes. I didn't fall down. I was still standing up, but I could not move anything. I didn't move my eyelashes, nothing, absolutely nothing. My daughter kept saying, "Mom, what's taking you so long? What's taking you so long?" I was rinsing my mouth in the bathroom sink. I couldn't answer. I could hear her. Then she said, "Oh, my God." She called the nurses, and they came in. My daughter was yelling and screaming, "What's wrong? Answer me! What's wrong? What's wrong? What's wrong?" My husband was there, and he kept saying, "What's wrong? Talk to me, what's wrong?" The nurse kept yelling, "Madeleine, talk to me, talk to me." I could not. I could see my husband going in and out of the room. I could see he was nervous and scared. He was going in, he was going out, he was going in, going out. My daughter kept yelling and crying. The nurses kept yelling, trying to get my attention, and all along I was thinking in my head, "Say something, talk, move, do something. Come on, you've got to move something to tell them that you can hear them."

At that point I realized something. I thought to myself, "This is what a person in a coma is going through. Maybe they hear you but they can't do anything about it." I tried and I tried and I tried. I said to myself, "Come on, move, move an eyelash, move your head, move your foot, move a finger, move something. No one knows that you hear them and you see them." I kept seeing them. I knew they were there, and I knew they were talking to me. I knew that they kept asking me, "Do you hear me?" But I could not say anything.

Then they put me in the bed. I tell you, that paralysis was probably the scariest thing that ever happened to me. They never found out why it happened. They actually thought that I'd had a stroke, or a heart attack, or something. But as soon as they disconnected me from the morphine, I came back. Thankfully, it cleared on its own and didn't recur.

I was discharged soon after.

After the initial shock and then after the chemotherapy, the bone marrow transplant, and stem cell transplant, I decided that I was going to take control. I always had a positive attitude. I never really let myself think negatively. One of the most important questions that I think anybody can ask is, "Am I going to live?" Every answer was always, "I don't know," which at the beginning I was reading as, "OK, then, I am going to die." But the more I was into the process, the more I realized that the doctors' words *I don't know* really meant they didn't know. They really don't know.

One of the most important questions that I think anybody can ask is, "Am I going to live?" Every answer was always, "I don't know," which at the beginning I was reading as, "OK, then, I am going to die." But the more I was into the process, the more I realized that the doctors' words I don't know *really meant they didn't know. They really don't know.*

I was tired when I returned home, but again I wanted to be back to a normal life so I just kind of ignored it. I just said, OK, I'm going to go back to work, the heck with it.

When I realized that I didn't know if I was going to live or not, and it didn't look good for me for a long time, I wasn't going to let any bad days get in my way. I was just happy to have a day, regardless of whether it was a painful day, whether it was a bad day, whether it was, you know, things didn't go right that day. I didn't care. It was a day. It was another day in my life.

When I got better and I was back at work, one of my customers came in, and she was having a bad day. I don't know if it was her marriage or something had happened in her life. She was just really moaning and groaning about it, and I said, "Come on back in the office. You want me to tell you about a bad day?" So I started telling her about what happened with me, and I said, "Your situation is very painful, but you know that you'll live the next day and you know that you can go on with your life if you choose to. You can negotiate with your life. You can go on." I said, "When I was going through this there was no negotiation. You cannot negotiate with God. He has total control. I could not negotiate for an extra day, so I would take any bad day. Give me any bad day, just so I'm gonna have an extra day in my life." So that's been my strength, I think, throughout all of this.

This experience began over ten years ago. The first three days I was looking at the worst picture, like everybody does. But then I realized that being pessimistic was not going to help me, so I figured I would be happy. That's the only way that I can live because living every day thinking I was going to die was not really living. So then I decided to think about it that way every day. I will live with pain. I am not going to look so pretty without any hair. I will not be looking good at all. I have always

> **But then I realized that being pessimistic was not going to help me, so I figured I would be happy.**

been a proud person, but I didn't let that bother me. I knew eventually I would get back, hopefully, to looking good again. But even looking good was not important to me.

Before I lost my hair, my hair had to be perfect all the time every day. If I had one little hair sticking out, I wouldn't go to work until I had it fixed. After I lost my hair I said, "If I can get a little bit of hair, believe me I won't care what it looks like." I won't care if it doesn't look good, I just will be happy to have hair.

I think when I turned around after those first three days and decided to be part of this (only because I needed to do that to live), it made everybody else around me feel better. It made everybody know that I was OK. Waking up in the morning, I knew I was going to live through the day because I wasn't going to let myself down. I never talked to people about cancer because I didn't feel enough strength from other people. I felt I was probably stronger than they were, and when I talk about what I went through, the pain that I went through, everything that I went through, sometimes I feel like it is not even me talking. I feel like it is someone else talking for me. Talking to people discouraged me. I didn't want to go to a group. Just leave me alone, and just let me do it. Just let me do it my way. I want to do it my way.

People would say, "I know somebody, and at least she lived for seven years." I don't want to hear that. Or someone else would say, "Well, she's had her six-month checkup, and so far she's been good." Well, what do you mean, "so far she has been good"? Don't tell me that. So then I stopped listening to people. I didn't read anything. As soon as I hear any comments about anything, I shut everything off. I said, "You know what? I am not like everybody else. I want to do it my way, with my own strength, and not depending on anybody else."

Today, I don't care if my hair's messed up, and I don't care if my clothes don't match. I am here today. I want to help other people and encourage them through all of this. That's my goal. Living every day with my husband and my kids and my grandkids and my family, playing music—that is my life. I am happy with myself. I am happy with my life. I am happy with my decisions in life. I am happy with the way my family came out. I am happy with the closeness we have with my brothers and my sister. I really don't have any regrets in my life, and if something doesn't make me happy, then I choose another way. I find another way.

PART FIVE

When Cancer Specialists Get Cancer

CHAPTER 23

A Professional and a Patient

Carole Seddon, LCSW-C, OSW-C

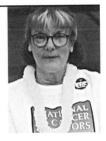

In January 1983, I started working as an oncology social worker with patients and their family members in the bone marrow transplant unit at the Johns Hopkins Hospital. I come from a family where most live to a very old age. Illness and death was not a major part of my background, so I had to come to terms, spiritually and emotionally, with knowing that all of the physical problems that were part of bone marrow transplant, those many years ago, could and did happen to people. I had to accept that people died. This included my friends, my family, and myself, as well as those patients on the bone marrow transplant unit.

My boss would come to the inpatient floor to see me and say, "How are you?" He was very concerned. I'd say, "A lot of people die." He'd say, "There are many living, Carole." And I'd say, "They're all dying." And he'd say, "No. I want you to see what the numbers are so you can keep some objectivity in this." I would watch the nurses coming back from vacation and by the time they had been back a day they looked as worn out and as tired as they had before their vacation. I learned a great deal about the ups and downs of cancer treatment, about death, and about coping from the many patients and families I met during my eight years working with the bone marrow transplant service.

I left that service in 1991 to develop and provide fee-for-service counseling services at Hopkins for cancer patients and family members. This was in January 1991. In December 1991, I had a mammogram. They kept me there for two and a half hours, looking, saying I had so many calcifications they couldn't tell what was what. They wanted me to come back in six months. A few weeks later, on my birthday in January, I came home and found blood in my bra; it had come from the nipple of my left breast. I had just been for my mammogram and thought that it could not be anything; I also remembered what a breast surgeon had told me two years earlier during a similar event involving my right breast. My gynecologist had sent me for a mammogram because she thought she had felt a lump in my right breast. During the mammogram, I had bled from the nipple of my right breast and had then been sent to a breast surgeon who said, "It could be a cyst. I don't feel anything. I really don't think it's anything."

Despite what I was thinking, I was anxious enough that I called the nurse practitioner in the breast center that same week of January 1992. She was someone I knew who had worked in oncology for some time. She did a full examination and felt a lump in the right breast where the gynecologist had felt something two years earlier. She said she thought I needed to see a breast surgeon.

Within a week, I went to another breast surgeon, someone I knew at Hopkins, and had a biopsy. It was malignant. It was recommended that I have the breast removed—have a mastectomy—because the tumor was poorly differentiated and was estrogen negative. It seems to me, thinking back, that we were just on the cusp of not having to do mammograms at the time of my diagnosis. One of the breast oncologists with whom I worked, when I told him about my diagnosis, very kindly, immediately went to read the pathology. He agreed with my breast surgeon's recommendations. It was a great feeling of belonging and being cared for by a team of nurses and physicians whom I respected greatly. It gave me whatever peace of mind I experienced in that early time of diagnosis.

I agreed to the mastectomy. My surgeon said to me, "You may want to think about a prophylactic mastectomy on the other side, because of the bleeding and because you have a chance of it spreading." It was just short of a two-centimeter tumor. And he said, "Don't decide now. Think about it. You don't have to do it now."

I didn't want reconstruction. I could not think of anything except doing whatever I could to ensure that I would live. What went through my mind at work was, "Am I going to wind up in one of these inpatient rooms like my bone marrow transplant patients?" At that time a woman who had been the director of nursing in oncology at Hopkins was dying from breast cancer; for confidentiality reasons, she was "housed" as an inpatient on the bone marrow transplant service at Hopkins. I walked past her room many times, thinking, "Is this going to be me?" I also experienced a time of hearing the voices and seeing the faces of many of the bone marrow transplant patients who had died. It happened several times with one face and voice after another, and I could not stop it. It didn't last very long. But it was very clear to me that I was on the other side, no longer just the professional but also the patient.

Following surgery, the surgeon recommended that I see the medical oncologist who had reviewed my pathology to discuss chemotherapy. I had an appointment in the medical oncology clinic at Hopkins, where my own patients also came for treatment. The aide who took patients' blood pressure and weight, without thinking, called out my name, to do the same for me. One of the nurses was walking by, and in a flash he realized that I was being called as a patient. The look of shock on his face mirrored the shock in my heart. I was close to tears as a woman, who also had heard my name called, came up to me. Her husband was my patient, and she said, "I won't tell him; I'll let you do that." And I thought, "I can't. I can't. This is just too much."

I was tearful when I saw the medical oncologist. He said, "What's wrong?" And I said, "I don't know," but I definitely knew. I couldn't even verbalize it to him; the boundary between professional relationship and my personal life had always been important to me. It was now being breached. When he finished, he said, "You don't need to be treated here, Carole. Your cancer is not that bad that you absolutely need to be treated at Hopkins. You can be treated elsewhere."

The breast cancer was stage II. It was estrogen negative and poorly differentiated, which indicated a greater risk of it reoccurring. I went to

A Professional and a Patient   351

see one of the Hopkins oncologists who also had a private practice in the community. He used the recommendations of the Hopkins breast oncology team but provided chemotherapy in his community office. I received six cycles of chemotherapy, which, unlike most adjuvant chemotherapies, was increased each cycle. It was during the time of clinical trials for stem cell transplants for advanced breast cancer. One of the nurses explained to me that some breast oncologists thought that the stem cell transplant, which even then was starting to show not great results, might do better with breast cancer patients in an earlier stage. Because there was no clinical trial for doing this, my oncologist did not do a stem cell transplant with me but did increase the dosage each cycle, and I'm very glad that he did it.

I kept doing administrative work. During treatments I stopped seeing patients at Johns Hopkins and in my part-time private practice in the community. I didn't do any clinical work during that time. It was a quick decision for me to make. In terms of cancer patients at Hopkins, I was too emotionally vulnerable to what any of my cancer patients might say that would hit too close to home. In terms of my private practice, I had a thought that was one of those things I didn't plan on thinking, but it was there immediately: if I was going to die from this disease, I didn't want to spend the rest of my life working all the time.

I told all of my patients that I would refer them to other people because I was getting treatment myself. I started seeing cancer patients and families again at Hopkins the year after my diagnosis; I did not see breast cancer patients for three years after my diagnosis. I told the Hopkins oncology center staff by going to a few of the medical staff I knew. I told them—and didn't tell them not to tell—and so they told others. I could not deal with saying, "I have cancer," over and over. As word got out, I felt very supported by the staff. On the days that I got treatment, I took a half-day, because I was going to the medical oncologist's office in the Baltimore community. I also was drugged after being given the antiemetics and would not have been able to concentrate sufficiently.

I had nausea from the beginning. I never was sick to my stomach, but I never was without nausea, that feeling and the awful taste in my mouth. I would feel like I was one big chemical; I felt drugged until shortly before my next cycle of treatments. Food tasted terrible, but I remembered the

When Cancer Specialists Get Cancer

team telling the bone marrow patients that they needed calories to help their bodies fight to regrow the good cells destroyed by their treatments. And so I ate.

I was exhausted, more so as each cycle went by. I was fortunate to have my office in one of the houses for patients and families who traveled from other states to be treated at Hopkins. Bedrooms were on the second and third floors, and there were television rooms on the first floor along with the offices. I would go into one of the television rooms and lie down for an hour nap, which helped a great deal. The "tireds" from chemotherapy are like nothing I have ever experienced before or since treatments; I was completely drained. Toward the end of treatment, my oncologist cut the dosage of Zofran in half. I am very susceptible to drugs. As my husband drove me home after that last cycle, my world was spinning.

One of the things my surgeon did early on in treatment was to say to me, "You know, you can take your professional hat off here." He literally said that to me, and I needed him to say that with all of the boundary confusion for me at that time. I said to him, "No, I don't know." He said, "You're a patient here." He had referred patients to me, and I had to him. I mean, it was really tangled, with me working in the cancer field. Another time, he said to me, "Do you know that breast cancer patients die from something other than breast cancer?" I said, "No, I don't." He said, "They do."

In terms of coping, I knew from my own work counseling cancer patients and what I had learned from them over the years that I had to hold onto the positives told to me by the oncologist and the surgeon. Fear and negative thoughts hold a great deal of power during this time. Remembering the positives said about one's prognosis and treatments is important and is sometimes hard work. It was for me as well. I talked with a friend of mine, saying I had worked for years with cancer patients about their feelings — the implication being that I should not be struggling with the feelings. She, wonderfully, said to me, "and I guess you thought you wouldn't have to go through those feelings just like everyone else does." I had to laugh because she was right on! She also went with me to my first breast cancer support group.

I was clear that I knew as much as I needed to know about cancer. I didn't pick up books. I got films that were funny. I didn't watch anything serious on television. My husband Frank was wonderful. He has a dry sense of humor, and in that crisis he used it a lot. I was so confused from chemo that if I was stopped halfway through a sentence, I wouldn't remember what I had just been saying. Frank would tease me, humming the music from *The Twilight Zone*. I would crack up laughing. We'd just really laugh and that was helpful in breaking our internal tension. It wasn't a matter of not dealing with it; it was just not making everything so serious.

But the fact was that I thought something else was wrong with me. I even said to my oncologist, "I think I've got Alzheimer's on top of every-thing else!" He said, "You do not have Alzheimer's. You know what you're trying to say, don't you?" and I said, "Yes." He said, "That's not Alz-heimer's, Carole." I am sure he said something about chemo, but I sure didn't remember for a while that this was "chemo brain."

My memory has never come back quite the same. If I'm meeting some new people, I cannot remember names. Sometimes, not always, when people are talking fast and I start to do the same, my brain just doesn't keep up. I know what I am trying to say, but I can see others do not. Of course, I am now fifteen years older and moving toward retirement, so many of my female contemporaries also say that they have the same prob-lem. I've learned to joke about it and say, "My brain's gone!" People just laugh, and then we'll go on. It was, however, upsetting and embarrass-ing to experience "chemo brain" throughout treatment and during the three years I was taking tamoxifen. I did not realize that it would get better, which it certainly did. I was embarrassed and thought, "They're going to figure this out." I felt so vulnerable that I spent time trying to cover all this up. I thought, "My God, I'm going to lose my job," and at that point, if you lost your job, your health insurance was gone. And I had cancer.

I went for counseling myself. The counselor was somebody that I knew. I went and just cried. I knew what I needed to do. I was in a safe place, and I liked her and so I could do it. My husband didn't tell me for two years that he had gone to a hospital across town that had a support group because he did not want to tell me that he was upset. He wanted to take care of me. In the group, they said, "Are you Carole Seddon's husband?"

It's like the preacher's spouse! I felt so bad for him. He never said another thing in the group and never went back.

I decided a year after diagnosis and four months after treatment ended that I wanted to have my other breast removed prophylactically and have reconstruction. All were difficult decisions, grievable losses, but decisions I have never regretted.

I am fifteen years out. I certainly do not think about my cancer on a daily, weekly, or even monthly regular basis. Yet I don't forget about it. I now have two small growths in my esophagus, which a new set of physicians are trying to biopsy. I'm told they do not think it is malignant, but I'll really relax when they can biopsy it.

At the international meeting of the association of oncology social work, we have a luncheon for those of us who are also cancer survivors. Several years ago, a woman who had just been diagnosed with breast cancer was at this luncheon in tears, saying, "Will this ever get any better? I'm terrified. I feel awful." The group facilitator, who was ten years out from her cancer at that time, said, "It gets better. I want to tell you it gets better. But it never is going to be the same as it was." And I've known that. I have said this to other patients. The facilitator said, "I'm ten years out and when my doctor says, 'I see something a little different. We need to check it. I don't think it's cancer, but we need to check,' my heart still goes." She said, "I'm all right afterward. It's not every day, it's not every month, but it's there."

As an oncology social worker, I probably have more empathy now. There always was caring, but I'm also tough in that I say things I would never have said prior to my cancer. My practice in the beginning was almost all newly diagnosed cancer patients and their families. Currently, it is mostly stage III, stage IV, and end-stage, death and dying. Now, I can say to these men and women, not during the first session or in the second but at some point, "You have an absolute right to be angry, to feel depressed," whatever, "but your cancer is not going to go away completely. You might want to think about what you want to do with whatever time you have. You are not dying today; you have time to do those things important to you so that you might have some peace in your heart when it is time to say good-bye." I would never have said that before, and it needs to be said because people can't sort that out and that's why they're coming to me — to talk about what they cannot say to family and close friends.

I don't think anybody ever feels absolutely safe again after a cancer diagnosis. I used to call it a loss of innocence. I would say to patients, after the first or second meeting, "If I had said to you five years ago that you were going to be diagnosed with leukemia in five years, I'll lay you odds that you would have said to me, 'I guess I could be,' but you would have thought I was a nut and you would never have believed it." None of us, unless there is a strong family history of cancer, believes he or she is going to ever be diagnosed with cancer. No one has disagreed with that statement. Upon diagnosis, however, Pandora's box has been opened and the lid cannot be put back; life is not as it was. However, that does not mean it is not good.

I have people recently diagnosed say to me, "You're going to think I'm crazy, but for the first three weeks I waited for the doctor to call back and say it was a mistake." They don't know that I've heard it from almost all of them. I offer to people that counseling is going to provide them with a place to vent their anger, cry their tears, and talk about their pain and sadness and struggles coping. The goal is that their lives are better, even with cancer, that there is some quality of life for cancer patient and family.

When a person calls asking for counseling, I talk with them about the cancer diagnosis, why they want to see me, and about the billing. Now I also say, "There's another thing I need to tell you, because I tell every-body. I'm a cancer survivor. I tell you this because many of the nurses and a lot of the doctors know, and I don't want you to hear this from someone else. I don't want it to be the elephant in the middle of the floor between us. And I want to ask you whether that's a problem for you. Is it all right and do you still want to come for counseling with me?" I have never had anybody say no, but it's a nice way of going into it. And then 99.9 percent of those coming to see me don't talk about my cancer; they come to talk about their cancer or their loved one's cancer and how scared and sad and depressed or angry they are. There may be a time, after we've known each other for a while and they have talked and now feel better, that they ask, "Did you ever feel like I felt?" and I say, "Oh, yes."

I say to people, "And I got my own counseling." You know, I couldn't counsel myself.

In the beginning when I first did the fee-for-service counseling, I wanted to do everything with everybody. I'm a bit wiser now. I don't want to try to do everything with everybody. Truthfully, no one can. It was my immaturity as a counselor to try. But, also, my life goals are different. Prior to being diagnosed with cancer, in my early fifties, I was ambitious and planning to get my doctorate. I wanted to be able to teach and write. I wanted to know all and try to do all. At some point, in the middle of the treatment, I knew that my ambitions had to be put aside to make sure I was all right and that this decision was really all right. What mattered most to me were the relationships I had with the important people in my life, my family and close friends. I did not need fame and all that comes with it. I did need to give of myself in this work with patients and families. I had to care and be involved in a relationship with them, to be open to their pain and the end results of their diagnosis and treatments, be that a time of no cancer or ongoing treatments to finally dying and death. Patients are not my friends, but it is a relationship, a working relationship. I get to meet them intensely at a certain level. There are many, many things in their lives about which I still do not know when they leave counseling, but I do know about who they are in this time of life and death.

I'm privileged that people share this. I have had people say to me many times, "Well, I thought I was going to be much braver. I feel like such a coward because I need to come and see you. I'm afraid." I will say to them, "It's very easy to be brave when there's nothing occurring about which one needs to be brave. When you're facing life and death, which is probably one of the most primitive fears anyone has, and you keep on going to treatment and doing all these things that aren't very pleasant, I think that's courage. If you decide to come in here and face your fears, I think that's courage."

I say this from my heart to, hopefully, their heart. They truly have been my mentors in dealing with "life on life's terms" and in learning to have courage. I believe that everything I have done at Hopkins and everything I am now doing in working with these incredible human beings teaches me and builds my strength and values. I've been told by my medical oncologist that there is a cost to my understanding so well what my patients are experiencing. And there has been in terms of understanding only too well what was about to happen when I was diagnosed. A little denial is okay! I found that difficult because of what I knew. But I have learned. Those of us who go to school to obtain a graduate degree in social work or psychology rightfully learn a great deal about emotional problems, distress, and psychiatric illness. There does not seem to be quite the same focus on the strength of the human animal. Part of what has kept me here is observing and being part of the journey cancer patients and their families take when told of a cancer diagnosis. I would not consider any other work.

CHAPTER 24

Lessons Learned

April Fritz, RHIT, CTR

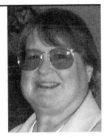

In December 1992, when I was diagnosed with breast cancer, I was 44. I had been involved in the cancer field for almost twenty years. I am a cancer registrar, a person who collects data and keeps statistics on cancer patients. I knew all about breast cancer anatomy, staging, treatment, and prognosis. In fact, I was training other data collectors. I've attended meetings (called tumor boards) where treatment decisions were made about cancer patients; I've attended breast cancer lectures; I've attended healthy lifestyle lectures . . . all that stuff. I'm also a large person. I knew I had a bunch of risk factors, but based on my experience and knowledge, I figured I wouldn't have to start worrying about cancer until I was in my sixties.

I grew up in a family that placed little emphasis on formal, regular medical care. My father was an orthopedist with little sympathy for injuries in his family. For a sprained ankle or knee strain, he'd say "Learn to walk on your hands." I was generally healthy. I married an army man, and we moved every two to three years. Army dependent care was free but a real hassle, and you never saw the same doc twice. Thus, my early life had not given me a good way to build up a lasting relationship with a physician.

I have a professional and personal friend who is a strong believer in preventive medicine, including breast self-examination and testicular self-examination for men. On our way home from a professional meeting in the fall of 1992, he started teasing me about getting mammograms, saying that my doctor would have to use extra large films, and imagining the physicians doing exams saying to each other, "Mark where you stopped—we'll continue the exam after the lunch break." I didn't admit to him that it had been over ten years since I'd had a physical or mammogram, but his teasing hit home, and I started paying more attention to breast self-exams (BSEs).

I used to do the exam haphazardly, you know, start around the nipple and work outward in circles . . . and on me, outward and outward. One morning, getting ready for a shower, I felt *it*. Way out at my right side, almost in my armpit, in the area of flesh called the axillary tail. Farther out than I had really examined well before. I shivered when I felt the mass, because it was just like the pea-sized mass I had learned to feel on the practice doll demonstration that the American Cancer Society had presented at an association meeting somewhere. Except it was bigger. It had the size and consistency of a "Snausage"—you know, the doggie treat. I immediately thought Clinical T2 (that's staging lingo). Oh, boy.

That morning, I called a gynecologist to set up an appointment so he could order the mammogram. That took a week, and all the time my mind was working overtime, speculating about this lump. The mammogram technician was nice, very concerned about causing me pain but careful to get the best picture possible. The radiologist was cool, too. He actually showed me what he saw on the films because he saw on the accompanying paperwork what my occupation was. He was nice but insisted that I get a biopsy.

The mammogram showed numerous densities bilaterally and a tiny ring of microcalcifications in the area of the right upper outer quadrant mass, which itself wasn't visible. Had I had previous mammograms? I had to request the old blue and white paper mammograms from the hospital where I had worked when they were taken. It turned out they had

When Cancer Specialists Get Cancer

been done seventeen years before, not ten. But without those old mammograms, I would have had to undergo bilateral, multiple biopsies.

LESSON LEARNED: Get a baseline mammogram if you are in your twenties or thirties, and remember where it was taken. If you are older than 40, get an annual mammogram.

The Biopsy

Because I was relatively new to the area where I was living, I had no idea who the good local docs were. My gynecologist referred me to a surgeon, whom I'll call Dr. Bill, who turned out to be very involved in hospital cancer programs around the country. He knew my profession, was familiar with what I do with cancer data, and was an all-around nice guy. We got along well immediately.

The surgeon examined me and recommended a mammographic needle localization (using a wire to identify the area where the possible tumor is, by means of a series of mammograms) and a biopsy of the microcalcifications. He thought the mass was a fibroadenoma, with an 80 percent chance of being benign.

LESSON LEARNED: Find a doctor you can be very comfortable with. You'll have a million questions, and you want someone who will pay attention to you.

On December ninth, I drove myself to the hospital, thinking that this biopsy was not going to be a big deal. The needle localization didn't hurt—not compared to all the times I'd stabbed my fingers with sewing needles. There are fewer pain nerves in breast tissue and the skin over it than in your fingers. But it was weird looking down and seeing this wire loop sticking out of my skin.

When they wheeled me into the operating room, I was awake, joking with the surgeon and surgical nurse. They asked me if my husband or boyfriend had accompanied me to the hospital; I said they were both out of town. But when I climbed onto the table, I freaked. It was so cold, I was shivering—partly from nervousness, too. They had to put a warming blanket over me. You don't get the full picture of what an operating room and a surgical procedure is like by simply watching TV shows or reading biopsy reports.

They put a drape up so I couldn't see what the surgeon was doing, but I could feel it. I felt the needle for the local anesthesia, and soon I felt the incision — not pain, but pressure. The surgeon kept talking to me as he was working. I heard him snipping — the sound was like scissors cutting your hair, but it was associated with tugging on my breast. As he cut deeper, the sound and feel made me more anxious, and I did begin to feel pain, so he gave me more local anesthesia.

He removed the mass and sent it to radiology to confirm that the microcalcifications were in the specimen, which they were. It seemed like forever before the surgeon received the call from the radiologist confirming that the specimen contained the microcalcifications. He closed the incision, put on a bulky dressing, and moved me back into the wheelchair for the trip back to the outpatient area where my clothes were.

Then the second phone call came just before we left the operating room. This outpatient procedure was supposed to be an excisional biopsy (cutting out the mass) without frozen section (a quick diagnostic procedure), so I knew from the surgeon's tone of voice as he talked with the pathologist that I was in deep doo-doo. The surgeon then calmly and kindly informed me that not only was the mass malignant (I was expecting maybe ductal carcinoma in situ — a minimally aggressive tumor — around the microcalcifications) but it was invasive and poorly differentiated (high on the aggressiveness scale). That kind of ruined my day. But I did have the presence of mind to give the surgeon the name and address of my favorite pathologist, to get a second opinion.

LESSON LEARNED: If it's your first procedure, insist on premedication, Valium or something, to remove the anxiety that made this procedure more arduous for me than it needed to be.

Needless to say, I was in shock at the news. My post-op blood pressure was 275 over something and the surgeon was concerned over my relatively difficult outpatient surgery and the bad news he'd just given me. He was so nice he even offered to drive me home. But that would have been awkward, leaving my car at the hospital with no easy way to get back and retrieve it.

I got some groceries and did a couple of errands on the way home. Hey—it's not every day that I can leave work while the stores are still open. As I shopped, the registrar in me kicked back in.

A long time ago, Elisabeth Kübler-Ross described the four phases of illness: denial (defiance), anger, bargaining, and acceptance (hope). There was no denial in my case. The Why Me? phase lasted about ten seconds as I checked off my risk factors for breast cancer:

✓ **Age over 30**
✓ **No children or first child after age 30**
✓ **Benign breast disease (fibrocystic disease)**
✓ **Obesity/high fat diet**

(The other breast cancer risk factors, which did not apply to me, are a family history of cancer, especially mother or sister with breast cancer; lower socioeconomic status; and early onset of menses.)

When I got home, I called Dr. Dave, the pathologist who had been my professional mentor and friend and asked for a sidewalk consultation. He was surprised to find out the consultation was on me. After he received the slides and reviewed them, instead of calling the pathologist back, he called me directly. The tumor was at the margin of excision and was very aggressive looking. He recommended—as gently as possible— a modified radical mastectomy.

The Surgery

As I said, the registrar in me had kicked back in at this point. Subconsciously, I had already thought through the next several steps. If my surgeon didn't recommend a modified radical, I would find one who would do it. I wanted any residual tumor out of my body. In addition to this personal belief (which I remember expressing to my sister-in-law some fifteen years previously), the following facts could not be disputed.

Lessons Learned

1. Location of the tumor. It was sitting right over the lymph nodes in my armpit, called the low axillary nodes. A lumpectomy would not have been effective treatment in my case.
2. Dr. Dave had told me that the tumor looked aggressive under the microscope.
3. He also said there was residual tumor at the biopsy site, and I wondered to myself: Where else might it be?
4. There were masses bilaterally, even if the mammograms were negative.

When I had my appointment with Dr. Bill to discuss surgery, I got the first piece of good news. My ERs (estrogen receptors) and PRs (progesterone receptors) were positive. That meant that the tumor was sensitive to changes in the hormone balance of my body and that I had one more cancer-fighting tool among my treatment choices. But the DNA analysis showed that the cancer was aneuploid (unfavorable/ aggressive), and the S-phase was quite high (the tumor was rapidly replicating itself). We agreed on going to surgery the next week — before Christmas — four days away.

By this time, I had gone into research mode, as many patients do when they're diagnosed. I was reading a brochure from the National Cancer Institute that I had gotten by calling 1-800-4-CANCER (the Internet hardly existed back then), and it said that large-breasted women often have back problems from being off-balance after mastectomy. I was also thinking about all those reconstruction discussions I had heard at tumor boards and professional meetings.

I decided I wanted to see a plastic surgeon prior to my mastectomy, so my surgeon referred me to a plastics guy in the same building who was able to see me the next day. It turned out that this conveniently located plastics guy had written one of the leading textbooks on breast reconstruction and had actually developed one of the major reconstructive procedures for breast cancer. He was cool, too. I asked him if it was possible to use the surplus part of my remaining breast to reconstruct the one I'd lose. (Waste not, want not.) Instead of laughing at me, he cited a study or case report where that approach had been tried and the results were not successful.

What I ultimately agreed to was his recommendation that I have a reduction on the left to reduce the unbalanced feeling, and reconstruction on the right beginning with placement of a tissue expander (similar to a balloon inserted under the chest wall muscle and gradually filled with fluid to stretch the muscle enough to fit a permanent prosthesis). His comment about the possibility of chest wall adhesions (tissue scarring) if the reconstruction were delayed convinced me to begin immediate reconstruction.

All of this was to be done under the same anesthesia as the modified radical—about five and a half hours' worth.

LESSON LEARNED: Talk to a plastics guy to find out what your options are *before* the surgeon makes his incision.

What I decided to do was not exactly what the surgeon recommended—or wanted—but he agreed to proceed according to my wishes. This was a lot of surgery for one sitting, but heck, I was going to be asleep the whole time.

By the time the surgeon, the plastics guy, and the operating-room scheduler could agree, the surgery was set for December 22. I was a little concerned, because my mother and sister were flying in on Christmas day to stay for a week.

By now, I had shared my diagnosis with my boss, with the human resources director at my company, with my family and a few close friends. In my office, I knew people were not the type to spray Lysol on their desks after I leaned against them. They were all wonderfully supportive, but I knew how the registrar grapevine worked. Though we are sworn to confidentiality about the patients in our databases, we still want to share information about our friends.

I made a conscious decision to share my news and ask for support from everyone. If my story were out in the open, people would talk openly to me, rather than discuss me behind my back with each other. I hate the idea of not talking to someone because you know something you think you shouldn't know and don't know whether the person knows you know. Furthermore, I could turn this into a teaching experience, and that is how I decided to deal with my diagnosis.

My husband Bob went to the hospital with me on December 22. I had to be there by 9:30 for a 12:30 surgery start. Pre-admission work had been done completely as an outpatient: blood work, EKG, bone scan, abdominal CT scan. While I was waiting for surgery, I finished the final touches on a manuscript that I had been working on. Bob took it to Federal Express while I was under anesthesia. (I wanted to keep him busy.)

In pre-op, the surgeon and plastics guy introduced me to their surgical residents as the most knowledgeable patient they'd ever met. As little as I knew about being a patient, that was a really scary thought. I didn't feel as nervous as before the biopsy, though, because I knew what to expect in the operating room now, and I had a plan for my treatment.

Much calmer this time, I made two requests of the surgeon before I went under: talk to me while I am asleep, and ask the pathologist to weigh the specimen. (Didn't you always want to know how much they weigh? I won't tell you how much that breast weighed, but I will say that, at the time, it would have cost $40.75 to send it anywhere by Federal Express.)

I woke up in my hospital room with my husband at my side, bless his heart. He said that the mastectomy and reconstruction took longer than expected and that I'd lost too much blood, so the reduction surgery was postponed. I was almost glad. I hurt so much on the right side that it was difficult to turn over in bed. I was on PCA (patient controlled analgesia), but the morphine sulfate they gave me the first day made me so sleepy I couldn't function, so they switched me to Demerol. That infiltrated from the vein into the skin on the second day. When I pressed the PCA button every ten minutes, my left wrist would sting. I was getting no relief. I had to tell the nurse that the IV was infiltrating. If I hadn't been in health care, I wouldn't have known what was happening. After that, I went to oral pain meds.

LESSON LEARNED: Have some idea what to expect before, during, and after your surgery, and be insistent that your pain be controlled adequately. There are lots of options to minimize the pain associated with a surgical procedure.

The plastics guy also told me that the surgery ran long because he had difficulty closing the mastectomy defect. Me, of all people, didn't have enough skin to close the wound, so he had to release the subcutaneous tissues nearly down to my waist to shift skin high enough to suture to the upper flap.

I got the best news of my life late on Christmas Eve. The surgeon called and said that all my lymph nodes were negative. All forty-eight of them. I have no idea how the pathologist found so many nodes, but I have a feeling that the surgeon called him and said, "This woman will not let me rest until you find and examine every single lymph node in that specimen." (To reward the pathologist for his patience and dissecting skills, I later baked four dozen cookies for him and his staff and sent them along with a note of thanks. He later responded that he was rarely if ever thanked for his part in the diagnostic process.)

Even though I was in and out of the hospital so fast, the registrars and the whole cancer program staff at that hospital were just wonderful. They were my first visitors, bearing a big plant and more than professional care and concern about my visit to their turf. The first thing I did was to "release" them from their professional confidentiality vows about my care. They were quite relieved that I gave them permission to talk about my patienthood in general terms when folks inquired about me. At least then they could admit that I was a patient at their hospital. Again, I felt that the more support I could get, the faster I would recuperate.

To reciprocate, the first time I ambulated with my husband, we walked over to the registry, which was on the same floor, and asked if they had any data that needed to be analyzed. Instead, they gave me a tour of their patient teaching area and library and told me to take whatever literature I needed. They also pressed into my hands two books, *Choices* and *Triumph*, both by Marion Morra and Eve Potts. I thought I didn't really need those books, but they turned out to be fantastic resources, much needed when I was at home. *Choices* is still in print in a revised and updated edition, and it covers all types of cancers in a question-and-answer format. (I heartily recommend *Choices* to patients and even to new registrars, who know about as much as patients do about things like different kinds of mastectomies, technical terms, staging, signs and symptoms, and so forth. They also need explanations in basic terms.)

Because of the holidays, the nurses were short staffed and couldn't spend a lot of time doing patient education. When I was about to be discharged, I requested patient education and got only about forty-five minutes worth from my assigned nurse. It wasn't really her fault. When the registrars and doctors introduced me or spoke of me as a registrar, people kind of assumed that I knew everything there was to know about cancer. I may know a fair amount about statistics, staging, data collection and analysis, but I didn't know much about being a patient. I had to keep reminding people to treat me like a patient and not skip over the details.

LESSON LEARNED: If you are a health professional, sometimes you have to remind other health professionals to treat you like a patient.

I went home on Christmas Day, three days post-op. My husband had gone to the airport to pick up my family, dropped them at home, then picked me up at the hospital. I fixed dinner for them that night. Then the pain meds wore off, and I crashed into bed early. My family was there for a week, and toward the end we were able to get out and do a little shopping, sightseeing, and visiting. Being mobile was slightly awkward because I left the hospital with two Jackson-Pratt (JP) drains dangling on long tubes from my chest. My sister suggested that I just tuck them into a fanny pack, and that worked perfectly.

LESSON LEARNED: Do your best not to let your diagnosis cause you to stop living your life as normally as possible.

I had to empty the JPs a couple of times a day and measure the output—lots of fun—but I was determined to recover as fast as I could. I did my exercises pretty religiously and spent some time at the computer writing thank-you notes for the dozens of flower arrangements, planters, books, and other get well wishes I had received. I am so grateful for those wishes and thoughts of support. They have become to this day my safety net.

I realize now that I wasn't told about some of the after-effects as part of my informed consent for the surgery. Yes, they told me all about the life-threatening stuff before I signed on the dotted line, but I'm still finding out about the life-aggravating stuff. For example:

- I have an 11.5 inch scar running transverse across my right chest from my breastbone (midsternum) to the middle of my side (midaxillary line).
- There is complete anesthesia for about an inch above and several inches below the scar. I can feel pressure but not heat or cold or gentle touch. This may last forever.
- There was complete anesthesia of the underside of my upper arm all the way to the elbow. A fellow registrar and patient had told me to anticipate that loss of feeling and that it might take a year to subside. It took closer to five years to get partial sensation back.
- Occasionally, I got phantom nipple pain—a weird sensation, especially when I knew it was only fluid, plastic, and pectoral muscle there.
- I had extreme weakness and limited range of motion in my arm, which took a lot of exercise to alleviate. The surgery requires that the big muscle between the chest and arm be stretched out of the way in order to gain access to those axillary lymph nodes. Imagine doing leg stretches or touching your toes when you are out of shape and how sore your calves are the next day. Multiply that by about fifty, and that's what it feels like when your shoulder muscles are snapping back into place. Thank God for oral pain meds.
- For quite a while, the center of my reconstruction was about two inches higher than the center of the breast that had been reduced. It made wearing vertical striped blouses OK, but horizontal stripes, checks, and plaids gave me problems.

Fortunately, nearly everything was covered in Morra and Potts's *Choices*. The book has a good section on exercises, which I typed up on

Lessons Learned   369

my computer when I got home. Finger walks, windmills, patting your-self on the back, flapping wings, all sorts of range-of-motion exercises to get me back on my feet quickly—well, back into arm's reach anyway.

Choices has an interesting section about using a prosthesis to fill out your form and getting your body image back to normal. The book rec-ommends using a soft form while the wound is still healing, such as a Dacron-filled contoured pillow or "puff." Other suggestions for tempo-rary prostheses included clean padding, cotton balls, lamb's wool, hand-kerchiefs, sanitary napkins, or padded bras during the period between the operation and being fitted for a regular prosthesis or the completion of the reconstruction.

What I really needed was a gym sock full of birdshot. I tried every-thing in the house to balance myself. I even checked out shoulder pads— regular, raglan sleeve, and ultimately even the football player type. For-tunately, because I sew, I had a variety on hand. The ones that worked best were the ones left over from the Linda Evans/Joan Collins fash-ions shown on *Dynasty*. Some days it was just a couple of my husband's gym socks rolled up in a ball.

For my size, there wasn't a good temporary prosthesis while the expander prosthesis was being pumped up. Whatever I used tended to migrate with a lot of arm motion. Even too much crossing and uncross-ing of arms, and I got into trouble some days. I'd look down and the puff would be almost up to my neck.

Post-Operative Treatment

OK so far—I made it through the surgery with nodes negative and ER and PR positive. But that nasty aneuploidy and high S-phase were lurk-ing out there. My surgeon asked me to think about chemotherapy. Also, I still wanted to get the reduction over with. I couldn't make up my mind about chemo. I was of the old school—negative nodes, negative addi-tional treatment, and the benefits of chemotherapy for node-negative breast cancer were just beginning to be explored in clinical trials. But aneuploidy and S-phase were relatively recently developed laboratory technologies and said something different. So I, and my surgeon, turned the decision over to the hospital's tumor board—a committee of cancer

When Cancer Specialists Get Cancer

experts from a variety of medical specialties who meet regularly to develop treatment recommendations for individual patients. I wanted to go as a visiting cancer registrar, but I was politely discouraged from doing so. I asked my friends the registrars to take good notes for me.

As I suspected, that august group recommended chemotherapy: six months of CMF (Cytoxan, methotrexate, and 5-FU). And I consented. My surgeon wrote out a referral to his buddy-oncologist who was his age and shared his background. I, on the other hand, went to my best-informed source, *my* professional friends, and asked them who the best oncologist on staff was. They gave me a different name, so I started setting up appointments to interview oncologists. I knew this would be a longer-term relationship than I had with the surgeon or plastics guy, and I wanted someone that I would get along with.

When I called the first office, I asked dozens of questions about the oncologist's treatment patterns. Did he use protocols? Which ones? Would he put a port in instead of use up my veins? Where were his offices? Who covers for him? And so forth. The nurse was quite patient with this unheard-of caller, so I made an appointment to meet and talk to her boss. He spent over an hour with me as I explained my story, asked him more questions, and talked about my options. In contrast to the Tumor Board recommendation of CMF, he recommended six months of CAF (Cytoxan, Adriamycin, and 5-FU), a far more aggressive treatment. And he went into extensive detail about why he felt it was better treatment in view of my age and extent of disease. He also said a port (direct venous access) was the best way to go. He was young, bright, and gave me his total attention when I was with him, even when I was asking what I thought were silly little questions. Needless to say, I did not bother with another oncologist interview.

LESSON LEARNED: You have a choice in doctors. Make sure you are comfortable with your oncologist because this relationship will last longer than the one with the surgeon.

The next step was to call the surgeon to set a date to put the port in and to see if he could coordinate with the plastics guy so I could have the reduction done under the same anesthesia. By this time — three weeks post-mastectomy—I was back at work full time, or as full time as possible with three to five appointments each week with the surgeon and plastic surgeon so they could check my progress. The people in my office were very supportive of my taking the necessary time off for doctor appointments.

Part of the reason I went back to work so fast was daytime TV. It was awful. (It still is.) Sally Jesse, Montel, Oprah, Donahue . . . aren't there any happy people in the world? At least it was good to know that somebody out there had worse problems than me.

My port placement and reduction surgery was set for late afternoon, so I worked a half-day. It was all supposed to be outpatient surgery, but I woke up in a hospital bed. The port placement hadn't gone well. They couldn't easily find a space between my clavicle and first rib to run the tube. But the reduction went fine. I hadn't been that perky since junior high (even though the firmness of the tissue went down as the bruising and wounds healed). Taking more time with the procedure, they placed the port the next afternoon. Two general anesthesias in two days, but at least I was discharged right from the recovery room.

At first the port felt weird, like something stuck in my throat where it crossed my esophagus, but within a couple of days I couldn't feel the tube at all. Now all I can feel is the bump under my skin where the Medi-Port is sutured. Everything is subcutaneous, so the nurse has to feel where to insert the IV needle to draw blood or to give me chemo.

About this time also, I decided to contact "Reach to Recovery" (a volunteer support and education network for people with breast cancer). I was already friends with the professional education director at our local American Cancer Society office, and she did a nice job of going over information with me. She gave me three puffs and other material, including a pulley contraption to help stretch my mastectomy arm.

I also took her suggestion that I find a wig before chemo started and get it while I still had my real hair for comparison. Adriamycin always causes hair loss. I set about finding a wig quickly because I had no idea how I would feel after my chemo started. Once again, I went back to my best source, the registrars. They recommended a lady who had been active in obtaining and styling wigs for their patients and who was also active in their "Look Good, Feel Better" program.

Because my husband is my toughest critic and because he would have to look at me more than I would, I took him with me to the wig lady. I think he wanted to get back the young girl with the waist-length blond hair that he married. (After all, I'd been threatening for a couple of years to trade him in for two twenty-two-year-olds.) I tried on a dozen or more wigs. Some we laughed at; some we groaned over. Just as I was about to give up, I tried one on, and he said, "You know, I'd try to pick you up in a bar if you wore that one." Guess which one I bought?

By the way, he was really cool through this whole process (notice I did not say *ordeal*). We talked about what was happening and expressed our concerns to each other. I knew I was going to be OK when he said, "When you start to worry, then I will worry, but I will take my lead from you."

It was my intent to have chemo on Friday late afternoon so I could be sick all weekend, and that was the appointment I made. I was so anxious that I burst into tears when the oncologist came into the room. I'd seen operations before, and I'd seen radiation machines before, but I just didn't know what to expect with chemo. Was I going to get sick right away, in the office? How much? How hard?

Well, he calmed me down, and we started dripping in the Zofran. I'll tell you that it is the oncology wonder drug of the late twentieth century. Rather than feeling sick, I just started feeling a little zoned-out. The nurse injected the clear 5-FU into my port, and the red Adriamycin went in the same way. And it was all over. No problem. We went home after hitting the grocery store. (By the way, the red in the Adriamycin stays red all the way through your system. Don't be surprised the first time you pee bright red if you take Adriamycin.)

I had more anti-emetics (anti-nausea drugs) to take when the Zofran wore off, but my husband said why not wait and see what my symptoms would be before doping myself up and masking them. Being empirical by nature, I went along with the experiment. What a lesson I learned.

In addition to the chemotherapy-induced vomiting, my main symptom from the spectrum of adverse effects was diarrhea. I was losing my fluids and nutrition from both ends. On Saturday night, Bob and I went out for dinner. I had to eat because you have to take Cytoxan with food. But all I wanted to do was sleep. I felt miserable and weak and tired, even after taking the oral anti-emetics and drinking fruit juices and so forth. I could barely drag myself to work on Monday. When I called the nurse, she offered to give me a bag of fluids, but I'd have to leave work and go to their office and spend more bucks. So I asked what Plan B was. She told me to go to the store and get some Gatorade. That's when I discovered the second-best wonder drug of the late twentieth century.

After drinking the first glass, I felt better within a half hour. One quart later, I was able to finish the workday. The diarrhea and vomiting had screwed up my electrolytes and the Gatorade replaced them, for about $1.25 a quart. Amazing. I continued to take the Cytoxan at night after dinner, as prescribed. I didn't have too many problems with that at first.

Day eight of chemo I was asked how things went, and I said pretty rough. So the nurse changed the Adriamycin to drip rather than push, to lessen the shock to my system. That worked much better, and I loaded up on anti-emetics before the Zofran wore off. I sailed through day eight and the weekend.

The nurse told me that it would take eighteen days for my hair to fall out. She was pretty close. About day fourteen, I started getting brush-fuls of hair after my morning shower and shampoo. By day sixteen, I could tug on a clump of hair and it would come out in my hand. The hair loss was getting messy, and I could no longer blame my golden retriever for all the loose hairs all over the floor and furniture.

The evening of day seventeen, I called the wig lady and asked for a buzz cut like army recruits get. Instead of taking that radical step, she compassionately cut my hair by hand, an inch or so at a time so I could get used to the feeling and the look in the mirror. She was right about taking this slowly because it was a shock. The next day, I went in to work with my new hair—my wig—which was just like my old hair only better. I think there are still some guys in my office who just think I got a new hairstyle. Well, as the commercial says, share the fantasy.

LESSON LEARNED: Support staff like the office nurse and the wig lady are not there to make your life miserable. They are there to help you along as much as they can. Express your needs and questions to them so they can use their experience to make your life better.

When Cancer Specialists Get Cancer

By the way, I lost hair everywhere, if you know what I mean, except for my eyelashes and eyebrows, which just thinned out. Some people lose them too. One of my friends said it was just like being twelve again.

As I approached the nadir (the midpoint of the chemotherapy cycle and the point at which a patient is most susceptible to infection), I put a sign up by my office door for people to let me know if they had colds, so I could keep my distance. They read the sign and cooperated, but apparently germs themselves can't read. I caught a nasty late-winter cold that nearly postponed my second cycle of chemo. I plunged ahead with it but had a miserable post-IV day. With the help of antibiotics, though, day eight wasn't as rough.

And so it went. Cycle three went OK, and part of cycle four had to be given in California because I was out there working when it was due to start. The main thing was that the chemo had to be given as close to schedule as possible, and there are helpful oncologists throughout the country.

By the middle of cycle three, I could see other effects on my body. Sores and hangnails healed very slowly. My skin tone had deteriorated, and my skin was very dry. I wasn't even producing earwax. I started paying attention to the cosmetics commercials aimed at the over-40 crowd whose skin had been messed up by too much suntanning. Now I was thinking about replenishing creams and moisturizers just to keep from itching.

At first, I was hoping to get a depressed appetite so I could lose some weight during chemotherapy. The nurses, cancer program people, and ACS staff urged me not to try to lose weight but didn't really give me a good reason why. I later read that if you insult your system or attempt to starve it, more of your cells go into the resting phase where chemo can't act on them. So I watched what I ate but did not attempt to lose weight. I also discovered that Cytoxan goes down much better with wine, Chunky Monkey ice cream, and margaritas, though not all at the same time. But wine, ice cream, and margaritas are not the only reasons to go through chemotherapy.

At the end of my chemotherapy, I had a party to celebrate with my friends who had formed my support group throughout my treatment. My general health, skin tone, and everything improved once chemo was over. My hair did grow back curly—at first. But my ovaries had shut down from the chemotherapy, and going on tamoxifen did not help them recover because it neutralizes the estrogen in your body. But tamoxifen reduces the likelihood that any residual tumor will grow in very low hormone conditions, and that's a good thing. It is still my "security blanket" against recurrence. Instant menopause was not a bad thing, in my opinion, but the hot flashes were difficult to deal with and took over a year to dissipate. My attitude changed somewhere along the way when I saw a cartoon over someone's desk that read: "Strong women do not have hot flashes—they have power surges."

At five years, I had another party. At ten years, an even bigger celebration. And I continue to celebrate a little each day. Like everyone, I have good days and bad, but the good ones far outnumber the bad. I try not to dwell on my disease or on whether I will have a recurrence because I refuse to become a slave to my diagnosis.

LESSON LEARNED: If you can't face a life-threatening—or at least life-changing—experience with a good sense of humor, the road will be much tougher than it has to be.

CHAPTER 25

"You're Going to Live"

Lillie Shockney, R.N., B.S., M.A.S.

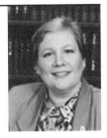

I'm in my early fifties. I was raised on the Eastern Shore of Maryland, on a farm where my folks still live. I had known I wanted to be a nurse, I think, since I was four. I actually have a photograph of me in a Sears catalogue Halloween costume that was a nursing uniform. In the picture I'm holding a baby doll on which I had performed a craniotomy and bandaged her head. I began working with brain tumor patients when I started my career here at the Johns Hopkins Avon Foundation Breast Center in 1983.

I went to nursing school at age 17, younger than most generally go today. I went to a three-year diploma program on the Eastern Shore. I have always had a passion for working with illnesses that are not just life threatening but life altering. When I first finished nursing school, before I got married, I worked for a few months in a doctor's office in this rural area, where there was one doctor for a fifty-mile radius who performed everything. It was like a MASH unit. We removed shards of glass from people's lungs, only giving them oral pills to take because we didn't have any anesthetic in the office. Often people didn't pay in money but in fish, chicken, eggs, or yard work. I held several other positions after that, and I came here to Hopkins twenty-four years ago.

It was an unusual fate. I found a lump in my right breast, which prompted me to get a mammogram. They also did a baseline on my left, and that's when they found the cancer. The lump ironically was benign on the right. I was a poster child for mammography. I was only 38. I had a cluster of microcalcifications that was highly suspicious, but I was in denial and preferred to think that I was going to fall into the 80 percent group that had benign biopsy results. The surgeon doing the biopsy dropped me hints that I was in big trouble. He said, "You have a very diseased breast, and there was a section of tissue much larger than I planned for."

I was in total denial. My surgeon told me he had to be out of town for five days. He said, "I would like to be the one to review the results with you rather than one of my colleagues who you don't know as well." That's the biggest thing because anyone could have told me it was benign. He said, "Will you have any trouble waiting?" I said, "No, Charlie, I won't have any trouble waiting."

My mother had trouble waiting. She called me often, saying, "Have you heard anything yet?" "No, Mom, the man's in Germany. He won't be back for five days." Next day, "Have you heard anything yet?" "No, Mom. He hasn't returned, he won't be back for four days."

I came into work the next day, and I thought, "I have access to the pathology data when I'm here. I will pull up my report, read it, and call my mom and tell her it was benign." I pulled up my report, and I read the word *carcinoma* twelve times—margin, margin, margin, all six margins dirty. I thought I had the Grim Reaper staring at me.

I didn't tell anybody. When I left that evening, I had to walk by the oncology center hallway, and I walked very fast because I was afraid it was going to suck me in through the double doors.

I went out past the statue of Christ to walk across the street to get to my car and avoided looking at the statue. (There is a large statue of Jesus Christ in the lobby of one of the entrances to the Johns Hopkins Hospital.) Usually, I always look at the statue, and I always touch his toes, always, always, always, coming and going. Nope, not tonight, not looking. I thought he was going, "You better come back here and talk to me."

I knew if I looked at him, I would break down. I wasn't ready for that. I thought, "I've got to get myself home. I've got to talk to my husband. My husband has no clue." He wasn't going to be home until 11:00.

I got home at 6:00 that evening, and, of course, my daughter was there. She didn't even know I had had the biopsy. I hadn't told her anything, and she was like, "Mom, what's wrong with you? Don't you feel all right?" And I said, "No, I don't feel all right, I must be getting a bug" and left it at that.

I got her to bed. The phone rang, and it was my mother. "Do you know anything yet?"

I said, "You know, Mom, I'd like to call you back after Al gets home." She said, "Oh, my God, you know something."

I said, "I can't talk to you right now, Mom. I'll call back when Al gets home. We didn't get the news that we wanted," and I hung up. I thought, "I know my mother's just lost it. I know she's lost it." I went into the bathroom, and I practiced in the mirror how I was going to tell my husband I had breast cancer.

When he came in the door at 11:00 that night, I said, "I have breast cancer." So much for rehearsing. And he said, "Wait, wait, what are you saying to me?" He said, "The doctor isn't back yet." I said, "I pulled up my own pathology report," and he said, "Does cancer mean it's malignant?" I said yes. He said, "OK." He got very, very focused, and he said, "OK." He said, "I don't care what the doctor tells you when he gets back. We're going to hold onto one another, and we'll overcome it together." I'm thinking, "You don't know what's going on in here." I said, "This can be a very sneaky disease and though I can look fine, I can really not be fine." He said, "Well, I know you. I know you. You're going to be fine."

I actually left a message for my surgeon. I left eight messages for him, saying, "Please prioritize me at the top of the pile. I've looked at my own pathology." When he came back, he said, "Oh, I didn't even think about you looking up your own pathology results while I was away. It didn't even cross my mind." And he said, "To think you've had three more days to have to worry and fret, not knowing what we need to do."

He said, "You have multicentric disease. Rather than cancer in one spot, it's kind of scattered through your breast like buckshot. The good news is that the invasive tumor you have is small. You have non-invasive ductal carcinoma in situ cancer scattered through probably two-thirds of your breast."

I had 44Ds, and so that was like a hell of a lot of scattering. He said, "The mammogram has really saved your life." He said, "You aren't a candidate for lumpectomy. You need to look at mastectomy." He said, "You're not a candidate for reconstruction because of your anesthesia history." I had had four previous abdominal surgeries, and in three out of four, I had serious respiratory problems with anesthesia.

I was disappointed about the reconstruction, but I said, "You can take my arms off, just tell me I'm going to live, because I have to raise my child." And he says, "You're going to live." I said, "OK, do whatever you have to do."

The nurses that were in the pre-op greeted me, "Oh, hello, Mrs. Shockney, how are you?" "Oh, I see you work here, oh." Then they look and see what you're having done, and they go, "Oh." They focus. They look straight at your chest, like this instinctive reaction. Patients complain about that also: "I'm so tired of people looking at my chest all the time! I feel like they're talking to my breasts, or talking to what *was* there rather than talking to me." So I say, "Please try to focus on a face." The circulating nurse came over and was holding my hand and looking at my chest and looking. The expression on her face was "I feel sorry for you, and I am so thankful I am not you." It was just all over her face.

The anesthesiologist was someone I knew, and she had been torn about whether to be my anesthesiologist. She was in my pre-op cubicle with me when I looked at my bra and said, "I will never be able to wear this again." She later told me, "I was speechless. I didn't know what to say. I just stood there feeling like an idiot and not knowing what to say."

In the recovery room I had a binder on, which they had not told me to expect. I put my hands on my chest, which patients also instinctively do, and I didn't feel anything because this side was gone and this one was flattened with the binder, and I thought something had gone wrong, and they had taken them both. I started yelling, "Oh, my God! Where did my other breast go?"

In the recovery room there was a patient to my left who was sobbing, and I could hear her saying, "My breast is gone, my breast is gone." I kept trying to sit up to see if I could reach over to touch her, but there

When Cancer Specialists Get Cancer

was too much space between us. I kept feeling that I needed to still be a nurse. I needed to get up. I needed to take care of this woman. And then I'm like, "Mine is gone too. Should I be shouting 'My breast is gone?'" It was so profound.

They kept me overnight, and I was throwing up to beat the band. I could not stop throwing up, and I wanted to be home, wanted to be home in bed with my husband. The nurse taking care of me on the evening shift—her name was Mikey—and I had heard her say out in the hallway that there was a patient that had crumped and had been moved to intensive care, and I felt like I was supposed to be taking care of that patient who had just come out. I heard all of that right there in the hallway. One of the nurses called in sick. There was no one to replace her, and it was chaotic. Mikey had been in and out of my room about every hour to empty my hemovac drains, replace my IV bag, and record my emesis, intake and output. Each time she came in she asked me how I was doing, and each time I said I was fine, when frankly I wasn't. But I didn't want to be a bother. There were far sicker patients on the unit than I. So I avoided eye contact with her each time she came in. At the end of the evening shift, Mikey came in one last time to record my IV amount and empty my drains, and she asked as she had each time that evening, "How are you?" At the same time she put the side rail down and sat beside me. This time we caught eye contact, and I lost it. I started crying, and I said, "I don't know how I ended up on this side of the side rail. I cannot tell you how difficult it is to be over here. You just don't know until you're over here." And I just rambled. I totally rambled about probably nothing and everything, and she sat there holding my hands and just nodding, saying she understood everything. I didn't know the status of my axillary node dissection yet nor the actual diameter of the invasive tumor, so in my mind my survival remained a question. There was a tear running down her face. I rambled for fifteen minutes, past 11 p.m., past the time for change-of-shift report to start. The unit clerk came to my door and said firmly, "Mikey, you are late for giving report." Mikey never turned around to acknowledge her. She never took her eyes off of mine. She replied, while still focusing all of her attention on me, "Tell them to wait; I am with a patient."

I tell nurses that the patient will remember you forever. She will remember if you are Mikey. Mikey just as easily could have not put that side rail down, could have said, "Oh, good, I'm glad you're fine." Or she could have seen me upset and said, "Let me go get you a sleeping pill," written a ledger, written her report, but she didn't. She gave me what she had the least of. She gave me her time.

I ended up, a year later to the day, needing to have a lumpectomy on my right breast, just performed as an outpatient, and then ten months after that I had another diagnostic mammogram and had a second mastectomy. After that I had hormonal therapy. I took tamoxifen, and on a clinical trial I took Megace, which now we don't use anymore. The Megace combined with tamoxifen was bad; it caused bad hair loss—the hair never did return—and terrible sexual dysfunction. I spent a lot of time talking to patients about how to overcome the side effects because they don't talk about it. The vaginal dryness was the worst.

After my second mastectomy I worked with the breast center to implement a program for our patients here called Waking up Transformed—a method to improve the surgical experience for women undergoing mastectomy surgery. My husband had said to me, "You're not having a mastectomy, you're not losing your breast. That's not what you're having done." He said, "You're having transformation surgery. It's a surgeon's mission to transform you from a victim to a survivor. So you're going to exchange your breast for another chance at life, and that's OK." He's a truck driver; his work has nothing to do with the health care field—go figure.

I have had people say to me, "If I had to lose my breasts and they couldn't be reconstructed, I would have refused to have the surgery. I'd rather die with my breasts." I had a patient tell me last week that the sight of lymphedema was enough for her to want to die. No one knows what they will do until it's their turn. You always think you know what you're going to do. You think you know how you are going to react. But you don't know until it's your turn. You have totally different thoughts when you're, you know, facing the music.

Not everything went smoothly. I had three nursing friends who stopped contacting me. People I knew well. My husband called them and said, "What's wrong with you?" Each of them said, "What happened to her could happen to me, and if I get her on the phone I'm going to cry." And one said, "I know I'm going to cry, and I don't want her to see that I'm upset about this and that I'm not dealing well with this."

So I thought about how to neutralize the discussion. When I got fitted for my breast prosthesis, I took my mother with me. On the way I said, "Mom, getting a prosthesis is like getting a puppy. She's going to be my bosom buddy. I'm going to take her everywhere I go, so she should have a name." We selected the name "Betty Boob," and I sent out adoption notices to these nurses and to my best friends that I had gotten "Betty Boob." I also took a photograph. Those three nurses each called me and said "How is Betty doing?" Really they were saying how are you doing with cancer. Betty did neutralize it. When I needed the second mastectomy, I called friends and said, "Betty Boob is getting a roommate, and I need your help in selecting a name for her." Perhaps one day I will learn ventriloquism and my breasts will speak to the public to promote breast cancer awareness. After all, it seems to work having crash dummies "talk" to us on public service announcements on television to inspire us to wear our seatbelts, right?

As I was going through treatment and after treatment was done, I started paying more attention to other aches and pains, and I felt very untrusting of everything but didn't show it, didn't want to scare my family, didn't want to scare my family. I saw one of the therapists here; it worried me so much. I thought, I know this is how patients are, but I don't want to be this way. I don't want to think these negative thoughts. I think that we underutilize therapists for patients. I really do. All these things became rapid learning lessons to me. I tell women, "You are going to have 'bomb' thoughts. You are going to have a headache and be convinced you have brain mets. If your knees hurt, you are going to feel that the cancer is in the bone."

You're doing an inventory of your body all the time because your breast didn't hurt and yet we found cancer in it. Now it's this "I don't trust my body" syndrome. I reassure women that this is a normal way to think because they're so tense.

When I learned that I had cancer in the other breast, my daughter was fourteen. When she was twelve, there were two questions I knew she would ask because these are questions that patients have told me their own children in this age group have asked. Sure enough, she said, "Mommy are you going to die?"

I said, "I don't think so. I technically have stage I breast cancer. The mammogram has saved my life. I do need to lose my breast, but I am going to be OK." And she was very relieved about that. And then she asked me a question children think but don't always verbalize: "Did you get breast cancer because you had me?"

I said, "Having you reduced my risk of getting this disease because I was 26 when you were born. If you are under the age of 30 when you have your first child, it helps reduce your risk." And she was like, "Oh. Well, then it was good to have me."

I said, "It was wonderful I had you."

Then she asked me, "Will the doctor let you bring your breast home? After all, it is yours. You could put it in Daddy's big pickle jar and have it down on the mantle, and when you're sad you can go down and look at it."

I said, "I don't think looking at it would make me feel better, and I am hoping maybe they can do research on the breast tissue and that research could result in someone else not needing the surgery one day." And she was content with that. When I needed the second mastectomy she said, "Good. I can stop worrying now. I've been worrying about this since you first got diagnosed. Now with both breasts gone, I won't worry about losing you." I had no idea she was fretting about this.

My mom handled things very well also. I didn't have to hold her together the second time around and use up my emotional energy on her as I had during my first diagnosis and treatment. Afterward she said, "I bet you that other mothers become a mess" and I said, "How come you weren't a mess the next time?" She said, "I knew how to help."

The Internet was young then. There were just a handful of web sites dedicated to cancer and none specifically for breast cancer. So I went onto six computer bulletin boards saying, "I am looking for an organization that provides support for mothers whose daughters have breast cancer. If you are aware of one can you privately mail me back." I did that on a Friday night, and on Monday afternoon I logged on and had 116 e-mails in my mailbox. I nearly had a heart attack. I called my mother and said, "I have found an organization to provide support to mothers of daughters with breast cancer."

She said, "That's great. Where is it?"

I said, "It's you, because there isn't one. Will you make one?"

And she said OK. So six weeks later, in March of 1995, with Senator Barbara Mikulski's help, we became a national nonprofit organization on a mission. Mothers Supporting Daughters with Breast Cancer (www.mothersdaughters.org) has worked with 25,000 mothers since that time. My mother has a team of thirty mother volunteers scattered across the United States that she matches to mothers based on the daughter's profile. So she has mothers whose daughters have died, some of them recently. She has mothers whose daughters are pregnant when diagnosed. The youngest she supported was a 41-year-old mother and a 19-year-old daughter. The oldest was a 97-year-old mother calling from a nursing home, collect. There was an article in the *Woman's Day* magazine about the organization. This elderly woman read it and called my mother and said, "I just found out my baby has breast cancer." She said, "How old is your daughter?" She said, "74."

As all of this was coming together, I thought, "I'm supposed to be doing this all the time. I'm supposed to be with breast cancer patients all the time." After my second mastectomy, I planned to do six hours a week as a volunteer, working with women with breast cancer. It quickly turned into twenty-four hours a week. I was writing patient education materials, working with the faculty in anesthesiology and surgery to implement changes in the breast cancer surgery program, and doing patient satisfaction surveys with patients over the phone. We need to hear the voice of the patient. And at the end of every survey, I would say, "By the way, I am also a breast cancer survivor. Is there anything else you want to tell me?" That's when I got the most valuable information and candid feedback from the patient—information that we would use to improve patient care for women coming to the breast center in the future.

After three years of volunteering for the breast center while continuing to work in my regular full-time nursing position at Hopkins, I transferred to the breast center as a full-time employee, dedicating myself personally and professionally to women who would end up "wearing my bra" in the future. As administrative director, I was able not only to provide medical care and oncology nursing expertise but also to serve as a patient advocate. Don't ever underestimate the importance of patient advocacy.

Several years ago I began thinking more about breast reconstruction. With the power of science and improvements in medicine I was finally eligible to undergo breast reconstruction if I wanted to do so. I went to Mo (Maurice) Nahabedian, then the chief of breast reconstruction at our breast center, and said, "There's a patient who's an employee here who is contemplating doing delayed reconstruction, and I wanted to arrange an appointment for her confidentially. I will be with her for her visit. Could she see you after work?" And he said absolutely, sure.

So Tuesday at 5:30, I went to his office and told him that we would be in exam room #3. So he comes in, and there I am in a gown, and he goes, "Gracious. It's you?"

"Yes."

"I've always assumed that you didn't want reconstruction."

"I wanted it but I wasn't able to do it, and now I found out I can," I told him. "I want to plan this for December."

And he said, "That'll be fine."

So I had six months to think about this, and I talked to my husband. My husband got very alarmed. He said, "What am I doing wrong? I'm doing something wrong. Oh, my God, I thought we were OK."

I said, "We are fine, but I want to do this."

And I would listen to Dr. Ted Tsangaris, who was our new medical director for the breast center. When he was with patients, he would say, "I want you to see a plastic surgeon. I want you to think about reconstruction."

Patients would say, "Just save my life, sir, please. I don't need any breasts."

He says, "You were born with two breasts; you have the right to have two breasts. I want you to meet with a plastic surgeon. If you tell me you don't like anything he has to offer, that's fine, but I still want you to meet with him." And I sat down with Ted his second week here and said, "I feel like you're pressuring patients into reconstruction."

He said, "No. I am giving them permission for them to pursue it because women are so focused on getting rid of the cancer."

When Cancer Specialists Get Cancer

I had lacked having a patient advocate when I was first treated, but now I realized that Ted Tsangaris had become my advocate. In reflecting back on my annual visits to my breast surgeon, I realized that the discussion of breast reconstruction never came up. The surgeon was waiting for me to initiate the conversation if I was interested, and I was waiting for him to bring it up on my behalf. The reality was that no one discussed it though it was certainly on my mind. I found this ironic because I am known for being an assertive, actually aggressive woman. I can speak up for myself. But when you become a cancer patient, things can change. You can lose the ability to be an advocate for yourself. A lesson I have remembered when taking care of other women, especially those also in the health care field, is that we cannot assume that they will be advocates for themselves. Everyone needs an advocate when confronted with a diagnosis of cancer. The diagnosis is too overwhelming to process all the information and decision making needed to be done by the patient.

My husband was very worried when I told him I was interested in pursuing DIEP flap reconstructive surgery and assumed he was doing something wrong. Ted reassured him, "You're not doing anything wrong. The choice has been restored. Let her choose." To me, Ted said, "One of the great things that will come out of this is that you're going to make it OK for women who can't do reconstruction, and you're going to make it OK for women to choose." So now I have a whole new experience to share with patients, which has been wonderful.

So I underwent another form of transformation surgery—DIEP flap reconstruction. Knowing my surgical team would be nervous operating on someone they worked with daily, I provided them comic relief that morning by typing up signs and taping them to my chest underneath my hospital gown. Once I was intubated, they lifted my gown to begin surgery to find messages like "I'm here for a front end realignment."

I had a patient sitting with me in clinic a few months ago, with her husband. Her husband called me in and said, "We would like to meet with you after our pre-op teaching is completed with the nurse practitioner to talk about our personal activities." The patient was scheduled for mastectomy with DIEP flap reconstruction later that week. And he said, "How soon before I can squeeze her new breasts?"

That's a good question. I told him that you should really wait six weeks until the blood vessels are all healed.

"When can we have intercourse?"

I said, "That's also six weeks." And I said, "You need to avoid lying on top of her because she's not going to want a lot of pressure on her new breast or abdominal incision." Then I asked her, "Do you ever get on top?" The husband replied for her, "No." I said, "Well, we're going to try that!" and she wrote down "Me on top six weeks." Of course, she writes all this down. So I said to him, "You can be up on your elbows. I just don't want you putting weight on her." He says, "OK, I can do that." And it was such a funny discussion but one I'm comfortable doing. I wish more health care professionals discussed these things with patients because sexual activity can be an important part of a woman's getting back to normal as well as feeling confident about her sexuality. For many patients that confidence has been threatened by having mastectomy surgery.

Well, she needed to go down and donate her blood, and I looked at my watch and said, "I better get you down to blood donation. Those people are really fussy about timing. They'll turn you away." So we stood up, and I said, "You're going to have a couple of weeks before you get active, and when you're in, see me. If you have other questions, you can call me, too."

Then I looked at her and said, "You will probably feel well feel enough to resume oral sex in three weeks. She looked at her husband, and she said, "Do you want me to write that down?" and he said, "Hell, yes." And she writes down, "Oral sex three weeks." He now looks like he's hit the lottery. I am serious. It was so intense. I mean, he is beaming, and so she went to the door. He said, "Honey, let me meet you at the eleva-tor. I have one more question I need to ask Lillie, and I'll meet you at the elevator." She says, "OK." So out the door she goes. He throws his arms around me and kisses me. He said, "I am so glad I called you and asked you if we could meet, and I am so glad that you did, and I am so glad that you said we could resume oral sex because we've been mar-ried eighteen years, and we've never had oral sex, and she wrote it down, so it's going to happen!" Oh, I think that's a great note to end on.

The Agony and the Opportunity of Choice

Kenneth D. Miller, M.D.

B ecause I am a medical oncologist, I know something about making medical decisions. Because of my personal experiences, I know something about the emotional toll that making medical decisions takes on an individual and a family. In this chapter I want to briefly share two of my experiences, the first when my daughter faced major brain surgery and the second when my wife was treated for acute leukemia.

Julie has always been one of my favorite names, both before and since we chose it for our second daughter, who was born in 1992. Julie was a happy child, though she occasionally complained of mild neck pain. When Julie was eight years old, her pediatrician suggested that she have an MRI scan to see what the trouble with her neck might be. The test took almost two hours to complete as I sat by Julie's side shouting encouragement to her between the loud bangs of the machine. The scan showed an abnormal collection of fluid that traveled down the entire spinal cord, a condition called *syringomyelia*. A renowned pediatric neurosurgeon came in and explained to us that Julie would need a six-hour operation on the back of her brain to relieve the pressure and to prevent progressive weakness and disability. I remember thinking that I might actually fall to the ground from the impact of hearing the news.

In spite of the sense of urgency for surgery, we delayed just a little so we could get a second opinion. A second brilliant neurosurgeon reviewed Julie's history, examined her, looked at the MRI, and concluded just the opposite—that surgery was not necessary and that Julie could be followed carefully with neurologic exams and MRI scans.

So who was right? Was one doctor smarter than the other? Did one have more experience with this type of problem? My wife and I were baffled and emotionally vulnerable, but we needed to make a decision that one way or the other could affect Julie's health throughout her life. I consulted a third neurosurgeon, who recommended surgery, but a much simpler procedure preceded by a special MRI scan. Just before the proposed surgery was to begin, the MRI scan was performed, and then the surgeon asked to speak to us in a consultation room, where he informed us that the flow of spinal fluid was better than expected. Julie didn't need the surgery, after all. It is now ten years later, and Julie is doing well. We have been fortunate.

Three years later my wife, Joan, was profoundly anemic and profoundly ill. The doctors offered differing opinions about whether she had acute leukemia, chronic leukemia, or a blood condition known as *myelodysplasia*. I found that it was easy to get caught up in the details about how the physicians' opinions differed, but I knew that it was important to focus on the consensus that Joan needed chemotherapy. I kept hoping that one of the oncologists would tell us that this was just a virus and that Joan didn't need treatment, like with our daughter Julie. Several oncologists offered different opinions about treatment with one chemotherapy protocol or another, a new antibody therapy, or bone marrow transplant. Unlike with Julie, this decision needed to be made quickly. Similarly to Julie's story, however, was the sense that there must be one "right" answer. Eventually, Joan and I came to the realization that we were not taking a "leap of faith" but rather a step with faith and hope. Joan and I decided on a course of treatment, she did obtain a remission, and, thankfully, she is doing well. I remain a believer that cancer is a treatable disease and that hope is a powerful prescription that doctors can give their patients.

In the treatment of some diseases there are few choices. Appendicitis requires surgery, and a fractured wrist requires casting. Breast cancer, however, often can be treated with lumpectomy or mastectomy; women can choose to have reconstructive surgery or not; and many women make a decision to receive adjuvant chemotherapy or hormonal therapy, or no therapy.

Making personal medical choices is a process often filled with uncertainty. Sometimes it seems that there is truly only one good therapeutic option, while at other times there are several good choices. Sometimes choices need to be made immediately—like in an emergency room—while at other times choices are made only after several consultations. In the treatment of breast cancer, many of the choices are between different options that are equally effective; these kinds of choices have less to do with medical science and more to do with personal preference.

Making medical choices can be empowering because it allows a person to feel some measure of control. Making decisions reinforces a person's individuality and independence. Her decisions reflect her personal perception of risk, risk tolerance, and balancing risks and benefits, and also her personality, background, and preferences. The process of healing during and after an illness is multifaceted: physical, emotional, social, and spiritual. Life usually feels turned upside down after the diagnosis of cancer. The decision-making process can begin the transformation of that sense of disorder into one of order. Making decisions about breast cancer treatment allows a woman to help direct the inevitable changes that life brings.

About the Contributors

Luther Ampey, M.D., is Assistant Professor of Radiation Oncology, University of Maryland School of Medicine, and Director of the Helen P. Denit Cancer Center in Olney, Maryland.

Robert Barnett, M.D., retired from an active practice of oncology surgery after forty years.

Nancy E. Davidson, M.D., is Professor and Breast Cancer Research Chair in Oncology and Director of the Breast Cancer Research Program at the Johns Hopkins University School of Medicine.

Peter J. Deckers, M.D., is Dean of the School of Medicine, University of Connecticut, and Executive Vice President for Health Affairs and Murray-Heilig Chair in Surgery at the Carole and Ray Neag Comprehensive Cancer Center, University of Connecticut Health Center.

Gregory O. Dick, M.D., is a plastic and reconstructive surgeon and former Chief of Surgery, Shady Grove Advent Hospital, as well as past President of the American Cancer Society, Montgomery County, Maryland.

Roger J. Friedman, M.D., is board certified by the American Board of Plastic Surgery and is a member of the American Society of Plastic and Reconstructive Surgery and the clinical faculties of George Washington and Georgetown Universities. He serves as the Chairman of the Sub-Section of Plastic Surgery at Suburban Hospital in Bethesda, Maryland.

April Fritz, RHIT, CTR, is a former Cancer Registrar at the National Cancer Institute. Until the spring of 2006, she was the Manager of Data Quality for the Surveillance, Epidemiology and End Results (SEER) Program of the National Cancer Institute in Rockville, Maryland.

Daniel F. Hayes, M.D., is Professor, Department of Internal Medicine; Co-Director of the Breast Care Center; and Clinical Director of the Breast Cancer Program at the University of Michigan School of Medicine.

Claudine Isaacs, M.D., is Associate Professor of Oncology and Medicine; Director of the Breast Cancer Program; and Medical Director of the Cancer Assessment and Risk Evaluation Program (CARE) at the Lombardi Comprehensive Cancer Center at Georgetown University.

Kenneth D. Miller, M.D., is Assistant Professor of Oncology, Yale School of Medicine, and Director of the Cancer Survivorship Program at Yale Cancer Center, Yale University.

Maurice Nahabedian, M.D., FACS, is Associate Professor of Plastic Surgery and Director of Microvascular Surgery at Georgetown University Hospital.

Chitra Rajagopal, M.D., is Clinical Assistant Professor of Medicine at Georgetown University.

Abram Recht, M.D., is Professor, Department of Radiation Oncology, Harvard Medical School, and Deputy Chief and Senior Radiation Oncologist, Department of Radiation Therapy, Beth Israel Deaconess Medical Center.

Mark Robson, M.D., is Clinical Director, Clinical Genetics Service, Memorial Sloan-Kettering Cancer Center.

Jerome Sandler, M.D., is Chairman of the Cancer Committee and a member of the Board of Directors of Shady Grove Adventist Hospital.

Carole Seddon, LCSW-C, OSW-C, is Director of the Cancer Counseling Center at the Johns Hopkins Breast Center, the Johns Hopkins University.

Lillie Shockney, R.N., B.S., M.A.S., is Director of Education and Outreach at the Johns Hopkins Breast Center, the Johns Hopkins University. She has written three books and fifty articles about her experiences. She was also the focus of the nursing documentary *A Touch of Mercy*, produced by Discovery Health.

Laura A. Siminoff, Ph.D., is Professor of Epidemiology at the Case Western Reserve School of Medicine.

Susan Stinson, M.D., is Medical Director at the Suburban Hospital Cancer Program, Bethesda, Maryland.

Sandra Swain, M.D., is Chief of the Breast Cancer Branch, National Cancer Institute, Bethesda, Maryland, and Professor of Medicine, Uniformed Services University of Health Sciences.

Theodore N. Tsangaris, M.D., is Medical Director and Chief of Breast Surgery at the Johns Hopkins Breast Center, the Johns Hopkins University.

Antonio C. Wolff, M.D., is Associate Professor of Oncology at the Johns Hopkins Medical School. He is a member of the Breast Cancer Core Committee of the Eastern Cooperative Oncology Group (ECOG) and of the Breast Cancer Guideline Panel of the National Comprehensive Cancer Center Network (NCCN) and is chair-elect of the Health Services Committee of the American Society of Clinical Oncology.

Index

Page numbers in *italics* refer to figures and tables.

locally advanced cancer, 36
local recurrence, 91–94, 186
local therapy: definition of, 187, 214; for metastatic cancer, 192–93. *See also* radiation treatment
Love, Susan, 265, 337
Love, Medicine, and Miracles (Siegel), 326
lumpectomy: choosing, 38; description of, *90*; mastectomy compared to, 37–38, 125–26, 128–29; modified radical mastectomy compared to, 47; radiation and, 39; without radiation, 94–95
lumpectomy stories: with chemotherapy, 281–85; with chemotherapy and radiation, 263–68, 293–95, 297–300, 323–27; without radiation, 258–62
lymphedema, 100, 121, 275
lymph node dissection, 96–97, 99–100, 114–15
lymph node involvement and TNM staging system, 34, *35*
lymph nodes: choice of treatment for, 54–55; examining, 39–40. *See also* lymph node dissection

magnetic resonance imaging (MRI), 68–69
mammographic needle localization, 361
mammography: after radiation therapy, 123; baseline, 361; description of, 204; early detection and, 91, 106; sensitivity of, 68
MammoSite, 130
margin, 32, 116
marital status and choice of treatment, 50
mastectomy: description of, 45; Halsted radical, 3, 46, *90*, 91–92; lumpectomy compared to, 37–38, 125–26, 128–29; modified radical, 39, 47, *90*, 92; prophylactic, 70–71; radiation therapy after, 118–19; radical, 3, 46; recommendation for,

101–2; skin sparing, 165, *166*, 257. *See also* breast reconstruction
mastectomy stories: bilateral, without tamoxifen, 240–49; with chemotherapy and hormonal therapy, 300–305; with preoperative chemotherapy, 285–89, 313–18; prophylactic surgery, 225–29, 305–13, 315, 355; with reconstruction and chemotherapy, 289–93, 295–97; without reconstruction, 268–71, 322–23
medical information, complexity of, 13–14
medical oncologists, 153–63; as members of treatment team, 77; systemic therapy and, 84–85
medical uncertainty, 14–15
MediPort, 294, 372
Megace, 382
members of treatment team, 75–78
menopause, early, 159, 331
metastasis, definition of, 186
metastatic cancer: bones and, 199–200; chemotherapy and, 196–99; choices in treatment and, 5; definition of, 45; diagnosis of, 187–88; endocrine therapy for, 194–96; local therapies for, 192–93; monitoring, 189–91; predictive factors in, 188–89; prognosis for, 188; risk of developing, 132–33; systemic therapies for, 193–94; in TNM staging system, 34, 36; treatment for, 187
metastatic cancer stories: chemotherapy, bone marrow transplant, stem cell transplant, and tamoxifen, 338–45; chemotherapy, stem cell transplant, then recurrence, 333–38; chemotherapy, then metastases, 329–33
Mikulski, Barbara, 385
milk glands, 27, *28*
modified radical mastectomy: choosing, 39; description of, *90*; lumpectomy compared to, 47; transition to, 92

moist desquamation, 120
Morra, Marion, *Choices*, 367–68, 369–70
Mothers Supporting Daughters with Breast Cancer, 385
mother with cancer, dealing with, 225–27, 273, 313–14
moving on to life after cancer, 221–22
MRI (magnetic resonance imaging), 68–69
myelodysplasia, 390
myocutaneous flaps, 164, *171*, 171–73, 180. *See also* TRAM (transverse rectus abdominis myocutaneous) flap

National Cancer Institute, 48, 364
neoadjuvant therapy, 151
nipple reconstruction: description of, 175–76, *176*; experience with, 257, 292; interest in, 182; timing of, 168
Nolvadex. *See* tamoxifen
non-invasive breast cancer: description of, 29; radiation therapy and, 129; risk of recurrence, 133; surgery for, 96, 105. *See also* ductal carcinoma in situ (DCIS)
non-invasive breast cancer stories: hormonal therapy, 238–40; lumpectomy without radiation, 258–62; mastectomy without tamoxifen, 240–49; recurrence, 249–58
nurses: communication with, 320, 381–82; as members of treatment team, 78, 81

oncologist, choosing, 371
oncologists. *See* medical oncologists; radiation oncologists
oncology social worker, counseling by, 355–57
Oncotype DX assay, 150–51, 159
ovarian cancer risk, 71
ovarian cancer screening, 69
ovarian suppression, 145

pain medication, 366
palliative treatment, 187
papule, 168, 175–76
parasthesias, 175
partial breast irradiation, 129–30
pathology findings, 32–33
physicians, choosing, 78–79
plastic surgeons, as members of treatment team, 78, 365. *See also* reconstructive surgeons
positive thinking, 163, 353
Potts, Eve, *Choices*, 367–68, 369–70
predictive markers, 150–51
preoperative systemic therapy, 151, 287–88
prevalence of breast cancer, 2, 26–27, *27*
prevention: of local recurrence, 91–94; methods of, 69–71
primary care physicians, as members of treatment team, 76
progesterone receptor (PR), 189
progesterone receptor (PR) positive disease, 136, 139
prophylactic mastectomy: decision to have, 225–29, 305–13, 315, 355; as prevention, 70–71
prostheses: being fitted for, 270; decision about, 303, 323; naming, 383; temporary, 370

race and choice of treatment, 51–52, *52*
radiation exposure, excessive, 63
radiation oncologists, 125–31; as members of treatment team, *77*–78
radiation pneumonitis, 122
radiation treatment: after mastectomy, 118–19; areas treated, 114–15; cancer recurrence and, 123–24; capsular contracture and, 177; chemotherapy and, *113*, 113–14; dealing with, 316; decision against, 258–62; description of, 37–38, 110–11, *112*; doses, 115–16; ductal carcinoma in situ and, 117–18; follow-up to, 123;